Lecture Notes in Artificial Intelligence 6889

Subseries of Lecture Notes in Computer Science

Bin Hu Jiming Liu Lin Chen
Ning Zhong (Eds.)

Brain Informatics

International Conference, BI 2011
Lanzhou, China, September 7-9, 2011
Proceedings

Springer

Volume Editors

Bin Hu
Lanzhou University, School of Information Science and Engineering
Lanzhou, Gansu, 730000, China
E-mail: bh@lzu.edu.cn

Jiming Liu
Hong Kong Baptist University, Department of Computer Science
Kowloon Tong, Hong Kong SAR
E-mail: jiming@comp.hkbu.edu.hk

Lin Chen
Chinese Academy of Sciences, Institute of Biophysics
Chaoyang District, Beijing, 100101, China
E-mail: linchen@bcslab.ibp.ac.cn

Ning Zhong
Maebashi Institute of Technology, Department of Life Science and Informatics
Maebashi-City 371-0816, Japan
E-mail: zhong@maebashi-it.ac.jp

ISSN 0302-9743
e-ISSN 1611-3349
ISBN 978-3-642-23604-4
ISBN 978-3-642-23605-1 (eBook)
DOI 10.1007/978-3-642-23605-1
Springer Heidelberg Dordrecht London New York

Library of Congress Control Number: 2011935139

CR Subject Classification (1998): I.2, H.3-5, F.1-2, H.2.8

LNCS Sublibrary: SL 7 – Artificial Intelligence

Typesetting: Camera-ready by author, data conversion by Scientific Publishing Services, Chennai, India

Printed on acid-free paper

Springer is part of Springer Science+Business Media (www.springer.com)

Preface

This volume contains the papers selected for presentation at the 2011 International Conference on Brain Informatics (BI 2011) held at Lanzhou University, Lanzhou, China, during September 7-9, 2011. It was organized by the Web Intelligence Consortium (WIC), the IEEE Computational Intelligence Society Task Force on Brain Informatics (IEEE-CIS TF-BI), and Lanzhou University. The conference was held jointly with the 2011 International Conference on Active Media Technology (AMT 2011).

Brain informatics (BI) has emerged as an interdisciplinary research field that focuses on studying the mechanisms underlying the human information processing system (HIPS). It investigates the essential functions of the brain, ranging from perception to thinking, and encompassing such areas as multi-perception, attention, memory, language, computation, heuristic search, reasoning, planning, decision-making, problem-solving, learning, discovery, and creativity. The goal of BI 2011 was to develop and demonstrate a systematic approach to achieving an integrated understanding of both macroscopic-and microscopic-level working principles of the brain, by means of experimental, computational, and cognitive neuroscience studies, as well as utilizing advanced Web intelligence (WI)-centric information technologies. BI 2011 represented a potentially revolutionary shift in the way that research is undertaken. It attempted to capture new forms of collaborative and interdisciplinary work. In this vision, new kinds of BI methods and global research communities will emerge, through infrastructure on the wisdom Web and knowledge grids that enable high-speed and distributed, large-scale analysis and computations, and radically new ways of sharing data/knowledge.

The Brain Informatics conferences started with the First WICI International Workshop on Web Intelligence meets Brain Informatics (WImBI 2006), held at Beijing, China, December 15-16, 2006. The second conference, Brain Informatics 2009, was held again in Beijing, China, October 22-24, 2009. The third conference, Brain Informatics 2010, was held in Toronto, Canada, August 28-30, 2010. This series is the first to be specifically dedicated to the interdisciplinary research in BI and provides an international forum to bring together researchers and practitioners from diverse fields, such as computer science, information technology, artificial intelligence, Web intelligence, cognitive science, neuroscience, medical science, life science, economics, data mining, data science and knowledge science, intelligent agent technology, human-computer interaction, complex systems, and systems science, to present the state of the art in the development of BI, to explore the main research problems in BI that lie in the interplay between the studies of human brain and the research of informatics. All the papers submitted to BI 2011 were rigorously reviewed by three committee members and external reviewers. The selected papers offered new insights into the research challenges and development of BI.

There are bidirectional mutual support directions in BI research. In one direction, one models and characterizes the functions of the human brain based on the notions of information processing systems. WI-centric information technologies are applied to support brain science studies. For instance, the wisdom Web, knowledge grids, and cloud computing enable high-speed, large-scale analysis, simulation, and computation as well as new ways of sharing research data and scientific discoveries. In another direction, informatics-enabled brain studies, e.g., based on fMRI, EEG, and MEG, significantly broaden the spectrum of theories and models of brain sciences and offer new insights into the development of human-level intelligence toward brain-inspired wisdom Web computing.

Here we would like to express our gratitude to all members of the Conference Committee for their instrumental and unfailing support. BI 2011 had a very exciting program with a number of features, ranging from keynote talks, technical sessions, workshops, and social programs. This would not have been possible without the generous dedication of the Program Committee members and the external reviewers in reviewing the papers submitted to BI 2011, of our keynote speakers, Ali Ghorbani of the University of New Bunswick, Toyoaki Nishida of Kyoto University, Lin Chen of the Chinese Academy of Sciences, Frank Hsu, Fordham University, Zhongtuo Wang of Dalian University of Technology (Xuesen Qian Memoriam Invited Talk), and Yulin Qin of Beijing University of Technology (Herbert Simon Memoriam Invited Talk), and the Organizing Chairs, Yuejia Luo, Mariano Alcaniz, Cristina Botella Arbona, as well as the organizer of the workshop, Xijin Tang. We thank them for their strong support and dedication. We would also like to thank the sponsors of this conference, ALDEBARAN Robotics Company, ShenZhen Hanix United, Inc., and ISEN TECH & TRADING Co., Ltd.

BI 2011 could not have taken place without the great team effort of the Local Organizing Committee, the support of the International WIC Institute, Beijing University of Technology, China, and Lanzhou University, China. Our special thanks go to Juzhen Dong, Li Liu, Yi Zeng, and Daniel Tao for organizing and promoting BI 2011 and coordinating with AMT 2011. We are grateful to Springer's *Lecture Notes in Computer Science* (LNCS/LNAI) team for their generous support. We thank Alfred Hofmann and Christine Reiss of Springer for their help in coordinating the publication of this special volume in an emerging and interdisciplinary research field.

June 2011

Bin Hu
Jiming Liu
Lin Chen
Ning Zhong

Organization

Conference General Chairs

Lin Chen	Chinese Academy of Sciences, China
Ning Zhong	International WIC Institute, Beijing University of Technology, China Maebashi Institute of Technology, Japan

Program Chairs

Bin Hu	Lanzhou University, China, and ETH Zurich, Switzerland
Jiming Liu	International WIC Institute, Beijing University of Technology, China Hong Kong Baptist University, Hong Kong

Organizing Chairs

Mariano Alcaniz	Universidad Politecnica de Valencia, Spain
Yuejia Luo	Beijing Normal University, China
Cristina Botella Arbona	University Jaume I, Spain

Publicity Chairs

Li Liu	Lanzhou University, China
Daniel Tao	Queensland University of Technology, Australia
Yi Zeng	Beijing University of Technology, China

WIC Chairs/Directors

Ning Zhong	Maebashi Institute of Technology, Japan
Jiming Liu	Hong Kong Baptist University, Hong Kong

IEEE-CIS TF-BI Chair

Ning Zhong	Maebashi Institute of Technology, Japan

WIC Advisory Board

Edward A. Feigenbaum	Stanford University, USA
Setsuo Ohsuga	University of Tokyo, Japan
Benjamin Wah	The Chinese University of Hong Kong, Hong Kong
Philip Yu	University of Illinois, Chicago, USA
L.A. Zadeh	University of California, Berkeley, USA

WIC Technical Committee

Jeffrey Bradshaw	UWF/Institute for Human and Machine Cognition, USA
Nick Cercone	York University, Canada
Dieter Fensel	University of Innsbruck, Austria
Georg Gottlob	Oxford University, UK
Lakhmi Jain	University of South Australia, Australia
Jianchang Mao	Yahoo! Inc., USA
Pierre Morizet-Mahoudeaux	Compiegne University of Technology, France
Hiroshi Motoda	Osaka University, Japan
Toyoaki Nishida	Kyoto University, Japan
Andrzej Skowron	Warsaw University, Poland
Jinglong Wu	Okayama University, Japan
Xindong Wu	University of Vermont, USA
Yiyu Yao	University of Regina, Canada

Program Committee

Ajith Abraham	Norwegian University of Science and Technology, Norway
Fabio Aloise	IRCCS Fondazione Santa Lucia, Italy
Xiaocong Fan	The Pennsylvania State University, USA
Anthony Finn	University of South Australia, USA
Philippe Fournier-Viger	National Cheng Kung University, China
Mohand-Said Hacid	Université Claude Bernard Lyon 1, France
Bin He	University of Minnesota, USA
Frank D. Hsu	Fordham University, USA
Kazuyuki Imamura	Maebashi Institute of Technology, Japan
Colin Johnson	University of Kent, UK
Hanmin Jung	Korea Institute of Science and Technology Information, Korea
Peipeng Liang	Xuanwu Hospital, Capital Medical University, China
Pawan Lingras	Saint Mary's University, Canada

Li Liu	Lanzhou University, China
Mariofanna Milanova	University of Arkansas at Little Rock, USA
Kazumi Nakamatsu	University of Hyogo, Japan
Mark Neerincx	The Netherlands Organization for Applied Scientific Research, The Netherlands
Vasile Palade	Oxford University, UK
Valentina Poggioni	University of Perugia, Italy
Hideyuki Sawada	Kagawa University, Japan
Lael Schooler	Max Planck Institute, Germany
Tomoaki Shirao	Gunma University, Japan
Andrzej Skowron	Warsaw University, Poland
Dominik Slezak	University of Warsaw and Infobright Inc., Poland
Diego Sona	Fondazione Bruno Kessler - Neuroinformatics Laboratory, Italy
Shanbao Tong	Shanghai Jiao Tong University, China
Shusaku Tsumoto	Shimane University, Japan
Sunil Vadera	University of Salford, UK
Frank van der Velde	Leiden University, The Netherlands
Jinglong Wu	Okayama University, Japan
Jian Yang	University of Science and Technology of China, China
Yiyu Yao	University of Regina, Canada
Yanqing Zhang	Georgia State University, USA
Ning Zhong	Maebashi Institute of Technology, Japan
Yangyong Zhu	Fudan University, China
George Zouridakis	University of Houston, USA
Kuan-Ching Li	Providence University, Taiwan

Table of Contents

Keynote Talks

Thinking and Perception-Centric Investigations of Human Information Processing Systems

Information Technologies for the Management, Analysis and Use of Brain Data

Cognition-Inspired Applications

Workshop on Meta-Synthesis and Complex Systems

The Global-First Topological Definition of Perceptual Objects, and Its Neural Correlation in Anterior Temporal Lobe

Lin Chen, Ke Zhou, Wenli Qian, and Qianli Meng

State Key Laboratory of Brain and Cognitive Science
Institute of Biophysics, Chinese Academy of Sciences
15 Datun Road, 100101 Beijing, China
linchen@bcslab.ibp.ac.cn

What is a perceptual object? This question seems to be straightforward yet its answer has become one of the most central and also controversial issues in many areas of cognitive sciences.

The"global-first" topological approach ties a formal definition of perceptual objects to invariance over topological transformation, and the core intuitive notion of a perceptual object - the holistic identity preserved over shape-changing transformations - may be precisely characterized as topological invariants, such as connectivity and holes.

The topological definition of objects has been verified by a fairly large set of behavioral experiments, including, for example, MOT and attention blink, which consistently demonstrated that while object identity can survive various non-topological changes, the topological change disturbs its object continuity, being perceived as an emergence of a new object. Companion fMRI experiments revealed the involvement of anterior temporal lobe, a late destination of the visual form pathway, in the topological perception and the formation of perceptual objects defined by topology. This contrast of global-first in behavior and late destination in neuroanatomy raises far-reaching issues regarding the formation of object representations in particular, and the fundamental question of "where to begin" in general.

B. Hu et al. (Eds.): BI 2011, LNAI 6889, p. 1, 2011.

Combinatorial Fusion Analysis in Brain Informatics: Gender Variation in Facial Attractiveness Judgment

D. Frank Hsu[1], Takehito Ito[2], Christina Schweikert[1], Tetsuya Matsuda[2], and Shinsuke Shimojo[3]

[1] Department of Computer and Information Science, Fordham University New York, NY 10023, USA
[2] Tamagawa University Brain Science Institute
6-1-1, Tamagawa Gakuen, Machida, Tokyo 194-8610, Japan
[3] Division of Biology/Computation and Neural Systems,
California Institute of Technology, Pasadena, CA 91125, USA

Abstract. Information processing in the brain or other decision making systems, such as in multimedia, involves fusion of information from multiple sensors, sources, and systems at the data, feature or decision level. Combinatorial Fusion Analysis (CFA), a recently developed information fusion paradigm, uses a combinatorial method to model the decision space and the Rank-Score Characteristic (RSC) function to measure cognitive diversity. In this paper, we first introduce CFA and its practice in a variety of application domains such as computer vision and target tracking, information retrieval and Internet search, and virtual screening and drug discovery. We then apply CFA to investigate gender variation in facial attractiveness judgment on three tasks: liking, beauty and mentalization using RSC function. It is demonstrated that the RSC function is useful in the differentiation of gender variation and task judgment, and hence can be used to complement the notion of correlation which is widely used in statistical decision making. In addition, it is shown that CFA is a viable approach to deal with various issues and problems in brain informatics.

1 Introduction

Using genomic profiles and biomarkers to diagnose and treat diseases and disorders, advances in biomedicine have made personalized medicine a possibility. Recent developments in molecular biology have made molecular networks a major focus for translational science [37]. Molecular networks, which connect molecular biology to clinical medicine, encompass metabolic pathways, gene regulatory networks, and protein-protein interaction networks. On the other hand, the Human Connectome Project aims to map all the brain connections in one thousand human subjects. Consequently, we will be able to understand more about the function of the brain at the systems and network levels [35]. So, the brain system and its connectivity are sure to translate research discoveries from the laboratory to the clinic. It will also contribute to the development of novel diagnosis and therapeutic treatment of neurodegenerative and psychiatric diseases and disorders.

B. Hu et al. (Eds.): BI 2011, LNAI 6889, pp. 2–20, 2011.

1.1 Brain System

The human brain is a complex system consisting of billions of neurons and tens or hundreds of billions of connections. Dowling [8] studies the brain system in terms of three levels: cellular and molecular, computational and systems, and cognitive and behavior. Each level represents each of the three layers of the brain's structure, function, and application, respectively. At the "Structure" layer, the brain consists of neurons and nerves, synapses and action potentials, anatomical areas and their connections. At the "Application" layer, the brain's activity controls real world cognition and behavior, including neurodegenerative diseases and disorders. The middle "Function" layer consists of perception, memory, neural circuits and networks and their connectivity. This layer serves as the glue between the cellular and molecular layer and the real world cognition and behavior layer. It is also the clue to the function of the brain including human information processing for learning, stimuli, reward, choice, and decision making, and functional mechanisms for sensing, motoring, and multi-perception (visual, auditory, tactile, and olfactory) (see Figure 1).

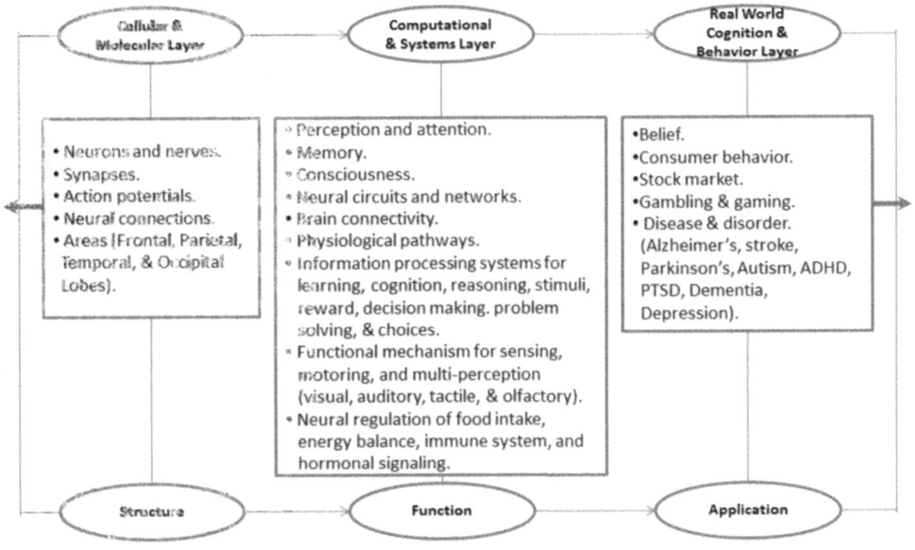

Fig. 1. Scope and Scale of the Brain System

1.2 Informatics

Over the last decade, since the debut of the World Wide Web in the 1990's, the number of information users and providers has increased exponentially. According to Norvig [32], the nature of information content has changed drastically from simple text to a mix of text, speech, still and video images and to histories of interactions with friends and colleagues, information sources and their automated proxies. Raw data sources now include sensor readings from GPS devices and GIS locations, medical devices such as EEG/MEG/fMRI, and other embedded sensors and robots in organizations and in the environment. Communication conduits include twisted pair, coaxial cables and optical fibers, wireline, wireless, satellite, the Internet, and more recently, information appliances such as smart phones and intelligent computing systems.

The word "Informatics" has been used in a variety of different contexts and disciplines. Webster's Dictionary (10th Edition) describes it as "Information science", and is stated as "the collection, classification, storage, retrieval, and dissemination of recorded knowledge treated both as a pure and as an applied science." Hsu et al [19] suggest the following:

"Informatics is the science that studies and investigates the acquisition, representation, processing, interpretation, and transformation of information in, for, and by living organisms, neuronal systems, interconnection networks, and other complex systems."

As an emerging scientific discipline consisting of methods, processes, practices, and applications, informatics serves as the crucial link between the domain data it acquires and the domain knowledge it will transform it to (see Figure 2).

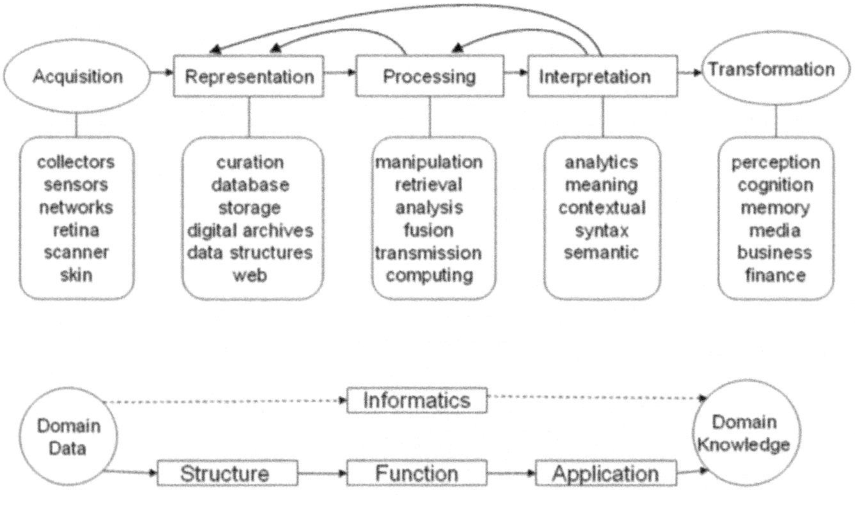

Fig. 2. Scope and Scale of Informatics (Hsu et al [19])

From Figure 2, we see that converting data into knowledge in an application domain is a complicated process of a serious information processing endeavor. As such, a pipeline of three layers has emerged where the "Information" layer serves as the connection and glue between the "Data" layer and the "Knowledge" layer.

Data ---> Information ---> Knowledge.

1.3 Brain Informatics

The brain system is a complex system with a complicated structure, dynamic function and a variety of diverse applications in cognition, behavior, diseases and disorders. To study the brain and to utilize the data obtained from such study or experiments requires a new kind of scientific discovery called the Fourth Paradigm by Jim Gray [14]. This emerging branch of contemporary scientific inquiry utilizes "data exploration" to coherently probe and/or unify experiment, theory, and simulation. In a similar fashion, experiments today increasingly involve very large datasets captured by instruments or generated by simulators and processed by software. Information and knowledge are stored in computers or data centers as databases. These databases are analyzed using mathematical, statistical and computational tools, reasoning, and techniques.

A point raised by Jim Gray is 'how to codify and represent knowledge in a given discipline X?'. Several generic problems include: data ingest and managing large datasets, identifying and enforcing common schema, how to organize and reorganize these data and their associated analyses, building and executing models, documenting experiments, curation and long-term preservation, interpretation of information, and transformation of information to knowledge. All these issues are complicated and hence require powerful computational and informatics methods, tools, and techniques. Hence the concept of "CompXinfor" is born which means computational-X and X-informatics for a given discipline X. One example is computational biology and bioinformatics. Another is computational brain and brain informatics. So, brain informatics is a data-driven science using a combination of experiment, theory, and modeling to analyze large structured (and unstructured) and normal (and peculiar) data sets. Simulation, modeling, and visualization techniques are also added to the process. This kind of e-science inquiry does need modern mathematical, computational and statistical techniques. It also requires a variety of methods and systems embedded in such fields as artificial intelligence, machine learning, data mining, information fusion, and knowledge discovery. Figure 3 gives the three levels of knowledge domain for informatics in general and for brain informatics in particular.

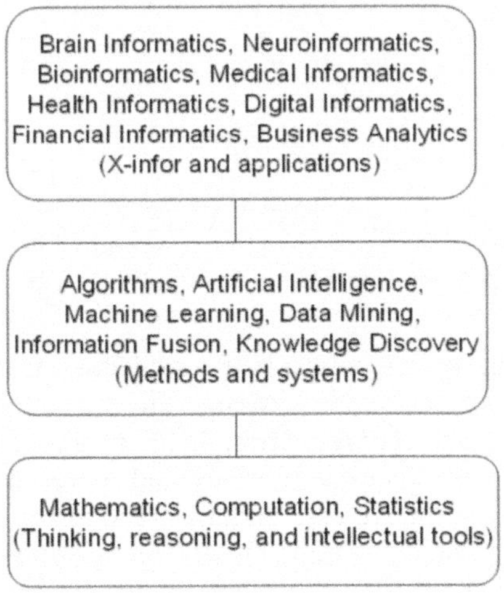

Fig. 3. The three levels of (Brain) Informatics knowledge domain (Hsu et al [19])

As illustrated in Figure 1, the field of "Brain Science" is evolving at the "Function" layer with neural circuits and brain connectivity as its main focus. These are complemented by other findings in genome-wide gene expression and epigenetic study. There have been many sources of databases resulting from multifaceted experiments and projects. The neuroscience information framework [1] is an example of efforts to integrate existing knowledge and databases in neuroscience. Combining the scope and scale of the brain system and informatics (see Figures 1 and 2), a brain information system framework (BISF) is needed to give a coherent approach in the integration of diverse knowledge and a variety of databases in studies and experiments related to the brain (see Figure 4).

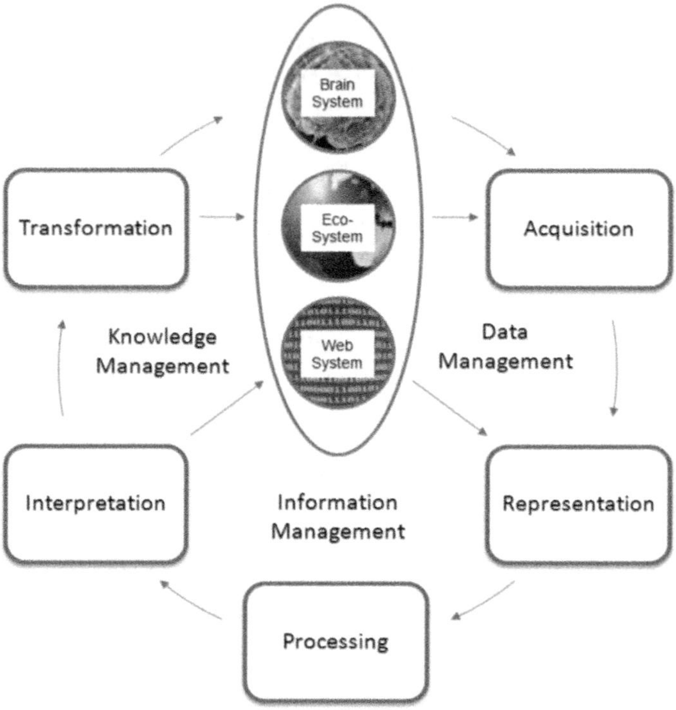

Fig. 4. Brain Information System Framework (BISF)

Other than the brain itself, data can be collected from the ecosystem in the environment and the various web systems on the Internet [11]. At the "data management" level, various data types from different sensors or imaging devices (e.g. fMRI/EEG) and sources are acquired, curated and represented as databases and data structures. Information extracted and patterns recognized from these data can be processed (retrieved, computed, transmitted, mined, fused, or analyzed) at the "information management" level. Further analysis and interpretation can be performed at the knowledge management level. Useful knowledge is extracted from the insightful interpretation of information and actionable data. This valuable knowledge is then transformed (in a feedback loop) to benefit the understanding of the brain system, the function of the ecosystem and the operation of various web systems.

1.4 Information Fusion

In each of the three levels of brain information system management – data, information, and knowledge, fusion is needed at the data, feature, and decision levels due to the following characteristics [2, 7, 18]:

- A variety of different sets of structured or unstructured data are collected from diverse devices or sources originated from different experiments and projects.
- A large group of different sets of features, attributes, indicators, or cues are used as parameters for different kinds of measurements.
- Different methods or decisions may be appropriate for different feature sets, data sets or temporal traces.
- Different methods or systems for decision and action may be combined to obtain innovative solutions for the same problem with diverse data and/or feature sets.

Information fusion is the combination or integration of information (at the data, feature, and decision level) from multiple sources or sensors, features or cues, classifiers or decisions so that efficiency and accuracy of situation analysis, evidence-based decision making, and actionable outcomes can be greatly enhanced [2, 18, 22, 39]. As shown in Figure 2, information fusion plays a central role in the informatics processing pipeline.

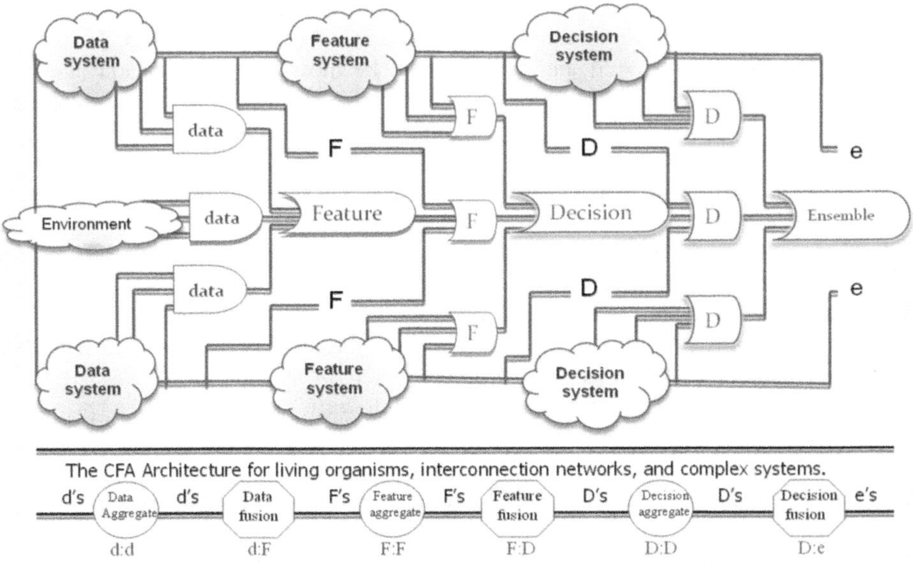

Fig. 5. The CFA Architecture and Workflow [19]

Combinatorial fusion analysis (CFA), a recently developed information fusion method and an informatics paradigm, consists of multiple scoring systems and uses a rank-score characteristic (RSC) function to measure the cognitive diversity between a pair of two scoring systems. The architecture and workflow of CFA is illustrated in Figure 5.

2 Combinatorial Fusion Analysis

2.1 Multiple Scoring Systems (MSS)

Let D be a set of documents, genes, molecules, tracks, hypotheses, or classes with $|D| = n$. Let $N = [1, n]$ be the set of integers from 1 to n and R be the set of real numbers. A set of p scoring systems $A_1, A_2, \ldots, A_p$ on D has each scoring system A consisting of a score function s_A, a rank function r_A derived by sorting the score function s_A, and a Rank-Score Characteristic (RSC) function f_A defined as $f_A: N \rightarrow R$ in Figure 6.

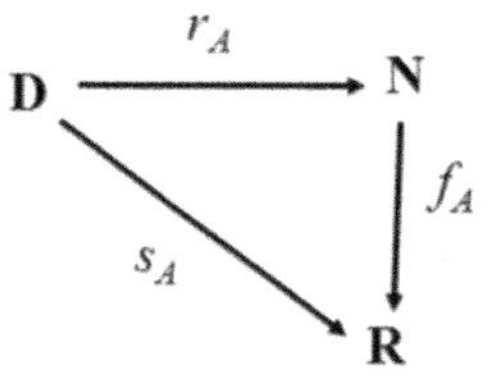

$$f_A(i) = (s_A \circ r_A^{-1})(i) = s_A(r_A^{-1}(i))$$

Fig. 6. Rank-Score Characteristic (RSC) Function

Given a set of p scoring systems $A_1, A_2, \ldots, A_p$, there are many different ways to combine these scoring systems into a single system A^* (e.g. see [15, 16, 18, 21, 25, 31, 40, 43]). Let $C_s(\sum A_i) = E$ and $C_r(\sum A_i) = F$ be the score combination and rank combination defined by $s_E(d) = (1/p) \sum s_{Ai}(d)$ and $s_F(d) = (1/p) \sum r_{Ai}(d)$, respectively, and let r_E and r_F be derived by sorting s_E and s_F in decreasing order and increasing order, respectively. Hsu and Taksa studied comparisons between score combination and rank combination [17] and showed that rank combination does perform better under certain conditions.

Performances can be evaluated in terms of true/false positives and true/false negatives, precision and recall, goodness of hit, specificity and sensitivity, etc. Once performance measurement P is agreed upon for the score combination $E = C_s(A,B)$ and rank combination $F = C_r(A,B)$ of two scoring systems A and B, the following two most fundamental problems in information fusion can be asked.

(a) When is $P(E)$ or $P(F)$ greater than or equal to $max\{P(A), P(B)\}$?

(b) When is $P(F)$ greater than or equal to $P(E)$?

2.2 Rank-Score Characteristic (RSC) Function and Cognitive Diversity

For a scoring system A with score function s_A, as stated before and shown in Figure 6, its rank function r_A can be derived by sorting the score values in decreasing order and assigning a rank value to replace the score value. The diagram in Figure 6 shows mathematically, for i in $N=[1,n]$: $f_A(i) = (s_A \circ r_A^{-1})(i) = s_A(r_A^{-1}(i))$. Computationally, f_A can be derived simply by sorting the score values by using the rank values as the keys. The example in Figure 7 illustrates a RSC function on $D = \{d_1, d_2, \ldots, d_{12}\}$ using the computational approach of sorting, reordering, and composition.

D	**Score function s:D→R**	**Rank function r:D→N**		**RSC function f:N→R**	
d_1	3	10		1	10
d_2	8.2	3		2	9.8
d_3	7	4		3	8.2
d_4	4.6	7		4	7
d_5	4	8		5	5.4
d_6	10	1		6	5
d_7	9.8	2		7	4.6
d_8	3.3	9		8	4
d_9	1	12		9	3.3
d_{10}	2.5	11		10	3
d_{11}	5	6		11	2.5
d_{12}	5.4	5		12	1

Fig. 7. Computational Derivation of RSC Function

Let D be a set of twenty figure skaters in an international figure skating competition, and consider the example of three judges A, B, C assigning scores to each of the skaters at the end of a contest. Figure 8 illustrates three potential RSC functions f_A, f_B, and f_C, respectively. In this case, each RSC function illustrates the scoring (or ranking) behavior of the scoring system, which is each of the three judges. The example shows that Judge A has a very evenly distributed scoring practice while Judge B gives less number of skaters high scores and Judge C gives more skaters high scores.

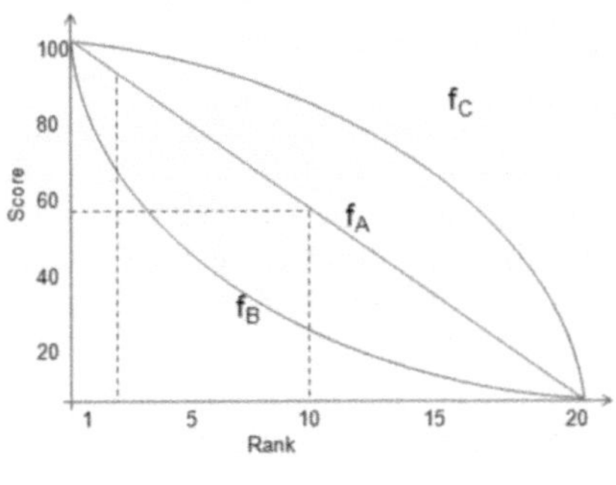

Fig. 8. Three RSC functions f_A, f_B, and f_C

This example highlights a use of multiple scoring systems, where each of the three scoring systems (judges) makes a judgment as to how good a given skater is.

In the case of two systems A and B, the concept of diversity $d(A,B)$ is defined (see [18]). For scoring systems A and B, the diversity $d(A,B)$ between A and B has the following three possibilities:

(a) $d(A,B)= 1-d(s_A,s_B)$, where $d(s_A,s_B)$ is the correlation (e.g. Pearson's z correlation) between score functions s_A and s_B,

(b) $d(A,B)=1-d(r_A,r_B)$, where $d(r_A,r_B)$ is the rank correlation (e.g. Kendall's tau τ or Spearman's rho ρ) between rank functions r_A and r_B, and

(c) $d(A,B)=d(f_A, f_B)$, the diversity between RSC functions f_A and f_B.

Correlation is one of the central concepts in statistics. It has been shown that correlation is very useful in many application domains which use statistical methods and tools. However, it remains a challenge to interpret correlations in a complex system or dynamic environment. For example, in the financial domain, Engle discussed the challenge of forecasting dynamic correlations which play an essential role in risk forecasting, portfolio management, and other financial activities [9]. Diversity, on the other hand, is a crucial concept in informatics. In computational approaches such as machine learning, data mining, and information fusion, it has been shown that when combining multiple classifier systems, multiple neural nets, and multiple scoring systems, higher diversity is a necessary condition for improvement [3, 18, 22, 39, 41]. Figure 9 shows some comparison on a variety of characteristics between correlation and diversity.

	Likely Target	Domain Rules	Reasoning / Method	Opposite Concept	Measurement / Judgment	Fusion Level
Correlation /Similarity	Object	Syntactic	Statistics	Difference	Data	Data
Diversity / Heterogeneity	Subject	Semantic	Informatics	Homogeneity	Decision	Feature / Decision

Fig. 9. Correlation/Similarity vs. Diversity/Heterogeneity (Hsu et al [19])

2.3 Examples of CFA Domain Applications

We exhibit six examples of domain applications using Combinatorial Fusion Analysis in information retrieval, virtual screening, target tracking, protein structure prediction, combining multiple text mining methods in biomedicine, and on-line learning where RSC function is used to define cognitive diversity [17, 25, 26, 27, 30, 42]. Other domains of application include bioinformatics, text mining and portfolio management [24, 29, 38, 40].

(a) Comparing Rank and Score Combination Methods

Using the symmetric group S_{500} as the sample space for rank functions with respect to five hundred documents, Hsu and Taksa [17] showed that under certain conditions, such as higher values of the diversity $d(f_A, f_B)$, the performance of rank combination is better than that of score combination, $P(F)\geq P(E)$, under both performance evaluation of precision and average precision.

(b) Improving Enrichment in Virtual Screening
Using five scoring systems with two genetic docking algorithms on four target proteins: thymidine kinase (TK), human dihydrofolate reductase (DHFR), and estrogen receptors of antagonists and agonists (ER antagonist and ER agonist), Yang et al [42] demonstrated that high performance ratio and high diversity are two conditions necessary for the fusion to be positive, i.e. combination performs better than each of the individual systems.

(c) Target Tracking Under Occlusion
Lyons and Hsu [27] applied a multisensory fusion approach, based on the CFA and the RSC function to study the problem of multisensory video tracking with occlusion. In particular, Lyons and Hsu [27] demonstrated that using RSC function as a diversity measure is an effective method to study target tracking video with occlusions.

(d) Combining Multiple Information Retrieval Models in Biomedical Literature
Li, Shi, and Hsu [25] compare seven systems of biomedical literature retrieval algorithms. They then use CFA to combine those systems and demonstrated that combination is better only when the performance of the original systems are good and they are different in terms of RSC diversity.

(e) Protein Structure Prediction
Lin et al [26] use CFA to select and combine multiple features in the process of protein structure prediction and showed that it improved accuracy.

(f) On-line Learning
Mesterharm and Hsu [30] showed that combining multiple sub-experts could improve the on-line learning process.

3 Facial Attractiveness Judgment

3.1 Neural Decision Making

Facial attractiveness judgment is a kind of neural decision making process related to perception. It consists of collection and representation of all sources of priors, evidence, and value into a single quantity which is then processed and interpreted by the decision rule to make a choice or commitment so that the decision can be transformed and used to take action [12]. Unlike information theory and a host of other biostatistical, econometric, and psychometric tools used for data analysis, we use the method and practice of combinatorial fusion analysis, which is related to the signal detection theory (SDT) defined by Green and Swets [13] (1966). SDT provides a conceptual framework for the process to convert single or multiple observations of noisy evidence into a categorical choice [10, 12, 13, 20, 23, 28, 34, 36]. As described in Section 2, CFA is a data-driven, evidence-based information fusion paradigm which uses multiple scoring systems and the RSC function to measure cognitive diversity between each pair of scoring systems [17, 24, 26, 27, 29, 30, 38, 40, 42].

3.2 Gender Variation in Facial Attractiveness Judgment

In the facial attractiveness judgment domain, people are asked to rate the beauty of a face image. We want to explore the factors which influence a person's decision. How much will personal perception or preference affect one's rating? Will the opinions of others influence the judgment? We are interested in examining these questions and, in particular, analyzing how the results vary for female and male subjects rating either female or male faces. In order to gain insight into the variations in attractiveness judgment for females and males, two face rating experiments were conducted. The experiments and their analysis are described below.

The subjects in the first and second experiments were divided into two and three groups, respectively, each with a mix of male and female subjects as follows:

Experiment 1	**Experiment 2**
Group 1: 60 subjects (12 males, 48 females)	Group 1: 61 subjects (32 males, 29 females)
Group 2: 68 subjects (29 males, 39 females)	Group 2: 101 subjects (58 males, 43 females)
	Group 3: 82 subjects (27 males, 55 females)

In the first experiment, the faces to be rated include two sets of images: 100 male faces and 100 female faces and in the second experiment there are two sets of faces, each with 50 male or 50 female faces. The subjects in the first experiment were asked to rate each face on a scale of 1 to 7 according to: (1) personal evaluation: How much do you like it? and (2) general evaluation: If 100 people are asked how much they like the face, how do you think they would evaluate it? We call these two tasks (1) "liking" and (2) "mentalization", respectively.

The subjects in the second experiment are asked to rate the faces on a scale of 1 to 7 according to the following three tasks:

(1) Judge the attractiveness: How much do you like it?
(2) Judge the beauty: How do you rate the face in terms of its beauty?
(3) Mentalization: If 100 people are asked how much they like the face, how do you think they would evaluate it?

We name these three tasks: (1) "liking", (2) "beauty", and (3) "mentalization". The task of beauty evaluation is added to this second experiment in order to see how judgments according to personal liking, beauty, and mentalization evaluation are related and how they may influence each other.

Experiment 1: Data Set Description:

Face	Task	Group	Subject
2(M/F)	2(L/M)	2(G1/G2)	2(M/F)
1:male	1:liking	1:group 1	1:male
2:female	2:mentalization	2:group 2	2:female

Since we are interested in comparing face genders, tasks, and subject genders, we integrate the two groups into one data set and categorize the data by Face (male / female), Task (liking / mentalization), and Subject (male / female) as outlined in the following table. We use "+" to denote integration of two groups. There are a total of 41 male subjects and 87 female subjects in this experiment.

Face	Task	Subject	Group 1 + Group2
male	liking	Male	A(1, 1, +, 1)
male	liking	female	A(1, 1, +, 2)
male	mentalization	male	A(1, 2, +, 1)
male	mentalization	female	A(1, 2, +, 2)
female	liking	male	A(2, 1, +, 1)
female	liking	female	A(2, 1, +, 2)
female	mentalization	male	A(2, 2, +, 1)
female	mentalization	female	A(2, 2, +, 2)

Experiment 2 - Data Set Description:

Face	**Task**	**Group**	**Subject**
2(M/F)	3(L/B/M)	3(G1/G2/G3)	2(M/F)
1:male	1:liking	1:group 1	1:male
2:female	2:beauty	2:group 2	2:female
	3:mentalization	3:group 3	

As in the first experiment, we then integrate all three groups into one larger data set. Here, we categorize the data according to: Face (male / female), Task (liking / beauty / mentalization), and Subject (male / female) and all combinations as shown in the following table. There are a total of 117 male subjects and 127 female subjects.

Face	Task	Subject	Groups 1, 2, and 3
male	liking	Male	A(1, 1, +, 1)
male	liking	female	A(1, 1, +, 2)
male	beauty	male	A(1, 2, +, 1)
male	beauty	female	A(1, 2, +, 2)
male	mentalization	male	A(1, 3, +, 1)
male	mentalization	female	A(1, 3, +, 2)
female	liking	male	A(2, 1, +, 1)
female	liking	female	A(2, 1, +, 2)
female	beauty	male	A(2, 2, +, 1)
female	beauty	female	A(2, 2, +, 2)
female	mentalization	male	A(2, 3, +, 1)
female	mentalization	female	A(2, 3, +, 2)

3.3 Experimental Results

There are many interesting observations that can be made on this data set; here we describe a few observations to demonstrate the potential of CFA analysis in this area. We observe that female subjects are more critical (more stringent) than male subjects, for the mentalization task when evaluating either female or male faces. The RSC graph in Figure 10 compares male and female subjects when judging male faces for the mentalization task, where the female RSC function is consistently lower than the male RSC function.

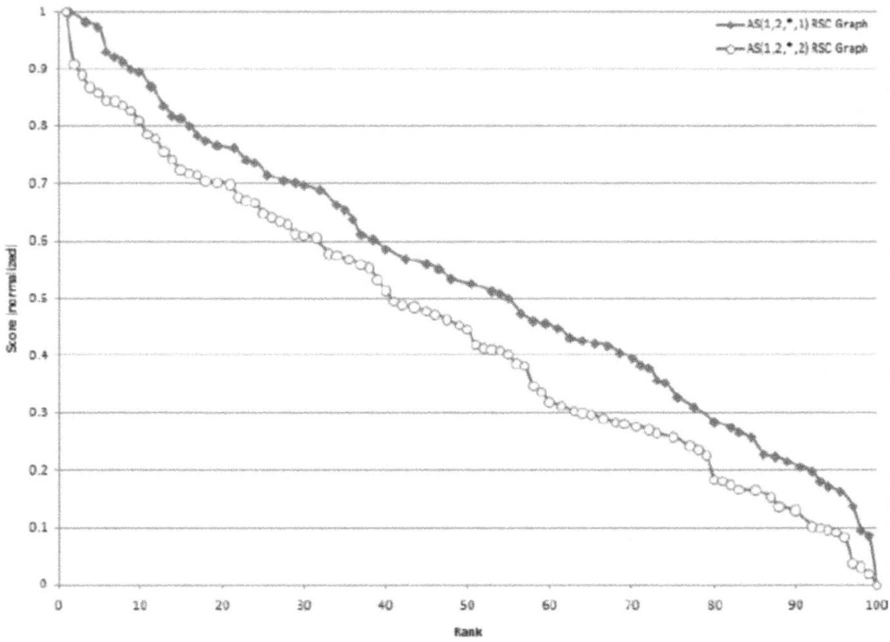

Fig. 10. RSC Graphs for male (blue) and female (red) subjects when evaluating male faces for the mentalization task (Experiment 1)

We observe that, in both data sets, there is little diversity between male and female subjects when judging female faces for the liking task. Figure 11 shows the RSC graph for male and female subjects evaluating male faces for the liking task. Comparing the RSC graphs in Figures 10 and 11, it is observed that male and female subjects demonstrated greater diversity in their scoring behavior for the mentalization task, compared to the liking task in this case; similar is true when evaluating female faces in the first experiment.

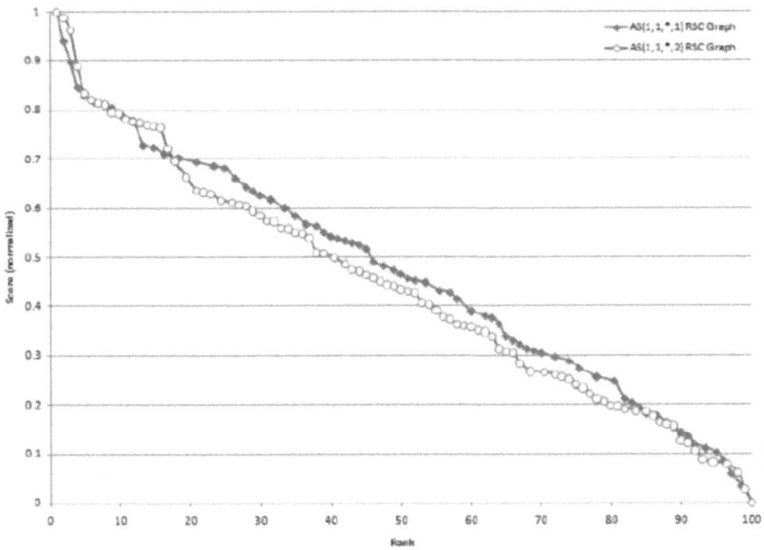

Fig. 11. RSC Graphs for male (blue) and female (red) subjects evaluating male faces under the liking task (Experiment 1)

When comparing face genders, it is observed in both experiments that there is very little diversity between male and female faces, in terms of how they are scored under the mentalization task; this is true for both male and female subjects. This is demonstrated in the following four figures (Figures 12, 13, 14, and 15).

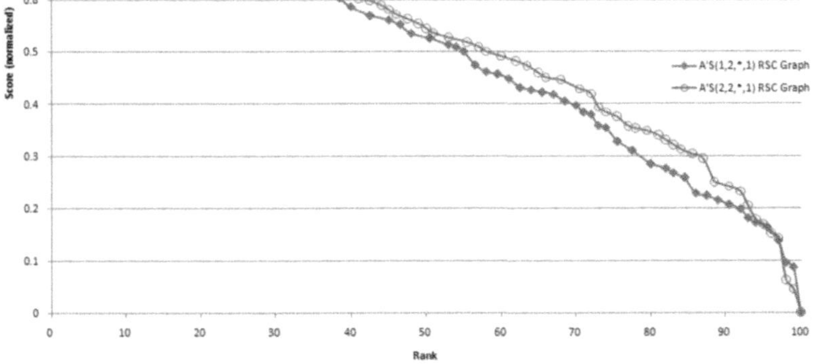

Fig. 12. RSC Graphs for male (blue) and female (red) faces when evaluated by male subjects under the mentalization task (Experiment 1)

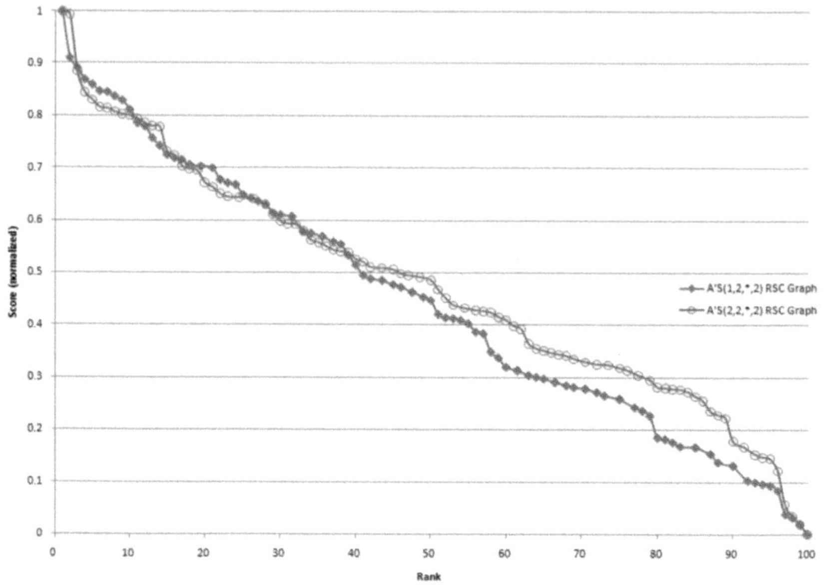

Fig. 13. RSC Graphs for male (blue) and female (red) faces when evaluated by female subjects under the mentalization task (Experiment 1)

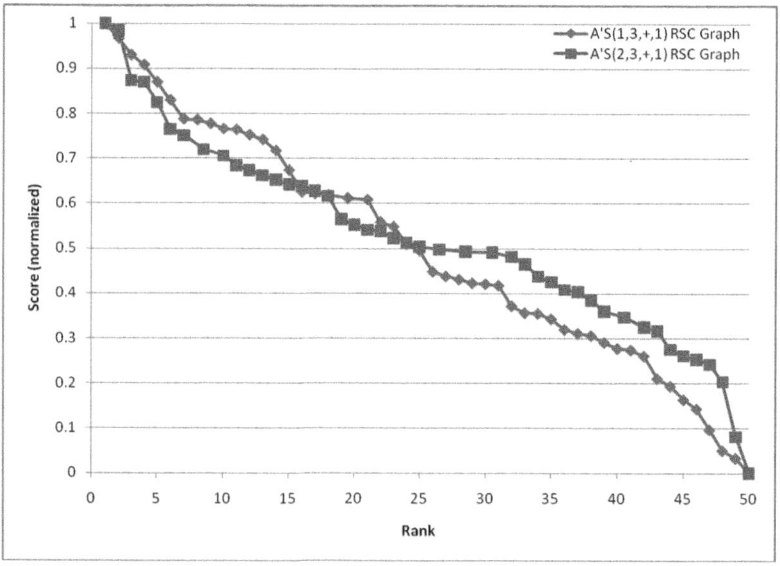

Fig. 14. RSC Graphs for male (blue) and female (red) faces when evaluated by male subjects under the mentalization task (Experiment 2)

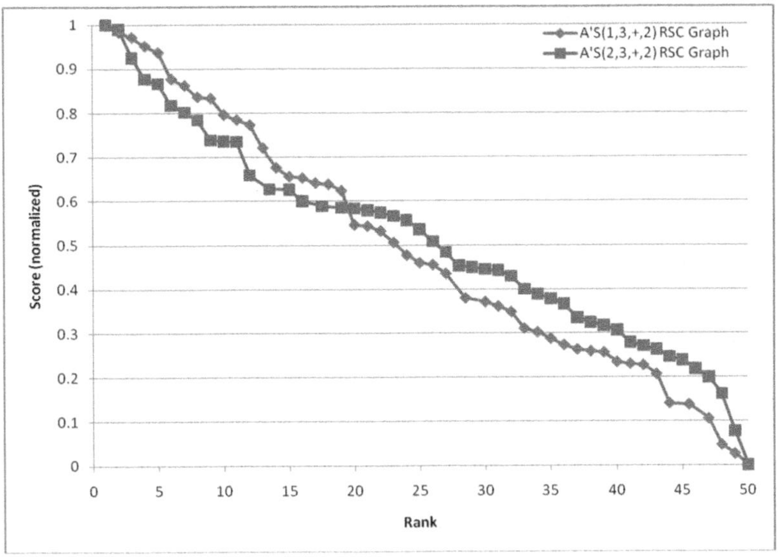

Fig. 15. RSC Graphs for male (blue) and female (red) faces when evaluated by female subjects under the mentalization task (Experiment 2)

3.4 Discussion

In our study, we use the Rank Score Characteristic function to measure the cognitive diversity between male and female subjects and between male and female faces. We have used the same technique to compare tasks among liking, beauty, and mentalization. This will be reported in the future. On the other hand, we have calculated rank correlation (Kendall's tau and Spearman rho) to study the variation between gender subjects and gender faces; this analysis will also be reported.

4 Conclusion and Remarks

4.1 Summary

In this paper, we cover brain systems, informatics, and brain informatics together with the new information paradigm: Combinatorial Fusion Analysis (CFA). CFA is then elaborated in more details using multiple scoring systems to score faces and the RSC function to measure cognitive diversity between subject genders and between face genders. We then describe the two experiments on facial attractiveness judgment and explore gender variation between male and female subjects and between male and female faces.

4.2 Further Work

Future work includes investigation into the relationship between the three tasks of liking, beauty, and mentalization for face judgment evaluation and experiments to determine what psychological and cognitive mechanisms lead to the evaluations subjects give in each of these tasks. We will develop and compare different diversity / similarity measurements, as well as compare our methods and findings to social psychology research.

Acknowledgement. TM was supported by the Japanese University Global Centers of Excellence Program of the Japanese Ministry of Education, Culture, Sports, and Technology. SS was supported by Core Research for Evolutional Science and Technology, the Japanese Science and Technology Agency.

References

[1] Akil, H., Martone, M.E., Van Essen, D.C.: Challenges and Opportunities in Mining Neuroscience Data. Science 331(6018), 708–712 (2011)
[2] Bleiholder, J., Naumann, F.: Data fusion. ACM Computing Surveys 41(1), 1–41 (2008)
[3] Brown, G., Wyatt, J.L., Harris, R., Yao, X.: Diversity creation methods: A survey and categorisation. Journal of Information Fusion 6(1), 5–20 (2005a)
[4] Chun, Y.S., Hsu, D.F., Tang, C.Y.: On the relationships among various diversity measures in multiple classifier systems. In: 2008 International Symposium on Parallel Architectures, Algorithms, and Networks (ISPAN 2008), pp. 184–190 (2008)
[5] Chung, Y. S., Hsu, D.F., Tang, C.Y.: On the diversity-performance relationship for majority voting in classifier ensembles. In: Haindl, M., Kittler, J., Roli, F. (eds.) MCS 2007. LNCS, vol. 4472, pp. 407–420. Springer, Heidelberg (2007)
[6] Chung, Y.S., Hsu, D.F., Liu, C.Y., Tang, C.Y.: Performance evaluation of classifier ensembles in terms of diversity and performance of individual systems. Inter. Journal of Pervasive Computing and Communications 6(4), 373–403 (2010)
[7] Dasarathy, B.V.: Elucidative fusion systems—an exposition. Information Fusion 1, 5–15 (2000)
[8] Dowling, J.E.: Neurons and Networks: An Introduction to Behavioral Neuroscience, 2nd edn. Belknap Press of Harvard University Press, Cambridge (2001)
[9] Engle, R.: Anticipating Correlations: A New Paradigm for Risk Management. Princeton University Press, Princeton (2009)
[10] Fleming, S.M., et al.: Relating introspective accuracy to individual differences in brain structure. Science 329, 1541–1543 (2010)
[11] Gewin, V.: Rack and Field. Nature 460, 944–946 (2009)
[12] Gold, J.I., Shadlen, M.N.: The neural basis of decision making. Annual Review of Neuroscience 30, 535–574 (2007)
[13] Green, D.M., Swets, J.A.: Signal Detection Theory and Psychophysics. John Wiley & Sons, New York (1966)
[14] Hey, T., et al. (eds.): Jim Gray on eScience: A Transformed Scientific Method, in the Fourth Paradigm. Microsoft Research, pp. 17–31 (2009)
[15] Ho, T.K.: Multiple classifier combination: Lessons and next steps. In: Bunke, H., Kandel, A. (eds.) Hybrid Methods in Pattern Recognition, pp. 171–198. World Scientific, Singapore (2002)
[16] Ho, T.K., Hull, J.J., Srihari, S.N.: Decision combination in multiple classifier system. IEEE Trans. on Pattern Analysis and Machine Intelligence 16(1), 66–75 (1994)

[17] Hsu, D.F., Taksa, I.: Comparing rank and score combination methods for data fusion in information retrieval. Information Retrieval 8(3), 449–480 (2005)

[18] Hsu, D.F., Chung, Y.S., Kristal, B.S.: Combinatorial fusion analysis: methods and practice of combining multiple scoring systems. In: Hsu, H.H. (ed.) Advanced Data Mining Technologies in Bioinformatics. Idea Group Inc., USA (2006)

[19] Hsu, D.F., Kristal, B.S., Schweikert, C.: Rank-Score Characteristics (RSC) Function and Cognitive Diversity. In: Yao, Y., Sun, R., Poggio, T., Liu, J., Zhong, N., Huang, J. (eds.) BI 2010. LNCS, vol. 6334, pp. 42–54. Springer, Heidelberg (2010)

[20] Kiani, R., Shadlen, M.N.: Representation of confidence associated with a decision by neurons in the parietal cortex. Science 324, 759–764 (2009)

[21] Krogh, A., Vedelsby, J.: Neural Network Ensembles, Cross Validation, and Active Learning. In: Advances in Neural Information Processing Systems, pp. 231–238. M.I.T. Press, Cambridge (1995)

[22] Kuncheva, L.I.: Combining Pattern Classifiers: Methods and Algorithms. Wiley-Interscience, Hoboken (2004)

[23] Lau, H., Maniscalco, B.: Should confidence be trusted? Science 329, 1478–1479 (2010)

[24] Li, Y., Hsu, D.F., Chung, S.M.: Combining Multiple Feature Selection Methods for Text Categorization by Using Rank-Score Characteristics. In: 21st IEEE International Conference on Tools with Artificial Intelligence, pp. 508–517 (2009)

[25] Li, Y., Shi, N., Hsu, D.F.: Fusion Analysis of Information Retrieval Models on Biomedical Collections. In: 14th International Conference on Information Fusion, Fusion 2011 (July 2011)

[26] Lin, K.-L., et al.: Feature Selection and Combination Criteria for Improving Accuracy in Protein Structure Prediction. IEEE Transactions on Nanobioscience 6, 186–196 (2007)

[27] Lyons, D.M., Hsu, D.F.: Combining multiple scoring systems for target tracking using rank-score characteristics. Information Fusion 10(2), 124–136 (2009)

[28] Macmillan, N.A., Creelman, C.D.: Detection Theory: A User's Guide, 2nd edn. Psychology Press, New York (2005)

[29] McMunn-Coffran, C., Schweikert, C., Hsu, D.F.: Microarray Gene Expression Analysis Using Combinatorial Fusion. In: BIBE, pp. 410–414 (2009)

[30] Mesterharm, C., Hsu, D.F.: Combinatorial Fusion with On-line Learning Algorithms. In: The 11th International Conference on Information Fusion, pp. 1117–1124 (2008)

[31] Ng, K.B., Kantor, P.B.: Predicting the effectiveness of naive data fusion on the basis of system characteristics. J. Am. Soc. Inform. Sci. 51(12), 1177–1189 (2000)

[32] Norvig, P.: Search. In "2020 vision". Nature 463, 26 (2010)

[33] Ohshima, M., Zhong, N., Yao, Y., Liu, C.: Relational peculiarity-oriented mining. Data Min. Knowl. Disc. 15, 249–273 (2007)

[34] Parker, A.J., Newsome, W.T.: Sense and the single neuron: Probing the physiology of perception. Annu. Rev. Neuroscience 21, 227–277 (1998)

[35] Pawela, C., Biswal, B.: Brain Connectivity: A new journal emerges. Brain Connectivity 1(1), 1–2 (2011)

[36] Rieke, F., Warland, D., de Ruyter van Steveninck, R., Bialek, W.: Spikes: Exploring the Neural Code. MIT Press, Cambridge (1997)

[37] Schadt, E.: Molecular networks as sensors and drivers of common human diseases. Nature 461, 218–223 (2009)

[38] Schweikert, C., Li, Y., Dayya, D., Yens, D., Torrents, M., Hsu, D.F.: Analysis of Autism Prevalence and Neurotoxins Using Combinatorial Fusion and Association Rule Mining. In: BIBE, pp. 400–404 (2009)

[39] Sharkey, A.J.C. (ed.): Combining Artificial Neural Nets: Ensemble and. Modular Multi-Net Systems. Perspectives in Neural Computing. Springer, London (1999)

[40] Vinod, H.D., Hsu, D.F., Tian, Y.: Combinatorial Fusion for Improving Portfolio Performance. Advances in Social Science Research Using R, pp. 95–105. Springer, Heidelberg (2010)

[41] Whittle, M., Gillet, V.J., Willett, P.: Analysis of data fusion methods in virtual screening: Theoretical model. Journal of Chemical Information and Modeling 46, 2193–2205 (2006)

[42] Yang, J.M., Chen, Y.F., Shen, T.W., Kristal, B.S., Hsu, D.F.: Consensus scoring for improving enrichment in virtual screening. Journal of Chemical Information and Modeling 45, 1134–1146 (2005)

[43] Zhong, N., Yao, Y., Ohshima, M.: Peculiarity oriented multidatabase mining. IEEE Trans. Knowl. Data Eng. 15(4), 952–960 (2003)

People's Opinion, People's Nexus, People's Security and Computational Intelligence: The Evolution Continues

Ali Ghorbani

Faculty of Computer Science, University of New Bunswick
Box 4400 Fredericton, N.B., Canada
ghorbani@unb.ca

The talk begins with a brief introduction to some of our research work in the past few years as well as the ongoing research. A new model on extending the flexibility and responsiveness of websites through automated learning for custom-tailoring and adaptive web to user usage patterns, interests, goals, knowledge and preferences will be presented. The second part of the talk will be devoted to the challenges that the Computational Intelligence communities are faced with in order to address issues related to people's nexus, opinion, and security on the Web, and our contributions to these topics. At the end, I will provide an overview of our current research focus on network security and intelligence information handling and disimination.

B. Hu et al. (Eds.): BI 2011, LNAI 6889, p. 21, 2011.

Towards Conversational Artifacts

Toyoaki Nishida

Graduate School of Informatics, Kyoto University, Yoshida-Honmachi Sakyo-ku
606-8501 Kyoto, Japan
nishdia@i.kyoto-u.ac.jp

Abstract. Conversation is a natural and powerful means of communication for people to collaboratively create and share information. People are skillful in expressing meaning by coordinating multiple modalities, interpreting utterances by integrating partial cues, and aligning their behavior to pursuing joint projects in conversation. A big challenge is to build conversational artifacts – such as intelligent virtual agents or conversational robots – that can participate in conversation so as to mediate the knowledge process in a community. In this article, I present an approach to building conversational artifacts. Firstly, I will highlight an immersive WOZ environment called ICIE (Immersive Collaborative Interaction Environment) that is designed to obtain detailed quantitative data about human-artifact interaction. Secondly, I will overview a suite of learning algorithms for enabling our robot to build and revise a competence of communication as a result of observation and experience. Thirdly, I will argue how conversational artifacts might be used to help people work together in multi-cultural knowledge creation environments.

Keywords: Conversational informatics, social intelligence design, information explosion.

1 Prologue

We are in the midst of Information explosion (*Info-plosion*). On the one hand, we often feel overloaded by the overwhelming amount of information, such as too many incoming e-mail messages including spams and unwanted ads. On the other hand, explosively increased information may also lead to a better support of our daily life [1]. Info-plosion has brought about an expectation that dense distribution of information and knowledge in our living space will eventually allow actors to maximally benefit from the given environment being guided by ubiquitous services.

Unfortunately, the latter benefit is not fully there, as one might be often trapped by real world problems, such as being unable to connect the screen of your laptop to the projector. From time to time, the actors might be forced to waste long time to recover from obsolete instructions or lose critical moments due to the lack of timely information provision. Should the knowledge actor fail to complete it in real-time, she or he may not benefit from the knowledge.

B. Hu et al. (Eds.): BI 2011, LNAI 6889, pp. 22–27, 2011.

A key issue in the information age is knowledge circulation [2]. It is not enough to just deliver knowledge to everybody who needs it. It is critical to keep knowledge updated, and have it evolve by incorporating ideas and opinions of people. Knowledge need to be circulated among proper people so that they can incorporate contribution from them. Although information and communication technologies provide us with potential keys to success, a wide range of issues need to be addressed, ranging from fundamental problems in communication to cultural sensitivity.

It is quite challenging to address what is called the knowledge grounding problem arising from the fact that information and knowledge on the web are essentially decoupled from the real world, in the sense that they cannot be applied to the real world problems unless the actor properly recognizes the situation and understand how knowledge is associated with it. Propositions decoupled from the real world may cause the "last 10 feet problem", i.e., one might not be able to reach the goal even though s/he is within the 10 feet from there. Computational models need to be built for accounting not only for the process of perceptual knowledge in action but also for the meaning and concept creation in general. We need to address the epistemological aspects of knowledge and build a computational theory of understanding perceptual knowledge we have to live in the real world. How can we do it?

2 Power of Conversation

Conversation plays a critical role in forming grounded knowledge by associating knowledge with real world situations [3]. People are skillful in aligning their behavior to pursuing joint projects in conversation, as Clark characterized conversation as an emergent joint action, to be carried by an ensemble of people [4]. Language use consists of multiple levels, from the signals to joint projects. Various kinds of social interactions are made at multiple levels of granularity. In the middle, speech acts such as requesting for information, proposing solution, or negotiating. In the micro, interaction is coordinated by quick actions such as head gesture, eye gaze, posture and paralinguistic actions. In the macro, long-term social relation building is going, trust-making, social network building, and developing social atmosphere. Occasionally, when they get deeply involved in a discussion, they may synchronize their behavior in an almost unconscious fashion, exhibiting empathy with each other to be convinced that they have established a common understanding.

People are skillful both in expressing meaning by coordinating multiple modalities and in interpreting utterances by integrating partial cues. People not only use signals to control the flow of a conversation, e.g., pass the turn of conversation from one to another but also create or add meaning by making utterances, indicating things in the real world, or demonstrating aspects of objects under discussion. Kendon regarded gestures as a part of speaker's utterances and conducted a descriptive analysis of gesture use by investigating in detail how speech and gesture function in relation to one another [5]. McNeill discussed the mental process for integrated production of gesture and words [6].

3 Conversational Artifacts

Conversational artifacts are autonomous software or hardware capable of talking with people by integrating verbal and nonverbal means of communication. The role of conversational artifacts is to mediate the flow of conversational content among people.

There is a long history of development for embodied conversational agents or intelligent virtual agents [7], [8]. Our group has been working on embodied conversational agents and conversational robots [9-14].

As the more sophisticated agents are being built, the methodology has shifted from the script/programming-based to data-driven approaches, for we need to gain more detailed understanding of communicative proficiency people show in conversation. The data-driven approach consists of two stages: the first stage for building a conversation corpus by gathering data about inter-human conversation and the second stage for generating the behavior of conversational artifacts from the corpus. WOZ (Wizard-of-Oz) is effective in collecting data in which a tele-operated synthetic character or robot are used to interact with experiment participants.

In order for this approach to be effective, two technical problems need to be solved. The first is to realize the "human-in-the-artifacts" feeling. In WOZ experiments, we employ experiment participants to operate conversational to collect how the conversational artifacts should act in various situations in conversation. In order for these WOZ experiments to be useful, the experiment participants should feel and behave as if she were the conversational artifact. Thus, the WOZ experiment environment should be able to provide experiment participants with the situational information the conversational artifact obtains and operate the conversational artifact without difficulty. The second is to develop a method of effectively producing the behaviors of the conversational artifact from the data collected in the WOZ experiments. I will address these issues in the following two sections.

4 Immersive WOZ Environment with ICIE

Our immersive WOZ environment provides the human operator with a feeling as if s/he stayed "inside" a conversational artifact to receive incoming visual and auditory signals and to create conversational behaviors in a natural fashion [15]. At the human-robot interaction site, a 360-degree camera is placed near the robot's head, which can acquire the image of all directions around it. The image captured by the 360-degree camera is sent to the operator's cabin using TCP/IP. The WOZ operator's cabin is in the cylindrical display, which is a set of large-sized displays which are circularly aligned. The current display system uses eight 64-inch display panels arranged in a circle with about 2.5 meters diameter. Eight surround speakers are used to reproduce the acoustic environment. The WOZ operator stands in the cylindrical display and controls the robot from there. The image around the robot is projected on an immersive cylindrical display around the WOZ operator. This setting gives the operator exactly the same view as the robot sees. When a scene is displayed on the full screen, it will provide a sense of immersion.

The WOZ operator's behavior, in turn, is captured by a range sensor to reproduce a mirrored behavior of the robot. We realize accurate and real-time capturing of the operator's motion by using a range sensor and enable the operator to intuitively control the robot according to the result of the capturing. We make the robot take the same poses as the operator does by calculating the angles of the operator's joints at every frame. We can control NAO's head, shoulders, elbows, wrists, fingers, hip joints, knees, and ankles, and we think they are enough to represent basic actions in communication. The sound on each side of the WOZ operator is gathered by microphones and communicated via network so that everyone can hear the sound of the other side.

5 Learning by Mimicking

Learning by mimicking is a computational framework for producing the interactive behaviors of conversational artifacts from a collection of data obtained from the WOZ experiments. In the framework of learning by mimicking, a human operator is guiding a robot (actor) to follow a predefined path in the ground using free hand gestures. Another learner robot watches the interaction using sensors attached to the operator and the actor and learns the action space of the actor, the command space of the operator and the associations between commands (gestures) and actions. This metaphor characterizes our approach to developing a fully autonomous learner, which might be contrasted with another approach to manually producing the behavior of conversational artifacts probably partially using data mining and machine learning techniques. Currently, we concentrate on nonverbal interactions though we have started on integrating verbal and nonverbal behaviors. We have developed a suite of unsupervised learning algorithms for this framework [16][17].

The learning algorithm can be divided into four stages:

1) the discovery stage on which the robot discovers the action and command space;
2) the association stage on which the robot associates discovered actions and commands generating a probabilistic model that can be used either for behavior understanding or generation;
3) the controller generation stage on which the behavioral model is converted into an actual controller to allow the robot to act in similar situations; and
4) the accumulation stage on which the robot combines the gestures and actions it learned from multiple interactions.

6 Application to Multi-cultural Knowledge Creation

Cultural factors might come into play in globalization. Based on the work on cross-cultural communication [18], we are currently investigating how difficulties in living in a different culture are caused by different patterns of thinking, feeling and potential actions. We are building a *simulated crowd*, a novel tool for allowing people to practice culture-specific nonverbal communication behaviors [19].

We have started a "cross-campus exploration" project aiming at prototyping a system that allows the user (e.g., in the Netherlands) to explore (probably in a RPG fashion) a virtualized university campus possibly in a different culture (e.g., in Japan), or use a tele-presence robot to meet people out there. It will permit the user to experience with interacting with people in a different culture or even actually. Technologies for conversational artifacts will play a significant role in these applications.

References

1. Kitsuregawa, M., Nishida, T.: Special Issue on Information Explosion. New Generation Computing 28(3), 207–215 (2010)
2. Nishida, T.: Social Intelligence Design for Cultivating Shared Situated Intelligence. In: GrC 2010, pp. 369–374 (2010)
3. Nishida, T. (ed.): Conversational Informatics: an Engineering Approach. John Wiley & Sons Ltd., London (2007)
4. Clark, H.H.: Using Language. Cambridge University Press, Cambridge (1996)
5. Kendon, A.: Gesture. Cambridge University Press, Cambridge (2004)
6. McNeill, D.: Gesture and Thought. The University of Chicago Press, Chicago (2005)
7. Cassell, J., Sullivan, J., Prevost, J., Churchill, E. (eds.): Embodied Conversational Agents. The MIT Press, Cambridge (2000)
8. Prendinger, H., Ishizuka, M. (eds.): Life-like Characters – Tools. Affective Functions and Applications. Springer, Heidelberg (2004)
9. Kubota, H., Nishida, T., Koda, T.: Exchanging Tacit Community Knowledge by Talking-virtualized-egos. In: Proceedings of Agent 2000, pp. 285–292 (2000)
10. Nishida, T.: Social Intelligence Design for Web Intelligence, Special Issue on Web Intelligence. IEEE Computer 35(11), 37–41 (2002)
11. Okamoto, M., Nakano, Y.I., Okamoto, K., Matsumura, K., Nishida, T.: Producing Effective Shot Transitions in CG Contents based on a Cognitive model of User Involvement. IEICE Transactions of Information and Systems Special Issue of Life-like Agent and Its Communication, IEICE Trans. Inf. & Syst. E88-D(11), 2532–2623 (2005)
12. Huang, H.H., Cerekovic, A., Pandzic, I., Nakano, Y., Nishida, T.: The Design of a Generic Framework for Integrating ECA Components. In: Proceedings of 7th International Conference of Autonomous Agents and Multiagent Systems (AAMAS 2008), Estoril, Portugal, pp. 128–135 (2008)
13. Huang, H.H., Furukawa, T., Ohashi, H., Nishida, T., Cerekovic, A., Pandzic, I.S., Nakano, Y.I.: How Multiple Concurrent Users React to a Quiz Agent Attentive to the Dynamics of their Game Participation. In: AAMAS 2010, pp. 1281–1288 (2010)
14. Nishida, T., Terada, K., Tajima, T., Hatakeyama, M., Ogasawara, Y., Sumi, Y., Yong, X., Mohammad, Y.F.O., Tarasenko, K., Ohya, T., Hiramatsu, T.: Towards Robots as an Embodied Knowledge Medium, Invited Paper, Special Section on Human Communication II. IEICE Transactions on Information and Systems E89-D(6), 1768–1780 (2006)
15. Ohashi, H., Okada, S., Ohmoto, Y., Nishida, T.: A Proposal of Novel WOZ Environment for Realizing Essence of Communication in Social Robots. Presented at: Social Intelligence Design 2010 (2010)

16. Mohammad, Y.F.O., Nishida, T., Okada, T.: Unsupervised Simultaneous Learning of Gestures, Actions and their Associations for Human-Robot Interaction. In: IROS 2009, pp. 2537–2544 (2009)
17. Mohammad, Y.F.O., Nishida, T.: Learning Interaction Protocols using Augmented Baysian Networks Applied to Guided Navigation. Presented at: IROS 2010, Taipei, Taiwan (2010)
18. Rehm, M., Nakano, Y.I., André, E., Nishida, T.: Culture-Specific First Meeting Encounters between Virtual Agents. In: Prendinger, H., Lester, J.C., Ishizuka, M. (eds.) IVA 2008. LNCS (LNAI), vol. 5208, pp. 223–236. Springer, Heidelberg (2008)
19. Thovuttikul, S., Lala, D., Ohashi, H., Okada, S., Ohmoto, Y., Nishida, T.: Simulated Crowd: Towards a Synthetic Culture for Engaging a Learner in Culture-dependent Nonverbal Interaction. Presented at: 2nd Workshop on Eye Gaze in Intelligent Human Machine Interaction, Stanford University, USA (2011)

Study of System Intuition by Noetic Science Founded by QIAN Xuesen

Zhongtuo Wang

Institute of Systems Engineering, Dalian University of Technology
116085 Dalian, China
wangzt@dlut.edu.cn

Abstract. This talk investigates the meaning, contents and characteristics of systems institution on the basis of Noetic Science, which was founded by Qian Xuesen. The systems intuition is the human capability to find the hidden system imagery of the object or to create an imagery of new system. The basic noetic foundation of system intuition and cultural influence to it are studied. The open problems are also listed.

Keywords: System intuition, Noetic Science, Imagery thinking, Inspiration, Tacit knowledge.

B. Hu et al. (Eds.): BI 2011, LNAI 6889, p. 28, 2011.

Study of Problem Solving Following Herbert Simon

Yulin Qin[1,2] and Ning Zhong[1,3]

[1] The International WIC Institute, Beijing University of Technology, China
[2] Dept. of Psychology, Carnegie Mellon University, USA
[3] Dept. of Life Science and Informatics, Maebashi Institute of Technology, Japan
yulinqin@gmail.com, zhong@maebashi-it.ac.jp

Herbert Simon (1916.6.15 - 2001.2.9) was one of the greatest pioneers in cognitive science and artificial intelligence, as well as in behavior economics and many other fields. Problem solving was his core work in artificial intelligence and cognitive psychology. He and Newell first postulated a general and systematic framework of human (and machine) problem solving as iteratively applying operators to transform the state of the problem from the starting state in problem state space to eventually achieve the goal state. Heuristic problem solving includes two basic components: heuristic searching (such as means-ends analysis) and heuristic rules (used to change the problem states). And then, he extended this framework in two dimensions. One is applying this framework to creative learning and scientific discovery (both were thought as specific ill-structured problem solving tasks); the other is to elaborate this general framework with more detailed models in memory (such as chunk structure in short term memory) and the knowledge (and problem) representations, including the knowledge structure difference between experts and naives, diagrammatic representation and mental imagery. To meet the challenge of Web intelligence and to pioneer the effective and efficient ways of information processing at Web scale, as the first step, we would learn this process from human brain, one of the greatest webs, based on Simon and Newell's framework in problem solving. We have found that, even in the basic application of heuristic rules, the processes are distributed in several major parts of brain and with certain areas for the communications across these networks. We have checked the brain activations in regard to working memory and mental imagery in problem solving. We have also found the evidences supporting the hypothesis that the scientific discovery is a specific problem solving from neural activations that central brain areas activated in scientific discovery overlapping with the areas in general problem solving tasks. These findings offer strong clues for how to solve problems at Web scale.

B. Hu et al. (Eds.): BI 2011, LNAI 6889, p. 29, 2011.

Cognition According to the Ouroboros Model

Knud Thomsen

Paul Scherrer Institut, CH-5232 Villigen PSI, Switzerland
knud.thomsen@psi.ch

Abstract. The Ouroboros Model is a novel proposal for a biologically inspired cognitive architecture. At its core lies a self-referential recursive process with alternating phases of data acquisition and evaluation. All memory entries are organized in junks, schemata. At any one time, the activation of part of a schema biases the whole structure and, in particular, missing features. Thus expectations are triggered. In the next step an iterative recursive monitor process termed 'consumption analysis' is checking how well these expectations fit with the unfolding activations. Mismatches between anticipations based on previous experience and actual current data are highlighted and used for controlling subsequent actions. In this short paper it will be sketched how the Ouroboros Model can shed light on selected cognitive functions including (human) reasoning, learning and emotions.

Keywords: Algorithm, Iterative, Recursive, Schema, Process, Consumption Analysis, Attention, Learning Problem solving Emotions.

1 Introduction

The Ouroboros Model as proposed recently in several papers describes an algorithmic architecture for cognitive agents. It can be seen as an attempt at following up on ideas and conceptions first articulated by Otto Selz about a 100 years ago [1]. The Ouroboros Model starts from two simple observations: animals and human beings are embodied, strongly interacting with their environment, and they can only survive if they maintain a minimum of consistency in their behavior. These conditions pose severe constraints but they also offer an indispensable foundation for a bootstrapping mechanism leading from simple to sophisticated behaviors. As for bodily movement, also for cognition, a minimum measure of coherence and consistency is essential, e.g. nobody can move a limb up and down simultaneously, and, at least in classical real-world settings, opposites cannot both be fully true at the same time.

A detailed description of the principal layout of the Ouroboros Model has been given together with a glimpse on how the proposed structures and processes can address many diverse questions distilled from 50 years of research into Artificial Intelligence [2]. In the following, after a brief conceptual outline of the Ouroboros Model, specifically topics related to learning, reasoning and emotions will be investigated. It will be shown how the Ouroboros Model offers a fresh unified, comprehensive and systematic account of these issues.

B. Hu et al. (Eds.): BI 2011, LNAI 6889, pp. 30–41, 2011.

2 Memory Structures

Otto Selz emphasized the importance of knowledge representation in the form of structured memories, for which he coined the term schema [1]. According to Selz and the Ouroboros Model, all neural representations in a brain can be bound together and preserved for later use. All new compound entities, here also called schemata, join diverse slots into cohesive memory structures. In a rather direct extension of conditioned reflexes, the processes and the resulting memory entries are the same in principle, irrespective of whether components of movements are combined into more elaborate choreographies, percepts into figures, or activations in many different brain areas into an entry for an episode. Existing junks are the material used to forge new and more elaborate entities. Stored data in brains are consequently organized into hierarchies of schemata, and an activation of any part promotes the selected concept and graded activation for each of the linked features.

As a direct consequence of these structures, every neural activation can trigger an expectation for the other associated constituents, which are usually active in the same context. Activation at a time of part of a schema biases the whole structure with all relevant slots and, in particular, also still missing features. It is important to note that in addition to old structures, which have been established well in advance, schemata can also be generated on the fly, assembled from parts and existing building blocks as the occasion or need arises [3].

3 Principal Architecture, Algorithmic Backbone

The core of the Ouroboros Model is established by a self-referential recursive process with two main alternating phases of data acquisition and evaluation. Input to this process can consist in sensory data or it can come as fragments of a memory, to give just two examples. A monitor process called 'consumption analysis' is then checking how well expectations triggered at one point in time fit with the successive activations; these principal stages are identified:

... anticipation,
action / perception,
evaluation,
anticipation,...

The sub-processes are linked into a full repeating circle, and the snake bites its end; the Ouroboros devours its tail as in the alchemists' serpent symbol. A general overview is presented in figure 1. A more detailed description of the flow of activity in cycles, together with a sketch of the gradual bootstrapping, which generates ever more sophisticated structures and processes has been given in recent papers [2,4]; here, only the most essential steps are presented.

Compared to the seemingly similar LIDA architecture, the main difference lies in the pivotal role of performance monitoring, which in an evolutionary approach is harnessed for bootstrapping and universal self-steered action [5].

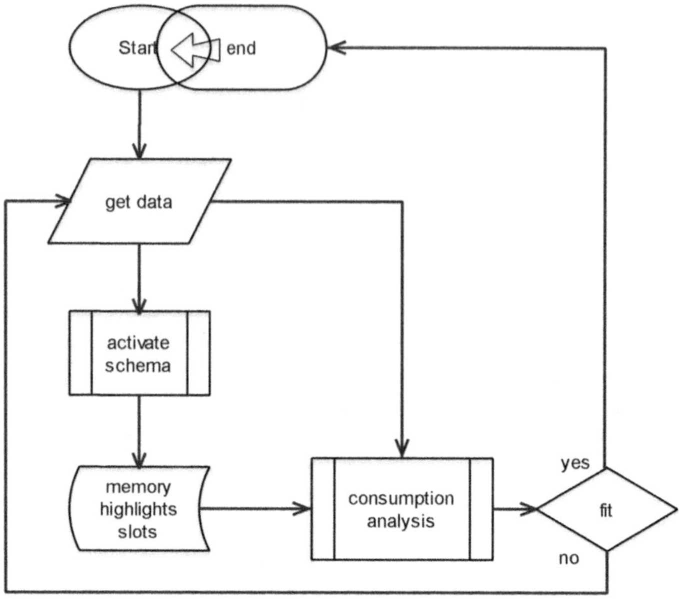

Fig. 1. Structure of the basic data processing loop in the Ouroboros Model (reprinted with permission from [2])

Start:
This is an almost arbitrary entry point.

Get data:
First (perceptional) data arrive as input.

Activate Schema:
Schemata are searched; the one with the strongest activation is selected.

Memory highlights Slots:
Features constituting the selected schema are activated to some extent; this biases all attributes belonging to this schema including ones which are not part of the current input.

Consumption Analysis:
Anticipations are compared to current actual data.

End / new Start…

3.1 Consumption Analysis

Any occurring activation possibly excites many associated schemata. All available memory entries are searched in parallel, the schema with the highest activation is selected first, and other, potentially also applicable, schemata are inhibited, suppressed [2]. Taking the first selected schema and ensuing anticipations as starting point, basis and reference, consumption analysis checks how successive activations fit into this activated frame, i.e. how well low level input data are "consumed" by the chosen schema. Features are assigned / attributes are "explained away" [6].

If everything fits perfectly the process comes to a momentary partly standstill and continues with new input data.

If discrepancies surface, they have an even more immediate impact on the following elicited actions. Empty slots stand out, attention is focused onto them, and fitting information is actively searched for in a well-directed manner.

In the case of severe mismatch, the first schema is discarded and another new conceptual frame is tried. The actual appropriateness of a schema can vary over a wide range. Under all circumstances, consumption analysis delivers a gradual measure for the goodness of fit between expectations and actual inputs, in sum, the quality and acceptability of an interpretation. Thresholds for this signal are set in terms of approval levels depending on the relevant experience in this context. A trade-off is required: in the real world nothing can always be perfect; nevertheless, a wrong schema has to be abandoned at some point.

4 Learning, Concept Formation

According to the Ouroboros Model, learning consists of forming and memorizing new associations, i.e. establishing new schemata from concurrent activations, which represent diverse content of all possible origin, i.e. ranging from primitive sensory features to self reflective monitoring signals [3].

Basically four different situations, in which novel concepts are formed and corresponding fresh memory entries are first created and shaped, can be distinguished.

Two types of occasions are directly marked in the Ouroboros Model as interesting by the outcome of the consumption analysis, and preferentially for them new records are laid down:

1. Events, when everything fits perfectly; i.e. associated neural representations are stored as kind of snapshots of all concurrent activity, - making them available for guidance in the future as they have proved useful once.
2. Constellations, which led to an impasse, are worthwhile remembering, too; in this case for future avoidance.

These new memories stand for junks, i.e. compound concepts, again as schemata, frames or scripts. Their building blocks include whatever representations are activated at the time when the "snapshot" is taken, including sensory signals, abstractions, previously laid down concepts, and prevalent emotions. They might but need not include / correspond to direct representation units like words. At later occasions they form the available basis for actions, and they will serve for controlling behavior, by guiding action to or away from the marked context and tracks. If a context is later encountered again, entries advantageously become malleable for possible corrections.

Knowledge is the very basis for these data processing steps, and its meaningful expansion is a prime outcome of its use as well; the available data-base of concepts / schemata is steadily enlarged and completed, especially in areas where the need for this surfaces and is felt most strongly as each new memory entry will add unexpected and highlighted dimensions to the previously existing structures.

Even without the strong motivation by an acute alert signal from consumption analysis, novel categories and concepts can be assembled on the spot:

3. New concepts are quickly built from existing structures.

We can rapidly establish new compound concepts of whole scenes from previously existing building blocks, i.e. by knitting together (parts of) other concepts; here is an example:

Let us assume that we hear about "the lady in the fur coat". Even without any further specification a figure is defined to a certain extent including many implicit details. Even in case we have heard this expression for the first time, the concept is established well enough for immediate use in a subsequent cycle of consumption analysis, expectations can effectively be triggered. When we now see a woman in this context, we are surprised if she is naked on her feet (...unless she is walking on a beach...). – A fur coat implies warm shoes or boots, and less so, if the wider frame already deviates from the associated defaults.

In parallel to the above described instant establishing of concepts and the recording of at least short time episodic memory entries, there exists a slower and rather independent process:

4. Associations and categorizations are gradually distilled from the statistics of co-occurrences.

In the sense that completely disadvantageous or fatal activity would not be repeated many times, also this grinding-in of associations can be understood as a result of successful and rewarded activations. In each case, remembered activity can pertain to many different, in fact, all possible, representations starting from low level sensory signals to the most abstracts data structures already available, and of course, their combination [3].

According to the Ouroboros Model, memories thus are laid down gradually when inconspicuous sequences are repeated often or, instantaneously at only one occasion, when sufficient activation has been triggered. In addition to the primary content, a measure of relevance and importance, which can naturally be derived from exactly the conditions under which the respective memory has been formed, will be included in the new schema as well. As another result of overlap between memory entries, similar ones will effectively be amalgamated in the course of time.

5 Problem Solving and Reasoning

Many different proposals concerning the principal working of cognition have been made. In front of this background, the Ouroboros Model offers a rather simple and unified account, which can shed light on different aspects pointed out so far and make previous conceptions appear as just distinct facets of one overall algorithmic architecture and its specific data processing steps. The Ouroboros Model can be seen as a common generalization, rendering extant approaches as special cases focusing on selected aspects of the overall puzzle. The following should be understood as a proposal for future investigations, working out the details of the proposed relations; for ease of reading, formulations are such as if this had already been achieved.

Consumption analysis can be understood as a particular algorithm for pattern-matching and -completion, which not only delivers a simple result, e.g. a perception, but also some meta-information relating to the overall performance, the quality of the results, and under what conditions progress unfolds. Suitable and promising next actions in a situation are highlighted, all of that based on the available concepts, i.e. schemata, which had been established earlier [7].

5.1 Attention

A basic feat of the data processing as described in the Ouroboros Model consists in the self-steered allocation of resources. The highlighting of special situations worth of creating a new memory entry as explained above produces concepts where they are required. The emphasis on activations, which will probably be useful in the future, is but one aspect of the feedback and monitor signal delivered by consumption analysis. On a smaller scale, within the frame of an activated schema, a general bias or deviations from expectations emphasize discrepancies and specifically allot resources to the points where they are needed most. These roles can directly be equated with the commonly understood functions of attention.

5.2 Production Systems

First order logic and rule-based behavior have attracted much attention in the past. Rules in production systems provide a means of knowledge representation and allow for its application. With existing implementations, difficulties have been encountered with respect to brittleness, consistency, generalization and learning.

The Ouroboros Model can be seen as offering a natural extension of production systems, with linear if→then rules turning out to be particular instances involving schemata with a single slot open. The Ouroboros Model thus subsumes good parts of symbolic approaches like SOAR and ACT-R on one side and also key features of connectionist models on the other side [8,9,10]. Since all of these approaches have been shown to be Turing equivalent, there is no doubt that the same holds true for the Ouroboros Model. Observing boundary conditions dictated by the implementation in a living body, which bears considerable heritage from its evolution, almost any combination of signals and responses can be learned and established in principle.

5.3 Constraint Satisfaction

Constraint satisfaction has been proposed as a general process for rational behavior and reasoning, applicable in a very wide range of settings [11]. A direct link to the Ouroboros Model is evident: maximizing the satisfaction of a set of constraints can be seen as maximizing coherence [12]. The Ouroboros Model not only is motivated by a principal striving for survival and consistency, it also offers a way to ensure and maintain maximum consistency, albeit within the accessible frames (and not necessarily to a truly global extent). This latter fact explains seemingly irrational behavior as being based upon limited data or frames, which do not encompass and consider all dimensions important in a wider and more complete context.

5.4 Bayesian Inference

In many circumstances, a Bayesian approach can be verified as the optimum way of considering all available evidence in order to arrive at a decision, e.g. in classification and learning [6,13]. In all cases, the decisive step is the proper combining of prior probabilities with current data. The interplay between a (partially) activated schema and newly observed features does just that, – presuming meaningful weight distributions. When certain combinations in general are much more likely than particular others, less additional evidence is required in the former case than in the latter. In practice, dimensions, which are activated first, have a more enduring impact, as new information is subsumed under the already prevailing interpretation; one and the same set of facts can thus give rise to somewhat different interpretations depending on their order and on the weight that the constituting slots are assigned.

5.5 Parallel versus Serial Accounts

Beyond the effectiveness of the proposed memory structures in the Ouroboros Model for the selection of interpretations and classifications of e.g. sensory percepts, the whole process of directed progress of activation in a mind is well adapted to more abstract problem solving, just involving more elaborate schemata.

The fundamental succession of parallel data acquisition and–evaluation phases interspersed with singular decision points in an overall serial repetitive process offers a natural explanation of purportedly contradictory observations concerning the prevalent character of human data processing: competing views stressing serial or parallel aspects can both be correct, depending on their focus.

As meaningful concepts are nested, so can be consumption analysis loops with several of them active at the same time, e.g. dealing with different levels of detail. Depending on the context, also diverse time scales can apply. Only at the top of the hierarchy, when the global activity is focused (and the actor´s self is involved to a high degree), strict seriality ensues. Thus, similar arguments as for known global workspace theories are applicable in an unaffected manner: activation actively spreads as a consequence of a well defined process whenever comprehensive resources are brought to bear in a demanding situation [14,15].

5.6 More General Remarks on Cognition

Similar to the parallel / serial distinction, another one between induction and deduction can be drawn. These two formal reasoning procedures can be mapped to the different aspects of concept generation and use, with generalizing from input (assuming consequences) versus the activation of already existing concepts, i.e. filling-in slots of extant schemata (employing established relations). When a schema has been selected and there still is significant uncertainty concerning its uniqueness and the unambiguousness of fitting fillers, the process corresponds more to abduction, which infers plausible causes for an event or result from available evidence. It dovetails nicely with the tenets of the Ouroboros Model that abductive evidential reasoning can be understood as form of Bayesian reasoning [16].

The potential mental processing power of an agent according to the Ouroboros Model is ground-laid in the number, complexity and elaboration of the concepts at her disposition. Schemata, their number of slots, the level of detail, the depth of hierarchies, degree of connection and interdependence of the building blocks, and the width, i.e. the extent of main schemata and their total coverage from the bodily grounding level to the most abstract summits, determine what can be thought of efficiently [7]. As but one example, knowledge guided perception and the organization of knowledge in useful chunks, i.e. meaningful schemata, was found to lie at the basis of expert performance [17].

Adequacy, coherence and consistency are crucial, with the first one actually based on and derived from the two latter. Sheer performance at a single point in time is possible as a result of the optimum interplay between these structured data and the effective execution of all the described processing steps, in particular, self-referential consumption analysis. At the same time, we do have a preference for simple models, which require only a minimum of necessary ingredients.
In the long run, memory efficiency comes on top as fundamental pre-condition.

One key feature of consumption analysis is that it is "relative", i.e. any evaluation rests at best on all available applicable experience at that point in time. It has been argued that an inherent ambivalence of the monitoring signal from consumption analysis is responsible for a principled opposition towards truly novel approaches as described by Thomas Kuhn [7,18].

Although the Ouroboros Model emphasizes the importance of embodiment and also of some implementation details in living agents, there is no reason why its key data structures and the procedures working in them could not be simulated in software and actually be built in other, artificial, hardware.

6 Emotions, the Other Side of the Coin

Monitoring the quality of congruence with experience as done by consumption analysis provides a very useful feedback signal for any actor under almost all circumstances. It is hypothesized that the "feeling", affective, component of emotions is primarily that: the feedback signal from the consumption analysis process to the actor. Progress can be as expected, better (feeling good) or worse (feeling bad).

Emotions are in a sense an extension to attention, they mark information; at first sight it appears that affect and emotion would last over a much longer time scales, much wider contexts and always comprise a value, good vs. bad, a measure of relevance and concernment of the affected individual, whereas attention is quick, automatic, possible also limited and completely unconscious, more abstract and often initially value free. The (personal) feeling component together with the specific content of an actual situation, make up affect and the respective different emotions; bodily, physiological signals are explicitly, most probably necessarily, included.

Consistency in the Ouroboros Model is checked globally, in parallel for all features, but as discrepancies are dealt with according to their weight, a rather fixed sequence of appraisal dimensions might be observed because of general similarities between schemata, i.e. shared parts for basic emotions [19]. The comprehensive inclusion of all prevalent activity, in particular prevailing affect, as information basis leads to many observed effects of "affect as information" [20].

Emotions occur as a consequence of a situation or an event and, most important, they set the stage for the activities following thereafter. Affects have motivational character; specific, most likely evolutionary appropriate, behavior is triggered or at least encouraged (while blocking other) in the respective affective states of an actor.

This picture combines well established and seemingly contradictory stances each purportedly explaining emotions [21,22]. Affects as information resulting from appraisal and motivational accounts stressing behavioral dispositions can easily be identified with different facets of the same basic processes in the Ouroboros Model.

When discrepancies become too big, an interruption, a kind of reset, of the ongoing activity will be triggered. Emotions appear to be tied to a particular event, object or situation; moods usually denote less focused affects or circumstances. In addition, these manifestations of one and the same monitoring, appraisal and motivational, signal differ in their time characteristics.

Emotions have an impact on the mode of cognitive processing and they exhibit a form of hysteresis: when everything runs smoothly, the requirements on control can be relaxed and new, creative and explorative behavior is encouraged; at the same time loosening the grip of consumption analysis enhances the likelihood of finding (novel) acceptable fits; spirits are high and stay high as an immediate result. In the case that there occur problems and pronounced discrepancies, stronger and more stringent control is the consequence; the tighter limits for acceptance in this detail-oriented mode of operation make it less likely that good fits result; consequently, the mood remains dampened. Wide versus narrow scopes of attention and thought-action repertoires are described by the "broaden-and-build theory" [23].

Many diverse and useful functions of emotions for humans and in artificial systems have been proposed; here, in addition to bodily adaption and the prioritizing of particular actions based on appraisal, only one more shall be addressed: actors are often not alone, any reaction based on evaluations and feedback, which is useful to one individual, certainly is of potential interest also to others in a group. This would explain the communication value of displayed emotions.

Similarly as claimed for the weight of dimensions for attracting attention, also emotions come in two versions (and various combinations, where they act additively, – with attention and also with each other). Emotions can be inherited, i.e. forming a constitutive part of a schema as an earlier associated feature; in this case they can be activated very directly and quickly. When novel circumstances give rise to a never before experienced situation and resulting evaluations, attention will be evoked and associated emotions will build up more slowly; they are incorporated into the memory of the event, – ready then for later fast use.

7 Discussion

It goes without saying that in a paper of a few pages only selected features of a complex data processing structure can be sketched. Still, starting from very simple beginnings, most sophisticated data structures, processing algorithms and efficient behavior and general intelligence can be naturally accounted for with just one unified global model. The single, most significant ingredient in the Ouroboros Model is self-reflectivity in a cyclic set-up, where all available knowledge at one point in time is brought to bear on a situation or problem, while preparations for the future are made by selectively enlarging the knowledge base, with a focus on areas for which (self-reflective) evaluation showed that current means did not fully suffice.

7.1 Against Simplistic Associationism

Hand in hand with the kindling and allocation of attention goes its restriction in the Ouroboros Model. Many features can be input and evaluated in parallel, embedded in an overall serial cyclic process. A selected concept biases its regular constituents and inhibits possible but apparently less probable alternatives. Technically, this means that often no truly global consistency of all stored knowledge is reached or demanded.

Elaborate structures can arise from humble beginnings. Following Hebb's law, already in quite simple animals neurons concurrently active often experience an enhancement of their link, raising the probability for later joint activation. Neural assemblies are permanently linked together when once co-activated in an approved manner. Later partial activation biases the whole associated neural population to fire together. Structured memories are laid down, and this especially effectively when they are associated with some reward markers for success.

Despite the plain fact that everything is connect to everything, knowledge is not stored or activated in an indiscriminate or pervasive manner. Context is recorded in the form of quite general concepts, which specify their constituents and at the same time confine their applicability. The features making up a schema are not all equal with respect of their centrality and importance to a concept.

One particular feature / dimension of many concepts again deserves special mention: time. Although at first sight the Ouroboros Model appears to retell the fairy tale of Baron Münchhausen who escaped from a swamp by pulling himself up on his own hair ("Schopf"), the here presented approach and arguments do not suffer from circularity. Any processing step relies solely on data and structures available from before. Still, the procedures work "backwards" in the sense that they have the power to influence this very basis, leading to changes, which then become effective for the same processes but only afterwards during subsequent process cycles.

In a self-consistent way, the Ouroboros Model first aims at providing a coarse and encompassing schema, which allows putting many different findings from a large variety of fields into a common framework. Relations inside and between the building blocks thus should become clearer and areas of specific demand for future work are outlined before dwelling on any level of intricate details. Only as a second step, formalizations and quantifications are worked out in case spending this effort looks promising.

7.2 The Next Step beyond Rationality and Emotions: Consciousness

Rationality and its inseparable companions, i.e. affect and emotions, are still considered by many as beyond the reach of understanding, let alone, their full realization in artificial minds. The Ouroboros Model claims that the same efficient algorithmic structure, which endows living beings with their mental capabilities, will allow artificial agents to exhibit significant general intelligence.

On a list of sublime features claimed to establish noble human uniqueness, consciousness comes next. It has been argued that consciousness can naturally be understood in the framework of the Ouroboros Model, successfully addressing well thought-of demands on what could count as a theory explaining consciousness [14]. Immediately relevant here, it can reasonably be claimed that a certain level of complexity and intelligence of any agent necessarily demands and actually also leads to the dawning of consciousness [14,24].

References

1. Selz, O.: Über die Gesetze des geordneten Denkverlaufs, erster Teil, Spemann, Stuttgart (1913)
2. Thomsen, K.: The Ouroboros Model in the light of venerable criteria. Neurocomputing 74, 121–128 (2010)
3. Thomsen, K.: Concept Formation in the Ouroboros Model. In: Third Conference on Artificial General Intelligence, AGI 2010, Lugano, Switzerland, March 5-8 (2010)
4. Thomsen, K.: The Ouroboros Model, Selected Facets, From Brains to Systems. Springer, Heidelberg (2011)
5. Franklin, S., Patterson, F.G.J.: The Lida Architecture: Adding New Modes of Learning to an Intelligent, Autonomous, Software Agent. In: Integrated Design and Process Technology, IDPT-2006. Society for Design and Process Science, San Diego (2006)
6. Yuille, A., Kersten, D.: Vision as Bayesian inference: analysis by synthesis? Trends in Cognitive Science 10, 301–308 (2006)
7. Thomsen, K.: Knowledge as a Basis and a Constraint for the Performance of the Ouroboros Mode. Presented at a Workshop at ZiF in Bielefeld, October 29-31 (2009)
8. Newell, A.: Unified Theories of Cognition. Harvard University Press, Cambridge (1990)
9. Anderson, J.R., Matessa, M.P.: A production system theory of serial memory. Psychological Review 104, 728–748 (1997)
10. Gnadt, W., Grossberg, S.: SOVEREIGN: An autonomous neural system for incrementally learning planned action sequences to navigate towards a rewarded goal. In: Neural Networks, vol. 21, pp. 699–758 (2008)
11. Thagard, P.: Coherence in Thought and Action. Bradford, MIT Press, Cambridge, London (2000)
12. Thagard, P., Verbeurgt, K.: Coherence as Constraint satisfaction. Cognitive Science 22, 1–24 (1998)
13. Tenenbaum, J.B., Griffiths, T.L., Kemp, C.: Theory-based Bayesian models of inductive learning and reasoning. Trends in Cognitive Science 10(7), 309–318 (2006)
14. Thomsen, K.: Consciousness for the Ouroboros Model. Int. Journal of Machine Consciousness 3, 163–175 (2011)
15. Baars, B.J.: A Cognitive Theory of Consciousness. Cambridge University Press, Cambridge (1998)
16. Poole, D.: Learning, Bayesian Probability, Graphical Models, and Abduction. In: Flach, P., Kakas, A. (eds.) Abduction and Induction: Essays on Their Relation and Integration. Springer, Netherlands (2000)
17. Ross, P.E.: The Expert Mind. Scientific American 295(2), 46–53 (2006)

18. Kuhn, T.S.: Die Struktur wissenschaftlicher Revolutionen. Suhrkamp, Frankfurt am Main (1978)
19. Sander, D., Grandjean, D., Scherer, K.R.: A systems approach to appraisal mechanisms in emotion. Neural Networks 18, 317–352 (2005)
20. Clore, G.L., Gasper, K., Garvin, E.: Affect as Information. In: Forgas, J.P. (ed.) Handbook of Affect and Social Cognition. Lawrence Erlbaum Associates, Mahwah (2001)
21. Scherer, K.R.: Appraisal Theory. In: Dalgleish, T., Power, M. (eds.) Handbook of Cognition and Emotion, pp. 637–663. Wiley, Chichester (1999)
22. Ekman, P.: Basic Emotions. In: Dalgleish, T., Power, M. (eds.) Handbook of Cognition and Emotion, pp. 45–60. Wiley, Chichester (1999)
23. Fredrickson, B.L., Branigan, C.: Positive emotions broaden the scope of attention and thought-action repertoires. Cognition and Emotion 19(3), 313–332 (2005)
24. Sanz, R., López, I., Rodríguez, M., Hernandéz, C.: Principles for consciousness in integrated cognitive control. Neural Networks 20, 938–946 (2007)

Dynamic Relations between Naming and Acting in Adult Mental Retardation

Sabine Metta and Josiane Caron-Pargue

Department of Psychology, University of Poitiers, Poitiers, France
sabinemetta@yahoo.fr, jcaron@univ-poitiers.fr

Abstract. Verbal reports obtained during the Tower of Hanoi puzzle were analyzed in the line of Culioli's enunciative operations, cognitively interpreted. It was produced by 20 Mentally Retarded during 6 trials on three consecutive days. For 10 of them, a perturbation occurred at the beginning of the fifth trial. The analysis focused on lexical choices referring to source objects (disks) and to goal objects (pegs) of the puzzle. Simple denominations were differentiated from double ones, and explicit denominations from implicit ones. The denominations were considered as marking, or not, elementary detachments from the object. The results allow to qualify the learning of the Mentally Retarded in terms of elementary processes of internalization, introducing flexibility through the external space. Two kinds of learning, one mechanical, the other strategic were differentiated. The introduction of the perturbation develops the strategic learning, increasing flexibility.

Keywords: external representation, lexical choice, verbal reports, problem solving, adult mental retardation, internalization.

1 Introduction

Mentally Retarded are generally characterized by failures in the access to abstraction and in mental flexibility. But, at the same time, their perceptive abilities are entirely preserved and remain very sensitive to environmental changes. Their mental representations are mainly externalized, restricted to concrete aspects of the situation [9]. Nevertheless, several researches show that the cognitive capacities of Mentally Retarded should be considered at first as underfunctioning rather than as non-existent or poorer. On the one hand, the under functioning should result from weaknesses at specific levels of the normative control, which ensures the executive functioning [3], [10]. The normative levels of control can be viewed as more or less involved in the access to abstraction, increasing or narrowing the executive flexibility and the cognitive management of the task. On the other hand, the underfunctioning should be due to a lack in the interaction between the internal representations and the external ones, the subject being stuck at one level of the generalization of contextual representations [9].

However, relations between internal and external representations are rather complex. While for the Piagetian school interactions involve the subject and the physical environment, for Vytgosky they involve the subject and the social

B. Hu et al. (Eds.): BI 2011, LNAI 6889, pp. 42–52, 2011.

environment, mediated notably by meanings constructed with language [7], [12]. These meanings have to be considered as local artefacts, which reify knowledge and information coming from the social environment. But for that they need a feedback to be interconnected and to gain some generalization.

In fact, current researches on cognitive linguistics, notably on Culioli's theory of enunciative operations [4], [5], [6], [8], and on cognitive processes involved in a problem solving task [1], [2], [10], [13], [14], allow to articulate the three kinds of interactions: internal-external representations, subjects-physical environment; subjects-social environment. The key point for that is to consider that knowledge and information have to be reconstructed as contextualized, local, time dependent, within the current situation. Their generalization has also to be reconstructed as the understanding of all the internal constraints of the situation.

Indeed, enunciative operations formalize different processes of detachment from the situation, some of them giving notably access to abstraction and to the reconstruction of knowledge within the task [1], [2], [5], [6]. Furthermore, in this line, the internal-external social interactions include also the contextual interactions between subjects and real world [13], [14]. Our assumption is that such an approach might improve not only the understanding of Mentally Retarded's cognitive processes, but general learning processes.

The aim of this paper is to show elementary detachments marked by lexical choices in the verbal protocols during the solving of the Tower of Hanoi puzzle by Mentally Retarded. Our intent is to analyze the naming of objects (disks and pegs) in relation with the acquisition of expertise, and with the introduction of a perturbation. Our general hypothesis is that elementary detachments, marked by the lexical choices, introduce reorganizations in the grasp of perceptive information, notably under the effect of the perturbation. Then, the learning of Mentally Retarded will be improved, some flexibility being introduced through their external representations.

2 Theoretical Background

Enunciative operations formalize several steps in the construction of the representation [4], [5], [6], [8]. These steps, all marked by linguistic markers, have to be considered as invariant among various inter-subjective activities of language. At first, the representation has to be viewed as local in space and time and dependent on the moment. Then, afterwards, in order to gain some stabilization, it has to be reconstructed by various operations of detachment as an abstract set of occurrences before being re-inserted into the situation. These two steps can be interpreted, in the context of a problem solving task, as the processes of internalization-externalization [1], [2].

The most basic of enunciative operations is the operation of location. It introduces a relation R between two entities a and b such as one of them, for example b is the locator relative to which the other a is located. The location of a relative to b is interpreted as an attentional focus bearing on b, and as the fact that a is coming with b. This operation may intervene at different levels of the construction of the representation.

The operation of location operates first to define an orientation of the predicative relation, the first argument being defined as the *Source*, and the second argument as the *Goal*. It may also operate between two utterances. Applied in the case of the verbalization of two consecutive actions, the operation of location accounts for a first step of the construction of a cognitive unit, i.e. of a *chunk* [1], [2].

Some enunciative operations introduce detachments from the situation. Some of these detachments, marked by modal expressions, are interpreted as reorganizations of planning activities. Some others, marked by starting terms[1], give rise to the characterization of the internal space and of its interactions with the external space as processes of internalization and externalization. Furthermore, the succession of these two kinds of detachments along a solving process is cognitively interpreted as the marker of an on-line identification of the constraints of the task [2].

Our intent in this paper is to consider operations of location, more elementary than above, which intervene within one action and which are implied in the naming of objects. Indeed, for Culioli, locations and detachments can be buried in the naming itself of objects, but can get working in specific contexts. Our assumption is that it will be in the case of external functioning.

Indeed, the denomination of an object implies first the construction of a domain of reference in which every object and every occurrence of it have common properties. Second, the function of the denomination is to demarcate this object, and its occurrence, from the others. For example, in the case of the Tower of Hanoi, an explicit denomination such as *disk 1* marks a larger distance between the subject and her or his action than an implicit denomination such as *this one* or than an absence of denomination. Our idea is that the detachment involved in an explicit denomination constitutes a first elementary step in the processes of external generalization of knowledge.

Furthermore, changes in thematic organization at the enunciative level [5] are marked by the construction of a constitutive locator, e.g. in the case of double denominations (*disk 1* and *the pink one*) in *disk 1 the pink one on disk 3*. As the explicit denomination integrates a detachment, the double denominations integrate a deeper detachment than simple denominations.

Such elementary processes need to be studied in the case of Mentally Retarded. We know that the restricted environment of Mentally Retarded has a strong effect on the limited and very familiar information they can grasp. Their cognitive work develops mainly in the external space and they have many difficulties with the processes of generalization of constraints. They remain very receptive to the slightest environmental change and to the slightest perturbation coming in that environment.

Our hypothesis is that such a perturbation entails a different way of grasping information, which can improve the process of detachment involved within the naming of objects.

---

1 A starting term is defined by the extraction of the first or second argument of the predicative relation, marked by an anaphora. This extraction introduces an operation of location, locating the predicative relation relative to the starting term. It controls the access to abstraction, contextualizing the predicative relation. For example, *disk 1* has the status of starting term in *disk 1 I put it on peg B*, marked by anaphora *it*.

3 Method

3.1 The Task

A 4-disks Tower of Hanoi, wooden made, is placed in front of the subject. Four disks of different size and of different color (the smallest disk, disk 1 is pink, disk 2 is green, disk 3 is yellow, the largest disk, disk 4, is black) are put on peg A in an ordered manner, disk 1 on the top, disk 4 at the bottom. The aim is to bring all disks on peg C in the same order, with the two usual constraints: “no bigger disk on a smaller one” and “no taking of several disks at the same time”.

Verbal reports are tape recorded and moves are noted in writing.

3.2 The Participants

The participants were adults, working in a specialized center for Mentally Retarded. They were chosen in two steps: a first selection was based on a IQ comprised between 50 and 75 at WAIS (Wechsler Adult Intelligent Scale); in a second time a verification of this selection was done with several subsets of the K. ACB which concern the problem solving area. They were from 25- to 45-years-old.

Two groups of 10 Mentally Retarded each solved 6 times the Tower of Hanoi puzzle, 2 consecutive times per day, during 3 consecutive days. For one of the two groups, the experimental group, a stranger was introduced in the room the third day, at the beginning of the fifth trial. No explicit interaction occurred between the stranger and the Mentally Retarded. In the other group, called the control group, no perburbation occurred.

3.3 Linguistic Markers

First of all we separated the objects *Source* (i.e. the disks) from the objects *Goal* (i.e. the pegs), see Table 1. Our idea is that the attentional focus of Mentally Retarded is a priori stuck in the immediate space and time, and that the goal enters in this focus only later.

Table 1. Denominations of the source object (disks) and of the goal object (pegs)

	Denominations source object			Denominations goal object		
	Simple	Double	Modified	Simple	Double	Modified
All	S_S	D_S	M_S	S_G	D_G	M_G
Implicit	I_S	I_{DS}	I_{MS}	I_G	I_{DG}	I_{MG}
Explicit	E_S	E_{DS}	E_{MS}	E_G	E_{DG}	E_{MG}

Second, for both kinds of objects, we differentiated the double naming from the simple one, and we studied the modified naming.

Third, we started the study of explicit naming versus implicit naming in the case of double and simple naming[2].

The categories studied in this paper are as follows:

E_S: *Explicit-Source.* Simple explicit denomination of the *source*, e.g. *the green one* in the example *the green one I put it here.*

E_G: *Explicit-Goal.* Simple explicit denomination of the *goal*, e.g. *peg C* in the example *this one on peg C.*

E_{DS}: *Double-Explicit-Source*. Double explicit denomination of the *source*, e.g. *disk 1 from peg A* in the example *disk 1 from peg A I put it on peg C.*

E_{DG}: *Double-Explicit-Goal*. Double explicit denomination of the goal, e.g. *peg B with disk 3* in the example *this one on peg B with disk 3.*

I_S: *Implicit-Source*. Simple implicit denomination of the *source*, e.g. *the other* in the example *the other on peg C.*

I_G: *Implicit-Goal*. Simple implicit denomination of the *goal*, e.g. *there* in the example *the green one I put it there.*

I_{DS}: *Double-Implicit-Source*. Double implicit denomination of the *source*, e.g. *this one that* in the example *this one that on peg A.*

I_{DG}: *Double-Implicit-Goal*. Double implicit denomination of the *goal*, e.g. *the other here* in the example *disk 3 I put it with the other here.*

Modified Denominations. Series of similar denominations can be often seen along a series of consecutive actions, either for the *source* or for the *goal.* For example the disks involved in the *source* are named by their number *disk 1, disk 2, disk 1, disk 3.* A *Modified-Denomination* will be defined by a sudden modification of the similar denominations appearing in the series either for the *source* or for the *goal.* For example *the yellow one* is a modified denomination for the *source* in the series *disk 1, disk 2, disk 1, the yellow one.*

M_S: *Modified-Source*. Modified denominations of the *source.*

M_G: *Modified-Goal*. Modified denominations of the *goal.*

3.4 Dependent Variables

Performance: Two dependent variables were defined as follows:

***Total Time*:** number of seconds for solving the puzzle during one trial

***Moves*:** number of moves for solving the puzzle during one trial

Linguistic Markers. A ratio to words was computed for each kind of linguistic marker: the total number of its occurrences for one trial was divided by the total number of words for this trial and multiplied by 1000.

---

[2] The study for the modified naming is an ongoing research. We present here only our first results. The criterion explicit versus implicit has yet to be considered for the modified denominations.

3.5 Hypotheses

Performance. One can expect an acquisition of expertise, marked by a decrease of *Total Time* and of *Moves*. The introduction of the perturbation will introduce a lower performance on trials 5 and 6 in the experimental group than for the control group.

Linguistic Markers. Mentally Retarded are strongly stuck to the external space, being focused on concrete aspects of the environment. Then one can expect that the conception of a goal needs a minimal detachment from concrete aspects in order to make anticipation. Then, the denominations of the *goal* will need a higher cognitive cost than the denominations of the *source*.

At the beginning of the solving process, the denomination will be more implicit than explicit. But, with the acquisition of expertise, the ratios of implicit denominations will decrease, while the ratios of explicit denominations will increase. Notably, one can expect that the learning of Mentally Retarded will be more explicit for the denominations of the *source* than for the denominations of the *goal* which already involve detachments. Furthermore, the representation gaining some stabilization by means of detachments linked to the increase of explicit denominations, one can expect a decrease of the proportion of modified denominations.

Mentally Retarded are also sensitive to every environmental modification. Then, one can expect that the introduction of a perturbation, here the presence of a stranger, will introduce a qualitative reorganization of their representation. That can be shown by an increase of the modified denominations, markers of reorganization, and an increase of detachments, marked especially by the double explicit denominations.

4 Results

4.1 Performance

As expected, there is an effect of trials for the *Total Time*, $F(5, 90) = 15.84$, $p < .0001$, which decreases with trials. The decrease appears particularly between trials 1 and 2, $F(1, 18) = 18.67$, $p < .0001$. There is no effect of group and no significant interaction.

As expected, the number of *Moves* decreases also with trials, $F(5, 90) = 10.46$, $p < .0001$. The decrease occurs notably between trials 1-2-3-4 and trials 5-6, $F(1, 18) = 10.46$, $p < .001$. There is no effect of group, and no significant interaction.

More precisely, there is a local effect of group for the number of *Moves* on trials 5 and 6, $F(1, 18) = 4.14$, $p < .05$, higher for the experimental group, perturbed by the introduction of the stranger, than for the control group.

Then, the study of performance shows two steps in the learning with trials. One is marked by a decrease of *Total Time*, but not of the number of *Moves*, in trial 2. It is common to both groups. The other is marked by a difference in the number of *Moves*, but not of *Total Time*, in trial 5. This second step is particularly marked for the experimental group, and characterizes the Mentally Retarded faced with a perturbation in their familiar environment.

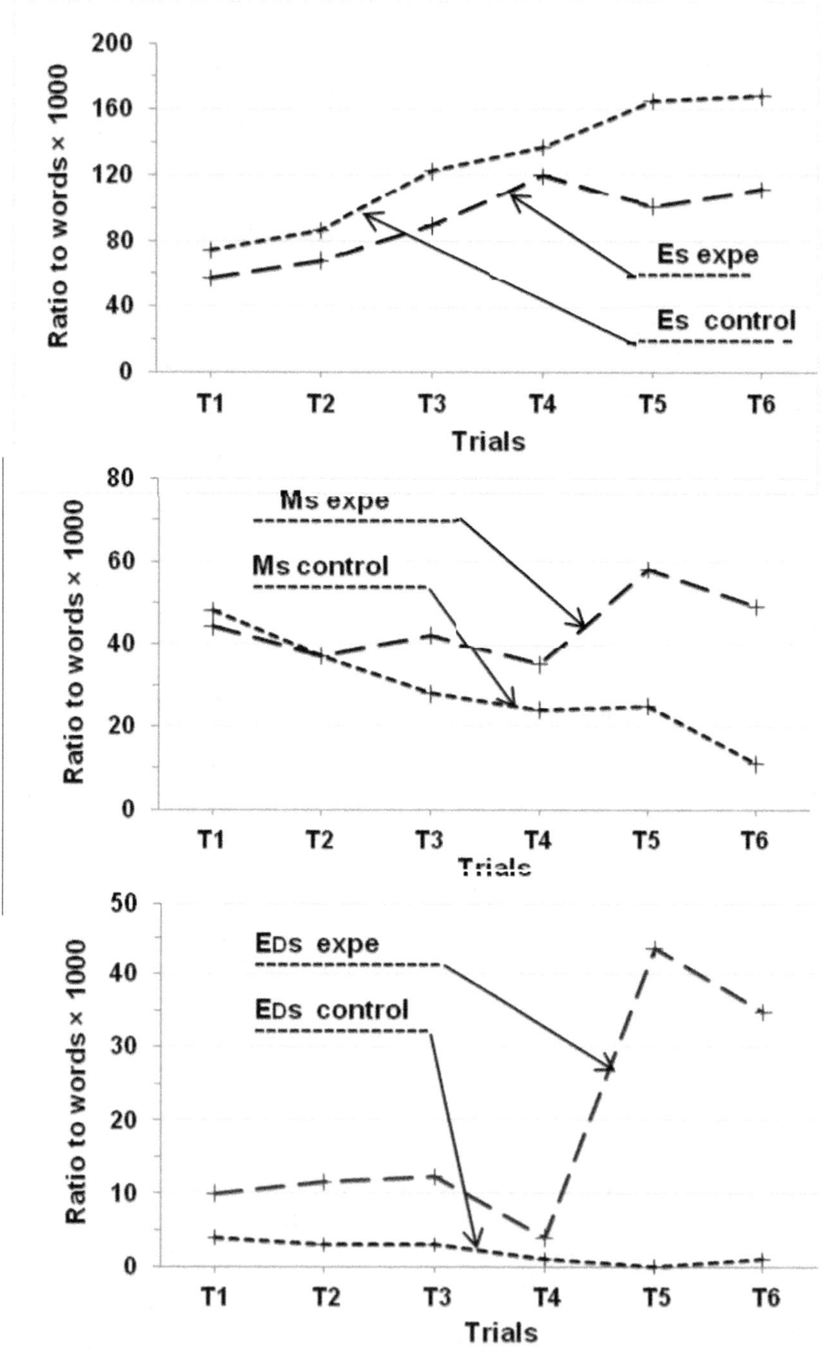

Fig. 1. Proportion of *Explicit-Source* (E_S), of *Double-Explicit-Source* (E_{DS}), and of *Modified-Source* (M_S) with trials for the two groups

4.2 Linguistic Markers (cf. Fig. 1)

The ratio of *Explicit-Source* (**E_S**) shows an effect of group, $F(1, 18) = 5.69$, $p < .02$, and an effect of trials, $F(5, 90) = 11.69$, $p < .0001$, without significant interaction. As expected, the effect of group concerns mainly the trials 5 and 6 for which the ratio of the experimental group remains lower for the experimental group than for the control group on trials 5 and 6 (respectively $F(1, 18) = 6.66(4.99)$, $p < .01(.03)$), when the perturbation is introduced. Furthermore, the ratio increases with trials in both groups, notably between trials 2 and 3, $F(1, 18) = 17.34$, $p < .0001$.

The ratio of *Double-Explicit-Source* (**E_{DS}**) shows no significant effect of group, nor of trials, nor interaction. Nevertheless, as expected, it shows a significant increase in the experimental group between trials 1 and 5, $F(1, 18) = 5.64$, $p < .03$. Then, the experimental group produces more E_{DS} in trials 5 and 6 than before.

Only a significant effect of trials is shown with the ratio of *Explicit-Goal* (**E_G**), $F(5, 90) = 9.40$, $p < .0001$, increasing with trials, and with the ratio of *Implicit-Source* (**I_S**), $F(5, 90) = 3.64$, $p < .01$, which decreases with trials. Furthermore, while the ratio of E_G begins to be higher than before at trial 3, $F(1, 18) = 17.34$, $p < .0001$, the ratio of I_S begins to be lower than before at trial 4, $F(1, 18) = 6.88$, $p < .02$.

There is no significant effect for the *Double-Explicit-Goal* (**E_{DG}**), for the *Implicit-Goal* (**I_G**), for the *Double-Implicit-Source* (**I_{DS}**), and for the *Double-Implicit-Goal* (**I_{DG}**).

Modified Denominations. The ratio of *Modified-Source* (**M_S**) shows no significant effect of group, but an effect of trials, $F(5, 90) = 5.73$, $p < .001$. It decreases with trials. Furthermore, a significant interaction *group × trials*, $F(5, 90) = 5.73$, $p < .001$, shows, as expected, an increase of this ratio for the experimental group on trials 5 and 6 (respectively $F(1, 18) = 5.23(12.57)$, $p < .03(.001)$, while it decreases in the control group.

No significant effect is shown for the *Modified-Goal*.

5 Discussion

5.1 The Different Steps of Learning

Our aim was to study elementary detachments marked by lexical choices, and to show their dynamic role in the learning of Mentally Retarded solving the tower of Hanoi puzzle. For that, we chose to study the distribution of denominations in their verbal reports in relation to their performance.

Our results allow a qualitative approach of the learning of Mentally Retarded. The main aspect is that our results on lexical choices allow the characterization of two kinds of processes underlying their learning.

An increase in performance shows that Mentally Retarded are able to gain expertise, as already attested [9], [11]. But it does not explain how.

No significant effect in lexical choices accompanies the first improvement in performance, between trials 1 and 2, due to a significant decrease in *Total Time*, but not in the number of *Moves*. Then, a *mechanical learning* develops first, at the beginning.

Later, a different kind of learning arises, qualified of *strategic learning*. It is accompanied by significant effects in lexical choices, and by the second improvement in performance between trials 4 and 5, marked by a decrease in the number of *Moves*, but not in *Total Time*. The *strategic learning* develops in several steps:

- In trial 3, with an increase in the proportion of *Explicit-Source* (E_S) and of *Explicit-Goal* (E_G).
- In trial 4, with a decrease in the proportion of *Implicit-Source* (I_S).

Then, before appearing in performance, two consecutive reorganizations of the representation arise: one introduces detachments marked by explicit denominations; the other develops the processes of detachment, getting the subjects less stuck to concrete environmental aspects.

Moreover, as expected, the introduction of a perturbation, here the presence of a stranger, leads to an increase in the number of *Moves* for the experimental group in trials 5 and 6, without significant effect on *Total Time*. This regression in performance seems like a return to a mechanical[3] learning. But the fact is not so clear, as shown by the effects on lexical choices. The perturbation introduces a decrease in the proportion of *Explicit-Source* (E_S) in the experimental group, but the detachments underlying this decrease are compensated by detachments underlying the increase of *Modified-Source* (M_S). Furthermore, the detachments underlying an increase of *Double-explicit-Source* (E_{DS}) enhance the flexibility in the experimental group. Besides, there is no significant interruption in the increase of *Explicit-Goal* (E_G) or in the decrease of *Implicit-Source*. Then, the introduction of the perturbation does not entail a return to a simple mechanical learning but improves the quality of the strategic learning. Indeed, it increases the number of detachments, decreasing the strength of the sticking previous mechanical learning. Then, this compensation improves the quality of the learning in spite of a decrease in performance. The introduction of the stranger entails an articulation between the two kinds of learning, mechanical and strategic.

5.2 Generalization Processes in the External Space

The results show a strong effect of elementary detachments in the acquisition of expertise. These operations account for some processes involved in the generalization of constraints. Bégoin-Augereau and Caron-Pargue [1] mentioned two kinds of processes of generalization, one within the external space, the other involving processes of internalization and externalization linked to an internal space identified by the presence of starting terms and anaphoras. The kind of generalization observed in this paper belongs to the external space [9], [14]. Nevertheless, elementary detachments shown in this paper are involved in this kind of generalization, specific of the external space, but they give rise to elementary processes of internalization [10].

Furthermore, these detachments bear mainly on the *source*, notably for the *Explicit-Source*, and constitute an elementary internalization at the declarative level, as advocated by Bégoin-Augereau and Caron-Pargue [2]. In fact, the authors identified the declarative level by semiotic relations between the *source* objects

[3] Only a marginally effect appears, at the limit of the non-significance, $F(1, 18) = 2.97$, $p < .10$. That does not contradict our argumentation.

(disks) in opposition to procedural semiotic relations between the *goal* objects (pegs). So, the detachments produced by the Mentally Retarded involved processes of internalization, i.e. of generalization, bearing on the conditions of actions.

Moreover, these effects are increased with the introduction of a stranger. Then, the processes marked by the *Double-Explicit-Source* and *Modified-Source* occurring at the same time as the increase of moves, without increase of time, appear as processes of reification, aiming at the externalization and stabilization of these conditions. These processes open the way toward improvements of the learning capacities for Mentally Retarded by means of provocations introducing perturbations. But further researches are needed in order to explain the different steps between these elementary processes and what Paour calls normative control [3], [11], which rather involves mechanisms of abstraction.

The elementary detachments we show are marked by linguistic forms, so some precisions can be given on what Vygosky called *artefacts* [7], [12]. They account for an active construction of knowledge, in his sense, even if they do not result from an interaction with other human beings[4].

More generally, beyond the case of Mentally Retarded, our account concerns as well the early learning of novices at the beginning of a task as the management of more or less automatized procedures in the external space.

6 Conclusion

The method presented in this paper allows a deeper analysis of processes underlying the performance in a problem solving task. The most important result of this research is to show progressive elementary structurations of the external space, involving several processes of internalization. Those processes are marked by several kinds of denominations, which involve implicit detachments usually buried, but getting to work in some specific contexts.

Beyond the case of Mentally Retarded, this research opens the way to a new approach of learning processes, understanding the processes of generalization at work in the external space, notably in the construction and the management of automatic processing.

Nevertheless, this study remains exploratory. Further research is needed, notably to make the articulation with previous and future studies based on a cognitive approach of Culioli's enunciative operations [2], [5].

This approach relies on a very general linguistic approach, based on a logical theory of relations, and an intersubjective view of language. It allows to consider complex interactions among a subject, the physical environment and the other human beings. Then, following Zhang [13], it is possible to extend this research to the study of interaction, notably in the case of intelligent agents' interactive learning.

---

[4] The stranger introduced as a perturbation did not intervene, but was only sitting at a table without talking and without looking at the subject.

References

1. Bégoin-Augereau, S., Caron-Pargue, J.: Linguistic markers of decision processes in a problem solving task. Cognitive Systems Research 10, 102–123 (2009)
2. Bégoin-Augereau, S., Caron-Pargue, J.: Modified decision processes marked by linguistic forms in a problem solving task. Cognitive Systems Research 11, 260–286 (2010)
3. Blaye, A., Chevalier, N., Paour, J.-L.: The development of intentional control of categorization behavior: A study of children's relational flexibility. Cognition, Brain, Behavior 11, 791–808 (2007)
4. Bearth, T.: Review of "Cognition and representation in linguistic theory" by Antoine Culioli. Pragmatics and Cognition 9, 135–147 (2001)
5. Culioli, A.: Cognition and representation in linguistic theory. J. Benjamins, Amsterdam (1995)
6. Culioli, A.: Representation, referential processes, and regulation. Language activity as form production and recognition. In: Montangero, J., Tryphon, A. (eds.) Language and Cognition. Archives Jean Piaget, Cahier, Genève, vol.10, pp. 178–213 (1989)
7. Daniels, H., Cole, M., Wertsch, J.V.: The Cambridge Companion to Vygotsky. Cambridge University Press, New-York (2007)
8. Groussier, M.-L.: On Antoine Culioli's theory of enunciative operations. Lingua 110, 157–182 (2000)
9. Inhelder, B.: The diagnosis of reasoning in the Mentally Retarded. John Day, New York (1968); Translation of: Inhelder, B.: Le diagnostic du raisonnement chez les débiles mentaux. Delachaux et Niestlé, Neuchâtel (1943)
10. Piaget, J.: The grasp of consciousness: Action and concept in the young child. Harvard University Press, Cambridge (1976); Translation of : Piaget, J.: La prise de conscience. PUF, Paris (1974)
11. Paour, J.-L.: From structural to functional diagnostic: A dynamic conception of mental retardation. In: Tryphon, A., Vonèche, J. (eds.) Working with Piaget: Essays in Honour of Bärbel Inhelder, pp. 13–38. Psychology Press Ltd., London (2001)
12. Vygotsky, L.S.: Mind in society: the development of higher psychological processes. Harvard University Press, Cambridge (1978)
13. Zhang, J.: A distributed representation approach to group problem solving. Journal of American Society of Information Science 49(9), 801–809 (1998)
14. Zhang, J.: External representations in complex information processing tasks. In: Kent, A., Williams, J.G. (eds.) Encyclopedia of Microcomputers. Marcel Dekker, Inc., New York (2001)

The Role of Lateral Inferior Prefrontal Cortex during Information Retrieval

Haiyan Zhou[1], Jieyu Liu[1], Wei Jing[1],
Yulin Qin[1,2], Shengfu Lu[1], Yiyu Yao[1,3], and Ning Zhong[1,4]

[1] International WIC Institute, Beijing University of Technology, China
[2] Dept. of Psychology, Carnegie Mellon University, USA
[3] Dept. of Computer Science, University of Regina, Canada
[4] Dept. of Life Science and Informatics, Maebashi Institute of Technology, Japan
zhouhaiyan@bjut.edu.cn, zhong@maebashi-it.ac.jp

Abstract. To investigate the role of lateral inferior prefrontal cortex (LIPFC) during information retrieval, we used two tasks based on the phenomenon of basic-level advantage and its reversal to examine the activities in this region across tasks. As expected, this region was involved in both tasks during the processing of information retrieval. ROI analysis showed there was a stronger activation in word-picture matching (WP) task in LIPFC than that in picture-word matching (PW) task. Moreover, although as for the behavioral performance, we observed a typical basic-level advantage effect in PW task and the reversal advantage effect to more general level in WP task, the activities in left LIPFC were similar across the tasks, which was not consistent with our expectation. The intensity was weakest in the condition of intermediate level, and the differences between intermediate and other two levels reached significant level in WP task. These results suggested the region of LIPFC controlled retrieval of knowledge information, and the activation in LIPFC depended more on internal memory system, not the external task demand.

1 Introduction

Human being was always sited in complex situations at any moment, and he had to make flexible response to adapt the world. For example, somebody A asked a person B where he was, if the querist A was relatively familiar with B's life, the person B might answer "In office"; while if the querist A was not so familiar with B, the person B might answer "In Beijing" or "In China". These answers were corresponded to a same question, but they were located in different level of specificity in the semantic system. This phenomenon suggested that people had the ability to select and retrieve information from memory system very flexibly. It's clear that retrieving suitable information from memory was a key ability to ensure the adaptation for human being.

Researchers of psychology examined this phenomenon in human. They found there was a basic-level advantage effect during information retrieval. For example, in a task a participant was shown a picture of collie and asked to name it,

B. Hu et al. (Eds.): BI 2011, LNAI 6889, pp. 53–63, 2011.

he would probably answer it with the concept of "dog" (an intermediate level of specificity), while not "collie" (more specific level) or "animal" (more general level). The result suggested although the several of category concepts could be right responses, (e.g. "collie", "dog", "animal", even "pet"), the intermediate level seems a preferred cognitive status in human mind. This phenomenon was first reported by Rosch in 1976 and named basic-level advantage [1]. The basic-level advantage effect could be a result of information processing history, including human experience, even the evolution in a long time. Researchers thought that the information in the basic-level was more frequently used than other terms [2], and usually the first nouns children typically acquired were also at this level [3]. So the information in this level seemed more readily to access than others and could be retrieved more quickly [3].

However it was another story for semantic dementia (SD). When SD patient was asked to name a picture of object, like a collie as before, the response was typically more general, such as animal [4, 5]. Patients with SD exhibited a deterioration of knowledge about meanings of world, together with a remarkable sparing of many other cognitive abilities. It can be seen from this that a damaged knowledge system led to the preferred cognitive status was changed from the intermediate level to more general level and thus a reversal of the basic-level advantage effect appeared. But to be noted, the reversal advantage effect to more general level was also appeared in healthy people. Rogers and his colleagues [3] asked college students to judge whether picture and object named match or not in a limited time, participants showed a general level advantage effect, which suggested the response times to the concepts in more general level were faster than that to the concepts in intermediate level. Some studies also found the reversal of basic-level advantage in similar or other tasks, such as categorization [6, 7]. The findings of reversal advantage effect in healthy people indicated the preferential status was not always located in the intermediate level, although the memory system was intact, the "ready" status might change to other levels according to task demands. We wondered how the brain modulated to these different processing during information retrieval. Because of the important role during information retrieval we investigated the activities of left lateral inferior prefrontal cortex (LIPFC) in this study.

Based on the theory of ACT-R (Adaptive Control of Thought-Rational) cognitive architecture and its relationship to brain regions, we defined the region of LIPFC associated with retrieval factors. In ACT-R, LIPFC was conceived serve as the role of maintaining the retrieval cues for accessing information stored elsewhere in the brain [8]. The research group of ACT-R found the longer it took to complete the retrieval successful, the longer the cues would have to be maintained and the greater the activation [8–13]. A lot of other brain imaging studies provided evidences about the role of this area in retrieval, especially in language task. A meta-analysis study [14] showed that LIPFC was related to semantic processing, which support a wealth of cognitive abilities ,including thinking and memory. Moreover, in the neuropsychological literature, LIPFC lesions had not typically resulted in semantic deficits [15]. It was argued this region supported processes that operate over semantic representations rather than the representations themselves [16–18]. Other researchers thought that this prefrontal region was activated in conditions that require difficult selections among retrieved information [16, 19, 20].

To investigate the role of LIPFC in information retrieval, we used two tasks, word-picture matching (WP) and picture-word matching (PW), to investigate basic-level advantage effect in human information retrieval. Researchers [6, 7] argued a possible explanation for the discrepancy between intermediate and general level precedence in the literatures, and suggested that might be related to the differences in processing demands of tasks used. In those tasks of object detection, perceptual processing of objects might be loaded upon more which led to a precedence of more general level; while in tasks of object naming, memory-based processing might be loaded more on and thus a basic-level advantage was oberverd.We expected in task of WP, the earlier presented words activated the semantic memory and participant would be guided to recognize the followed picture, and a reversal advantage to general level would appear in this task. But in task of PW, the processing was more similar with naming task and more semantic memory would loaded on, then a basic-level advantage effect would be observed. We expected LIPFC would be involved in these two tasks because of the important processing of retrieving and maintaining knowledge of words or object in the tasks. But based on their behavioral performances, the activation in LIPFC would change according to the basic-level advantage effect or its reversal. That is to say, activation in LIPFC in the condition of general level would be weakest in PW and activation in the condition of intermediate level in WP would be the weakest.

2 Method

2.1 Participants and Tasks

15 college students from Beijing University of Technology finished the WP task and 17 students finished the PW task. Details of the participants please see reference [21].

Same materials were used in WP and PW tasks. Pictures were 32 color photographs of animals and vehicles in superordinate level. 4 different photographs for each of eight specific categories in subordinate level: water buffalo, milk cows, goat, jumbuckgoat, bus, truck, sailboat and steamboat. They made up to 4 sets of cows, sheep, cars and boats for classification at intermediate level. For the two tasks, the only difference between them was the present orders of pictures and concept words. In WP task, word was presented earlier for 1000ms, and then followed by the picture; while in PW task, picture was presented first for 1000ms and then concept word. Participants were demanded to respond in 2000 ms with pressing index finger to matching response and pressing middle finger to non-matching response. The details of the tasks, materials and procedures please also see the reference [21].

2.2 Imaging Scanning and Data Processing

Images were acquired from a 3.0 Tesla MRI system (Siemens Trio Tim; Siemens Medical System, Erlangen, Germany). Both EPI and T1 weighted 3D images were acquired. Functional images were sequenced from bottom to top in a whole brain EPI acquisition. The following scan parameters were used: TE = 31 ms, flip angle = 90, matrix size = 64 by 64, field of view = 200 mm by 200 mm, slice thickness = 3.2 mm, number of slices = 32, TR =2000 ms. In addition, a high resolution, T1 weighted 3D image was acquired (SPGR, TR = 1600 ms, TE = 3.28 ms, flip angle = 9, matrix size =256 by 256, field of view = 256 mm by 256 mm, slice thickness = 1 mm, number of slices = 192). The orientation of the 3D image was identical to the functional slices.

We use SPM2 (Statistical Parametric Mapping, Institute of Neurology at University College London, UK. http://www.fil.ion.ucl.ac.uk/spm) to analyze the imaging data. After preprocessing (see details in reference [21]), we did t-test to determine whether activation in human brain regions was significant or not in the tasks. All reported areas of activation were significant using $P < 0.001$ uncorrected for the voxel level and contained a cluster size greater than 0 voxels. And then we did a ROI (regions of interest) analysis of LIPFC. ROI was defined by the definition function in Marsbar and the percentage of signal change was calculated. Only the left LIPFC was investigated. The center point of LIPFC was X= -40, y=21, z=21 in Talairach coordinates, with 5 voxels wide, 5 voxels long and 4 voxels high (a voxel was 3.125 mm long and wide and 3.2 mm high)(see Figure 3). ROI analysis included two parts, first was the comparison between two tasks (WP vs. PW), and the second was analysis of the advantage effect within conditions of 3 levels across WP and PW.

3 Results

3.1 Behavioral Performance

As reported in reference [21], in PW task a significant basic-level advantage effect was observed, and the response time to the concepts in intermediate level was the fastest (832 ms for intermediate, 869 ms for superordinate and 897 ms for subordinate; pairwise comparison between intermediate level and other two levels indicated both $P < 0.001$); while in WP task there was a reversal advantage effect to general level, which meant response times to the concepts in superordinate level were faster than the times to the concepts in intermediate level(762 ms for superordinate, 802 ms for intermediate and 882 ms for subordinate;pairwise comparison between superordinate level and other two levels indicated both $P < 0.01$). (details see reference [21]). Figure 1 showed the behavioral performance across the two tasks. The behavioral performances suggested people retrieving information flexibly according to task demands and exhibited different advantage effects, although stimuli were same in the tasks.

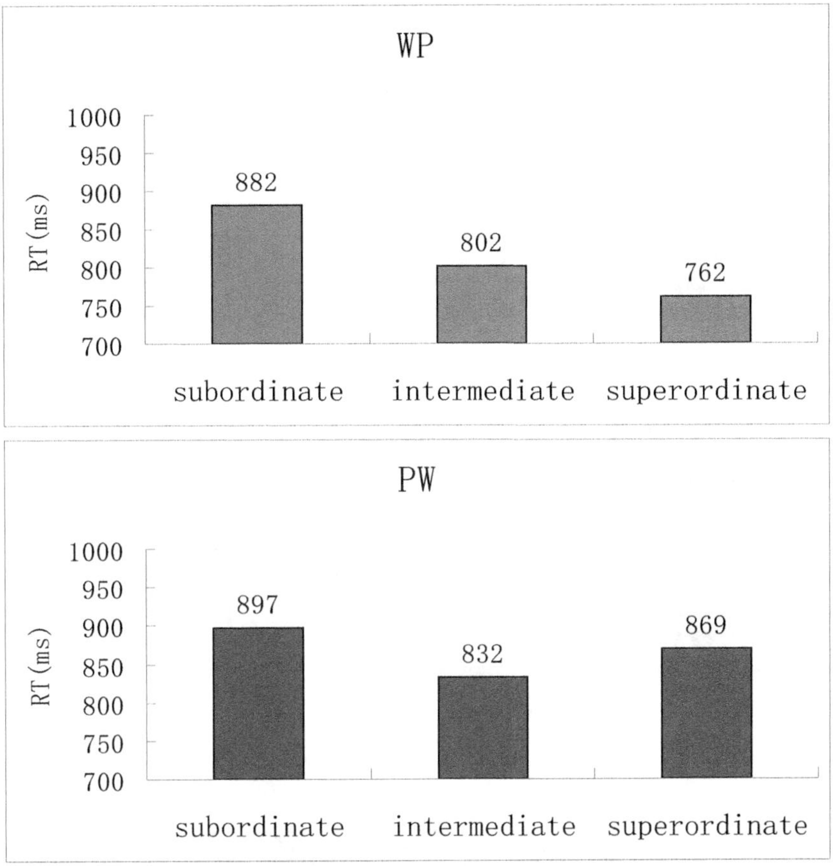

Fig. 1. Response times in WP and PW tasks

3.2 Brain Activities in Tasks

The brain activities were similar in WP and PW task. The most significant activated areas were located in the bilateral middle occipital gyrus (BA 18/19), superior frontal gyrus (BA 10/11), middle frontal gyrus (BA 9/10), inferior frontal gyrus (BA 45/47), inferior parietal lobe (BA 40), anterior cingulate gyrus (BA 24) and fusiform gyrus (BA 37). Top of Figure 2 showed the brain activities in WP task, and the bottom was activities in PW task. The results were consistent with previous studies [14, 16], the activation in the regions of occipital, parietal and frontal gyrus suggested visual word and picture recognition and higher semantic processing were involved in both tasks.

3.3 Activation in Left LIPFC

Figure 3 showed the region of LIPFC in brain and figure 4 indicated the BOLD (blood-oxygen-level dependent) response in this region in different conditions

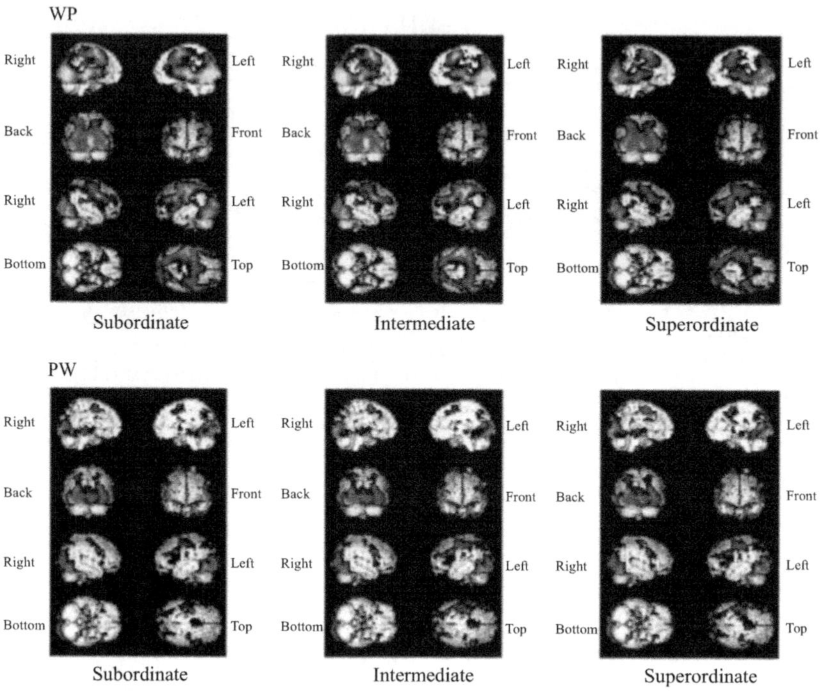

Fig. 2. Brain activities in WP and PW tasks

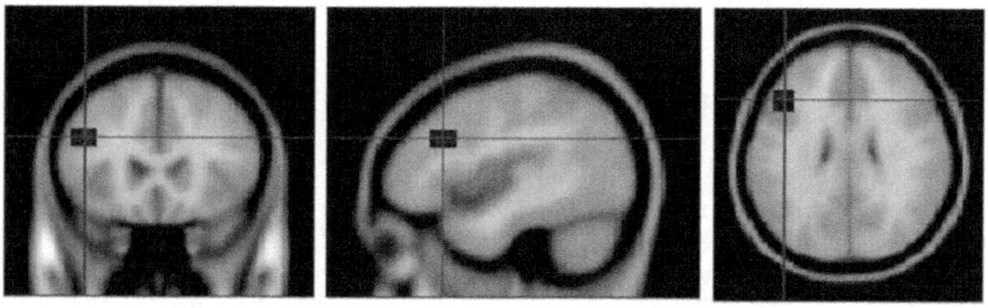

Fig. 3. Location of LIPFC in brain

across the two tasks. Comparison between tasks revealed the activation in WP task was stronger than that in PW task. ANOVA showed the difference were significant ($F(1,30)=166.090$, $P=0.000$). The result will be discussed later.

Moreover, the analysis of advantage effect within conditions of 3 levels in both WP and PW was quite interesting. For the two tasks, both the activation in the condition of intermediate level was weakest. A repeated measures ANOVA revealed a significant effect of concept level in WP task ($F(2,28)=12.660$, $P=0.000$), and pairwise comparison showed the intensity was weaker in the intermediate level than those in both the subordinate and superordinate levels ($P=0.000$ for

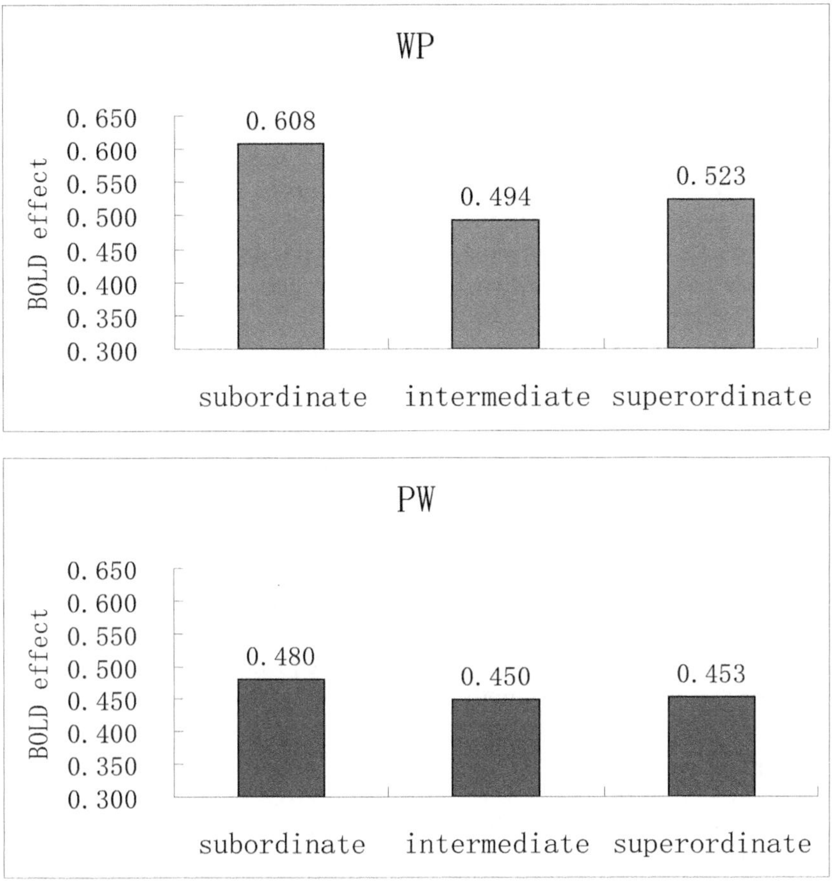

Fig. 4. BOLD effects in left LIPFC in tasks of WP and PW

the comparison between intermediate and subordinate, and P=0.032 for the comparison between intermediate and superordinate). And for the task of PW, although the intensity pattern was similar to that in task of WP, the main effect of concept level did not reach the significant level ($F(2,32)=1.850$, $P=0.174$).

4 Discussions

4.1 Task Analysis

In this study, we used fMRI to investigate the role of left LIPFC during human information retrieval. Based on the phenomenon of basic-level advantage, two tasks were used to examine the processing of information retrieval. As expected and reported before [21], in WP task, the behavioral performance showed the advantage effect reversing to general level and the response times to the concepts in the superordinate level was the fastest; and in PW task, we observed a typical basic-level advantage effect in behavior, which meant response times to the concepts in intermediate level was quite faster than that to concepts in other levels. The behavioral performance provide new evidences to explain basic-level advantage and its reversal. In WP task, the precede presented word activated the memory system and guided the following picture recognition, so more perceptual processing was loaded on and recognition in the general level was the most easy and quickly, which led to a reversal advantage effect to general level. But in PW task, the precede presented picture guided participants to recognize the object based on memory system first, and those corresponding concepts most familiar or most easy to access would had the strongest activation in working memory, which led to the judgement in the intermediate level fastest. These results were consistent with the researcher's views [6, 7]. The behavior pattern suggested human being could respond according to external world condition, and retrieve information from internal knowledge memory flexibly. Those information most familiar as well as satisfying task demands best would be the most easy to access and be retrieved most quickly.

Obviously, for these two tasks, participants needed to recognize the concept words and pictures first, and then compare them to judge whether match or not. fMRI results showed both tasks activated similar regions in brain, and wide areas in the occipital, parietal and frontal lobes were activated in tasks, suggesting the visual recognition, semantic retrieving and maintaining, and information competition were involved in the processing of tasks. All the processing should be considered when exploring how human brain modulated to behavior performances.

4.2 Role of LIPFC

Left LIPFC was examined in this study because of the key role during information retrieval. As expected, whether in WP or PW task, we observed the activation in left LIPFC across three conditions of concepts levels. For both tasks, participants would access knowledge in memory about concepts or semantic of pictures and words, by comparing them to finish the tasks. This processing might depend on the involvement of LIPFC activity. The activities in LIPFC were consistent with many studies before [8–14, 17, 19].

We also noted that there was a stronger activation in this region in task of WP than that in PW based on ROI analysis. For WP task, the earlier presented words would activate a concept first, and then to finish the comparison between word and pictures participants would maintain the concepts semantic as retrieval cues in working memory. Thus the pre-retrieved words would add the maintaining load and lead to a stronger activation in LIPFC. While for PW task, the earlier presented pictures certainly would active its corresponding semantic knowledge in mind and maintain it in working memory as well, but the representation of imaging would be involved more in the posterior parietal cortex, which region was related to visual and spatial processing. So the activation in LIPFC was weaker in this task. To test our hypothesis, we further analyzed the region of posterior parietal cortex based on ACT-R theory, and found there was a stronger activation in this region in PW than that in WP ($F(1,30)=153.008$,

P=0.000). We would further discuss the relationship between the two tasks and brain activities in other papers.

ROI analysis also showed there were highest activations in condition of subordinate level both in WP and PW tasks as expected; because it contains the most specific information, and it is hard to access concepts and semantic knowledge in this condition. According to previous studies, more cognitive load needed in a task, more activation would be in LIPFC [8]. But we also expected the intensity of LIPFC activity would change corresponding to the behavioral patterns. That is to say, in this study there would be a weakest activation in the condition of intermediate level in PW task according to the basic-level advantage effect, and a weakest activation in the condition of superordinate level in WP task because of the reversal of basic-level advantage. It is very interesting there was a similar activation pattern across the two task as figure 4 showed, and both the intensities in the condition of intermediate level in WP and PW were the weakest. That was not consistent with our expectations. Further ANOVA revealed that the intensity in the condition of intermediate level was significant weaker than those in other two conditions in the task of WP. Although the intensity differences between intermediate and other two conditions did not reach the significant level in PW, the nonsignificant result could not support the expectation either.

The dissociation of behavior and LIPFC activity suggested that although LIPFC played a role during retrieving information from memory, the activity might depended more on the knowledge memory system. There were some studies providing evidences to support the view. For example, there was a stronger activation in low frequency words comparing to high frequency words [19, 22, 23]. Because the inferior frontal gyrus was involved to compute and access the word information, the low frequency word was not so familiar with the high frequency words, so the activation for low frequency was quite stronger. In our study, the concepts or information in intermediate level was the most familiar [2], and that was most easy to access in human status [1, 3], so the LIPFC activation in this condition was the weakest. Some researchers suggested that LIPFC was involved in the selecting among competing alternatives [16, 20]. Information in the basic-level achieved the optimal balance between informativeness and distinctiveness [24], which might reduced the weakest selection conflict. In addition, some researchers thought this region supported the control of retrieval from knowledge information [17, 25].Controlled behaviors, in contrast to automatic behaviors, including the strategic interrogation of conceptual knowledge to generater specific pieces of information for a given task, were attention-demanding and driven by internal goals and knowledge [16, 26]. The prefrontal cortex was a source of top-down source. From above we might considered the activation of the region of LIPFC was depended more on the internal memory system, while not the external task condition. So we observed a similar activity patterns in LIPFC in WP and PW, although the behavior performances in the tasks were different. The results in this paper further suggested that how human brain modulated the advantage effect during information retrieval might be charged by other regions in the brain [21], which need more investigation. We are going to investigate the difference of brain networks between the two tasks to further explore how human brain modulates to basic-level advantage effect and its reversal.

4.3 Summary

Left lateral inferior prefrontal cortex (LIPFC) is a key region in human brain related to information retrieval. In this paper, we focused on the activity of this region in two tasks which demanded retrieving information about pictures and concepts from memory. This region was activated in both task, and the intensity was stronger in WP, indicating a stronger semantic memory load upon in this task. Although the behavioral performances was different, a typical basic-level advantage in PW and a reversal advantage effect to more general level in WP, the brain activity patterns were similar in the area of LIPFC across the two tasks. The results might suggest the region of LIPFC is related to controlled retrieval, and the activation in this region might depend more on internal memory system, but not the external task demands. It is still need more investigation to understand how brain modulate to different behaviors.

Acknowledgments. This study was supported by the National Science Foundation of China (No.60875075 and No.60905027), Beijing University of Technology Doctoral Foundation Project (No. 52007999200701) and Beijing Natural Science Foundation (No. 4102007).

References

1. Rosch, E., Mervis, C.B., Gray, W., Johnson, D., Boyes-Braem, P.: Basic objects in natural categories. Cognitive Psychology 8, 382–439 (1976)
2. Wisniewski, E.J., Murphy, G.L.: Superordinate and basic category names in discourse: A textual analysis. Discourse Processing 12, 245–261 (1989)
3. Rogers, T., Patterson, K.: Object categorization: Reversals and explanations of the basic-levle advantage. Journal of Experimental Psychology: Gerneral 136(3), 451–469 (2007)
4. Hodges, J.R., Graham, N., Patterson, K.: Charting the progression in semantic dementia: Implications for the organisation of semantic memory. Memory 3, 463–495 (1995)
5. Warrington, E.: Selective impairment of semantic memory. Quoterly Journal of Experimental Psychology 27, 635–657 (1975)
6. VanRullen, R., Thorpe, S.J.: Is it a bird? is it a plane? ultra-rapid visual categorization of natural and artifactual objects. Perception 30, 655–688 (2001)
7. Large, M., Kiss, I., McMullen, P.: Electrophysiological correlates of objects categorization: Back to basics. Cognitive Brain Research 20, 415–426 (2004)
8. Anderson, J., Byrne, D., Fincham, J.M., Gunn, P.: Role of prefrontal and parietal cortices in associative learning. Cerebral Cortex 18, 904–914 (2008)
9. Sohn, M.H., Goode, A., Stenger, V.A., Carter, C.S., Anderson, J.R.: Competition and representation during memory retrieval: Roles of the prefrontal cortex and the posterior parietal cortex. Proceedings of National Academy of Sciences 100, 7412–7417 (2003)

10. Sohn, M.H., Goode, A., Stenger, V.A., Jung, K.J., Carter, C., Anderson, J.R.: An information-processing model of three cortical regions: Evidence in episodic memory retrieval. Neuroimage 25, 21–33 (2005)
11. Qin, Y.L., Carter, C.S., Silk, E.M., Stenger, V.A., Fissell, K., Goode, A., Anderson, J.R.: The change of the brain activation patterns as children learn algebra equation solving. Proceedings of the National Academy Sciences 101(15), 5686–5691 (2004)
12. Ravizza, S.M., Anderson, J.R., Carter, C.S.: Errors of mathematical processing: The relationship of accuracy to neural regions associated with retrieval or representation of the problem state. Brain Research 1238, 118–126 (2008)
13. Anderson, J.R., Anderson, J.F., Ferris, J.L., Fincham, J.M., Jung, K.J.: The lateral inferior prefrontal cortex and anterior cingulate cortex are engaged at different stages in the solution of insight problems. Proceedings of the National Academy Sciences 106(26), 10799–10804 (2009)
14. Binder, J.R., Desai, R.H., Graves, W.W., Conant, L.L.: Where is the semantic system? a critical review and meta-analysis of 120 functional neuroimaging studies. Cerebral Cortex 19, 2767–2796 (2009)
15. Grodzinsky, Y.: The neurology of syntax: language use without broca's area. Behavioural and Brain Sciences 23, 47–117 (2000)
16. Moss, H.E., Abdallah, S., Fletcher, P., Bright, P., Pilgrim, L., Acres, K., Tyler, L.K.: Selecting among competing alternatives: selection and controlled retrieval in the left prefrontal cortex. Cerebral Cortex 15, 1723–1735 (2005)
17. Poldrack, R.A., Wagner, A.D., Prull, M.W., Desmond, J.E., Glover, G.H., Gabrieli, J.D.E.: Functional specialization for semantic and phonological processing in the left inferior frontal cortex. Neuroimage 10, 15–35 (1999)
18. Fletcher, P.C., Henson, R.N.A.: Frontal lobes and human memory: insights from neuroimaging. Brain 124, 849–881 (2001)
19. Hofmann, M.J., Herrmann, M.J., Dan, I., Obrig, H., Conrad, M., Kunchinke, L., Jacobs, A.M., Fallgatter, A.J.: Differential activation of frontal and parietal regions during visual word recognition: An optical topography study. Neuroimage 40, 1340–1349 (2008)
20. Thompson-Schill, S., D'Esposito, M., Aguirre, G., Farah, M.: Role of left inferior prefrontal cortex in retrieval of semantic knowledge: A reevaluation. Proceedings of National Academic Science 94, 14792–14797 (1997)
21. Zhou, H., Liu, J., Jing, W., Qin, Y., Lu, S., Yao, Y., Zhong, N.: Basic level advantage and its switching during information retrieval: An fMRI study. In: Yao, Y., Sun, R., Poggio, T., Liu, J., Zhong, N., Huang, J. (eds.) BI 2010. LNCS, vol. 6334, pp. 427–436. Springer, Heidelberg (2010)
22. Fiebach, C., Friederici, A., Mueller, K., Von Cramon, D., Hernandez, A.: Distinct brain representations for early and late learned words. Neuroimage 19, 1627–1637 (2003)
23. Fiebach, C., Friederici, A., Mueller, K., Von Cramon, D.: fmri evidence for dual routes to the mental lexicon in visual word recognition. Journal of Cognitive Neuroscience 14, 11–23 (2002)
24. Murphy, G.: Parts in object concepts: Experiments with artificial categories. Memory and Cognition 19, 423–438 (1991)
25. Fiez, J.A.: Phonology, semantcis and the role of the left inferior prefrontal cortex. Human Brain Mapping 5, 79–83 (1997)
26. Miller, E.K., Freedman, D.J., Wallis, J.D.: The prefrontal cortex: categories, concepts and cognition. Philosophical Transactions of the Royal Society B: Biological Science 357, 1123–1136 (2002)

Dissociations in Limbic Lobe and Sub-lobar Contributions to Memory Encoding and Retrieval of Social Statistical Information

Mi Li[1,2], Shengfu Lu[1], Jiaojiao Li[1], and Ning Zhong[1,3]

[1] International WIC Institute, Beijing University of Technology
Beijing 100024, P.R. China
lusf@bjut.edu.cn

[2] Liaoning ShiHua University, Liaoning, 113001, P.R. China
limi135@gmail.com

[3] Dept. of Life Science and Informatics, Maebashi Institute of Technology
Maebashi-City 371-0816, Japan
zhong@maebashi-it.ac.jp

Abstract. Social statistical information is the quantitative description of social phenomenon, which is widely used in our daily life. However, the neural activity during encoding and retrieval of social statistical information remains unclear. We examined this issue in an fMRI study by measuring the brain activity of 36 normal subjects. The tasks consisted of encoding and retrieval the social statistical information visually presented in three forms: text, statistical graph and statistical graph with text. At encoding, subjects were required to try to read and comprehend the meaning of social statistical information presented in any of the three forms; at retrieval, they were asked to make judgments in regard to the content of reading comprehension. The direct comparison between encoding and retrieval showed that encoding more significantly activated the limbic lobe than retrieval; in contrast, retrieval significantly activated the sub-lobar than encoding. The results suggest that the limbic lobe is more involved in memory encoding of social statistical information, whereas the sub-lobar is more involved in memory retrieval.

Keywords: Limbic lobe, Sub-lobar, Social statistical information, Memory encoding, Memory retrieval.

1 Introduction

Social statistical information is the quantitative description of social phenomenon in our daily life. However, the neural activity during encoding and retrieval of social statistical information remains unclear.

Social statistical information describes social phenomenon, which is related to the self, hence, its encoding (understanding) involves self-reference. The limbic lobe, especially the cingulate cortex is involved in regulating emotional and processing of associative information [1]. In the last decade, the researches about

B. Hu et al. (Eds.): BI 2011, LNAI 6889, pp. 64–75, 2011.

the neural correlates of self have indicated that the cingulate cortex is involved in processing of 'self-relevant' [2,3,4,5]. These regions are more activated during both judgments of self-description and thinking about similar others [6,7,8]. Thus subjects will compare self-related things with ourselves [9,10]. Because the social statistical information is closely related to 'self-relevant', its encoding may require the involvement of the cingulate cortex.

Numerous studies reported that both anterior cingulate cortex [11,12]and posterior cingulate cortex [13,14,15]are engaged by the tasks which are related to emotion. The process of self-reference will lead to the change of emotion, because the social phenomenon is described by social statistical information may be consistent with our existing knowledge or not. Therefore, the cingulate cortex should be engaged during the encoding.

The statistical information is highly associative information, which includes items and their relationships, and each item itself has a name and a value. The basic operation is associative processing to link item's name to its value. The studies about the neural substrates of narrative comprehension have showed that, posterior cingulate cortex is involved in associative processing, which is at narrative-level, not at word-level or sentence-level [16,17]. Otherwise, the same results are also observed in the researches of context. The posterior cingulated cortex is activated during the tasks involving highly associative stimuli, and consistently more active for an increased level of associativity [18,19,20,21]. Thus, the encoding of social statistical information may activate the limbic lobe including the cingulated cortex.

Sub-lobar includes nuclear cluster which all around insula and basal ganglia, such as caudate, lentiform lucleus and claustrum. Some studies reported that caudate is related to memory retrieval [22], abstract reasoning [23], decision making [24,25], as well as rule-based category learning [26,27,28,29]. Moreover, lentiform lucleus is significant activated during the retrieval related tasks [30]. Thus, the retrieval of social statistical information may activate the sub-lobar which includes the caudate, lentiform lucleus and claustrum regions.

In our study, we focus on the neural activity during encoding and retrieval of social statistical information. The social statistical information was visually presented in three forms: text, statistical graph and statistical graph with text. At encoding, subjects were required to try to read and comprehend the meaning of social statistical information presented in any of the three forms; at retrieval, they were asked to make judgments in regard to the content of reading comprehension. We explore the brain activity of social statistical information through the direct comparison between encoding and retrieval.

2 Methods

2.1 Participants

Thirty-six volunteers (eighteen female and eighteen male; mean age $\pm$ standard deviation (S.D.) = 22.5 $\pm$ 1.7) participated in this study. All of the subjects were right-handed and native-Chinese speaking. The subjects had no history of neurological or psychiatric illness, and no developmental disorders, including reading disablities. All of the participants gave their written informed consent, and the protocol was approved by the Ethical Committee of Xuanwu Hospital of Capital Medical University and the institutional Review Board of the Beijing University of Technology.

2.2 Materials and Procedure

In our study, the stimulus materials were selected with the content about the common concerned information in daily life, such as "In 2007, five top countries of the global transgenic crop area include: first is USA 57.7 million hectares; second is Argentina 19.1; third is Brazil 11.5; then Canada 6.1 and India 3.8". The same content of social statistical information was described in three forms: text, statistical graph and statistical graph with text. We presented six kinds of stimuli to subjects: text encoding, text retrieval, statistical graph encoding and statistical graph retrieval, statistical graph with text encoding and statistical graph with text retrieval. At the stage of encoding, each text was presented for a period of 14 seconds, each statistical graph was presented for 16 seconds, each statistical graph with text was presented for 18 seconds, and subjects were required to try to read and comprehend the graphic information. Then, at the stage of retrieval, subjects were required to make judgments in regard to the content of previous reading, and press the corresponding button in which right or left, as quickly as possible. The experiment consisted of four sessions. The order of different type stimuli within the sessions was presented randomly in an event-related design. The participants were instructed to read text, statistical graph and statistical graph with text information attentively. Four sessions were collected per each participant.

2.3 Image Acquisition

Blood oxygenation level-dependent fMRI signal data were collected from each participant using a Siemens 3-T Trio scanner (Trio system; Siemens Magnetom scanner, Erlangen, Germany). Functional data were acquired using a gradient-echo echo-planar pulse sequence (TR = 2000 ms, TE = 31 ms, FA = 90°,the matrix size = 64× 64 mm, 30 axial slices parallel to the AC-PC plane, Voxel = 4 × 4 × 4 mm, 0.8 mm inter-slice gap, FOV = 240 × 240 mm). High-resolution T1-weighted anatomical images were collected in the same plane as the functional image using a spin echo sequence with the following parameters (TR = 130 ms, TE = 2.89 ms, FA = 70°, the matrix size = 320 × 320 mm, 30 axial slices parallel to the AC-PC plane, Voxel = 0.8 × 0.8 × 4 mm, FOV = 240 × 240 mm).

2.4 Data Analysis

Data analysis was performed with SPM2 from the Welcome Department of Cognitive Neurology, London, UK implemented in Matlab 7.0 from the Mathworks, Sherborne, MA, USA. MNI coordinates were transferred into Talairach coordinates (Talairach and Tournoux, 1988). The first two scans were discarded from the analysis to eliminate nonequilibrium effects of magnetization. The functional images of each participant were corrected for slice timing, and all volumes were spatially realigned to the first volume (head movement was < 2 mm in all cases). A mean image created from the realigned volumes was coregistered with the structural T1 volume and the structural volumes spatially normalized to the Montreal Neurological Institute (MNI) EPI temple using nonlinear basis functions. Images were resampled into 2-mm cubic voxels and then spatially smoothed with a Gaussian kernel of 8 mm full-width at half-maximum (FWHM). The stimulus onsets of the trials for each condition were convolved with the canonical form of the hemodynamic response function (hrf) as defined in SPM 2. Statistical inferences were drawn on the basis of the general linear modal as it is implemented in SPM 2. Linear contrasts were calculated for the comparisons between conditions. The contrast images were then entered into a second level analysis (random effects model) to extend statistical inference about activity differences to the population from which the participants were drawn. Activations are reported for clusters of 50 contiguous voxels (400 mm^3) that surpassed a corrected threshold of $p < .05$ on cluster level.

3 Results

3.1 Behavioral Results of the fMRI Study

Behavioral accuracy was larger than 0.75 in each of the memory retrieval tasks under scanning, indicating that the brain activity being measured was associated with successful memory encoding and retrieval in all tasks (Table 1). The accuracy from the fMRI experiment showed that there was no significant difference among the three forms (Analysis of variance between the forms showed that: ST vs. SG $[F(1,71) = 0.03, p = 0.87]$; ST vs. SGT $[F(1,60) = 0.01, p = 0.90]$; SG vs. SGT $[F(1,60) = 0.07, p = 0.80)]$). These results suggest that the three forms of social statistical information have no significant effect on the comprehension of the content of social statistical information.

Table 1. Behavioral results during the fMRI experiment

	Accuracy (%correct)	Reaction time (s)
Text(ST)	78.62 ± 8.76	3.88 ± 0.57
Statistical graph (SG)	78.96 ± 9.29	4.17 ± 0.61
Statistical graph with text (SGT)	78.76 ± 10.98	4.20 ± 0.67

3.2 fMRI Results

In order to examine the neural activity during encoding and retrieval of social statistical information, we did the direct comparison between encoding and retrieval tasks. The results in detail were shown in Fig. 1, Table 2 and Table 3.

Memory Encoding vs. Memory Retrieval. As shown in Table 2, the limbic lobe was activated when encoding task was compared with the retrieval task. The anterior cinglate gyrus (BA32) and cinglate gyrus (BA31) were more activated during the encoding of social statistical information from text compared with its retrieval (STR vs. STA). The anterior cinglate gyrus (BA32/24), cinglate gyrus (BA31/23/24) and posterior cinglate gyrus (BA31) were more activated during the encoding of social statistical information from statistical graph compared with its retrieval (SGR vs. SGA). Morever, the anterior cinglate gyrus (BA24) and cinglate gyrus (BA31) were more activated during the encoding of social statistical information from statistical graph with text compared with its retrieval (SGTR vs. SGTA). Through the conjunction analysis (as shown in Table 2 and Fig. 1(a)), we found that the conjunction of (STR vs. STA), (SGR vs. SGA) and (SGTR vs. SGTA) significantly activated the limbic lobe, which suggests that irrespective of the forms, the limbic lobe is more involved in the encoding of social statistical information.

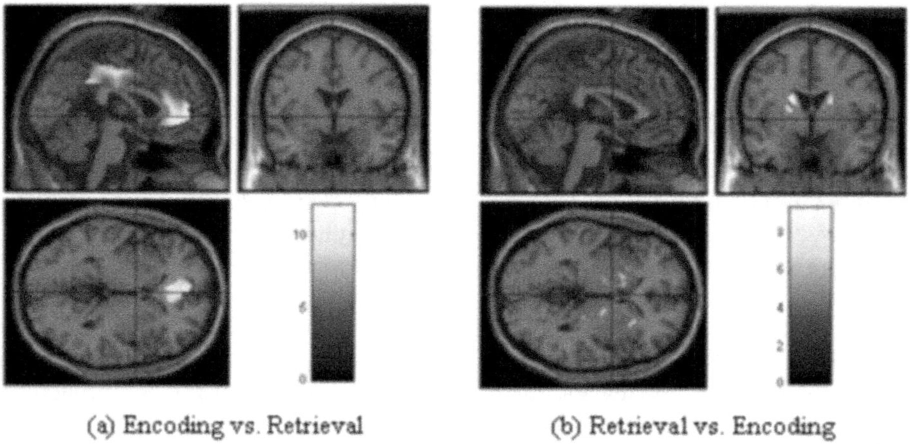

Fig. 1. Statistical parametric map (SPM) through the subjects normalized averaged brains of the limbic lobe and sub-lobar for comparisons of encoding and retrieval.(a) encoding vs. retrieval (b) retrieval vs. encoding. All of the Statistical Parametric Mapping t of the contrasts was thresholded at $t > 5.63$ ($p < 0.05$, corrected) and an 400 mm^3.

Memory Retrieval vs. Memory Encoding. As shown in Table 3, the sub-lobar was more activated when retrieval task was compared with the encoding task. The caudate (caudate body), lentiform lucleus and thalamus were more activated during the retrieval of social statistical information from text compared with its encoding (STA vs. STR). The lentiform nucleus (putamen), caudate (caudate body and caudate tail) and thalamus were more activated during the retrieval of social statistical information from statistical graph compared with its encoding (SGA vs. SGR).Thalamus, caudate (body) and claustrum were more

Table 2. Brain activations within limbic lobe related to memory encoding vs. retrieval ($p < 0.05$, *corrected*)

Anatomical regions	Coordinates[a] x	y	z	t	Cluster size (mm^3)
STR vs. STA					
Anterior Cingulate (BA32)	-8	33	-3	11.90	648
Cingulate Gyrus (BA31)	-2	-43	32	11.14	3112
SGR vs. SGA					
Anterior Cingulate (BA32)	-6	48	-2	9.92	456
Cingulate Gyrus (BA31)	-8	-45	32	8.59	3624
Posterior Cingulate (BA31)	-8	-57	21	9.24	5008
Cingulate Gyrus (BA23)	0	-34	24	8.97	2400
Cingulate Gyrus (BA24)	2	-15	41	10.20	8328
Anterior Cingulate (BA24)	6	31	6	9.95	2264
SGTR vs. SGTA					
Anterior Cingulate (BA24)	-8	31	-2	9.82	1560
Cingulate Gyrus (BA31)	-4	-51	27	11.70	1432
Anterior Cingulate (BA24)	8	31	-5	9.50	2656
Cingulate Gyrus (BA31)	6	-45	28	10.95	456
Conjunction analysis					
Anterior Cingulate (BA32)	-4	33	-2	10.83	2048
Cingulate Gyrus (BA31)	-4	-45	30	10.78	4104
Anterior Cingulate (BA32)	0	41	-5	10.45	408

[a] The Talairach coordinates of the centroid and associated maximum t within contiguous regions are reported.
STR: text reading; STA: text answering; SGR: statistical graph reading; SGA: statistical graph answering; SGTR: statistical graph with text reading; SGTA: statistical graph with text answering; BA: Brodmann area.

Table 3. Brain activations within sub-lobar related to memory encoding vs. retrieval ($p < 0.05, corrected$)

Anatomical regions	Coordinates[a] x	y	z	t	Cluster size (mm^3)
STA vs. STR					
Caudate Body	-18	-7	19	10.73	4352
Lentiform Nucleus	-12	-8	-2	8.21	680
Lentiform Nucleus	16	-4	-3	9.05	1944
Thalamus	22	-19	18	8.31	432
Caudate Body	20	-5	21	8.03	1048
SGA vs. SGR					
Lentiform Nucleus	-18	2	11	8.44	2464
Caudate Body	-18	-5	19	8.04	592
Thalamus	-18	-15	19	7.71	408
Caudate Tail	30	-31	9	8.71	408
Thalamus	24	-25	12	8.68	592
SGTA vs. SGTR					
Thalamus	-22	-29	12	9.16	1176
Caudate Body	-18	-11	23	8.67	2376
Claustrum	-30	21	-1	13.02	5640
Thalamus	22	-22	18	10.16	1760
Conjunction analysis					
Caudate Body	-18	-7	19	9.28	3456
Lentiform Nucleus	-16	-6	-5	8.13	1240
Lentiform Nucleus	16	-3	-3	9.30	504
Thalamus	22	-18	19	7.30	1176
Caudate Body	20	-5	21	7.62	1160

[a] The Talairach coordinates of the centroid and associated maximum t within contiguous regions are reported.
STR: text reading; STA: text answering; SGR: statistical graph reading; SGA: statistical graph answering; SGTR: statistical graph with text reading; SGTA: statistical graph with text answering; BA: Brodmann area.

activated during the retrieval of social statistical information from statistical graph with text compared with its encoding (SGTA vs. SGTR). We also did the conjunction analysis (as shown in Table 3 and Fig. 1(b)), the conjunction of (STA vs. STR), (SGA vs. SGR) and (SGTA vs. SGTR) significantly activated the sub-lobar, which suggests that irrespective of the forms, the sub-lobar is more involved in the retrieval.

4 Discussion

The aim of this study was to determine the neural activity during encoding and retrieval of social statistical information. The social statistical information was visually presented in three forms: text, statistical graph and statistical graph with text. The direct comparison between encoding and retrieval showed that encoding more significantly activated the limbic lobe including cingulate cortex than retrieval; in contrast, retrieval significantly activated the sub-lobar including the caudate, thalamus, lentiform lucleus and claustrum than encoding.

In encoding vs. retrieval, the anterior cingulate gyrus showed greater activation. This result suggests that the anterior cingulate gyrus plays a critical role during the encoding of social statistical information. The anterior cingulate gyrus was considered to be a high-level regulated structure in executive function neural network [31]. The changes of emotion will affect our normal cognition [32], which requires self-regulation to adopt the right way of thinking. Various studies showed that the anterior cingulate gyrus was involved in emotional processing [11,12], executing of attention [33], monitoring of conflict [34,35,36], processing of reward [37]and error detection [38]. Executing of attention serves as one basis for the self-regulation [39], and monitoring of conflict, error detection and emotional reactions are the results of self-regulation. In a review of ACC, Posner et al. [39]considered that self-regulation might be a natural function of brain networks, designed to avoid conflicting responses in behavior through controlling the information obtained [40]. In our opinion, when we are in conflict during the understanding of social statistical information, the anterior cinglate gyrus will regulate brain activation to allow us to carry out normal cognition.

In encoding vs. retrieval, we also found activation in posterior cinglate gyrus. The study of associative processing showed the significant activation in posterior cinglate gyrus during tasks involving highly associative stimuli [18]. Ferstl et al. [17]presented a quantitative review of 23 relevant text comprehension studies using a meta-analysis. Their results suggested that the processing in context recruited the posterior cinglate gyrus. In the study of viewing famous faces by Bar et al. [18], strong activation was observed in the posterior cinglate gyrus when the subjects viewing personal familiar faces. They considered that the response to personal familiar faces was modulated not only by the degree of visual familiarity but importantly by the concomitant associations involved, because viewing personally familiar faces elicits spontaneous retrieval of social and personal knowledge associated with close friends and family members. The posterior cinglate gyrus showed significant activation not merely in viewing familiar faces, but also in viewing personal familiar names [41]. Social statistical information is likewise familiar to us, and thus spontaneously gave rise to personal knowledge and experience retrieval during the comprehending to associate with our background knowledge, which activated the posterior cinglate gyrus.

In retrieval vs. encoding, the caudate was more activated. Abdullaev et al. using PET investigated the role of the caudate nucleus in cognitive tasks, and found that the firing rate of caudate cells was increased when the semantic processing was required, which suggest that the regions subserve more semantic judgements and processing [22]. Similarly, the study investigated by Verney et al. found that the caudate was more activated during success-related task, and the result suggested that the region was related to the decision making [24]. Consistent with these findings, the lesions study also suggested that damage to the region causes abstract reasoning deficits [23]. Moreover, some studies have indicated that the caudate was involved in the rewarded related tasks [42,43], as well as rule-based category learning [26,27,28,29]. In the present study, during the process of retrieval, subjects were required to retrieve and make judgments in regard to the content of memory encoding. Thus, it needs the involvement of caudate.

In retrieval vs. encoding, we also found activation in thalamus, lentiform lucleus and claustrum. The lesions study about thalamus found that damage to the region causes recognition memory deficits [44]. Moreover, Volz et al. investigated the neural substrates of prediction under varying uncertainty based on a natural sampling approach, predictions under uncertainty elicited activations in thalamus, which suggested that the region was related to prediction [45]. Moreover, the lesions study suggested that damage to the region causes rule-based category learning deficits [30]. A PET study investigated by Turner shown that the lentiform lucleus with adjacent cortex contributes to the control of movement extent [46]. DeLong et al. reported that lentiform lucleus, thalamus and claustrum have functional connectively [47]. A review study about claustrum showed that the region was involved in integrating conscious percepts [48]. Thus, in our study, caudate, thalamus, lentiform lucleus and claustrum are contributes to retrieval of social statistical information.

5 Conclusion

This study investigated the neural substrates of encoding and retrieval of social statistical information. The results showed that irrespective of the social statistical information visually presented in any of three forms, encoding more significantly activated the limbic lobe than retrieval; in contrast, retrieval significantly activated the sub-lobar than encoding. Our results suggest that the limbic lobe is more involved in the encoding of social statistical information, whereas the sub-lobar is more involved in the retrieval.

Acknowledgements. This work is partially supported by the National Natural Science Foundation of China (No. 60905027), the Beijing Natural Science Foundation (No. 4102007) and the grant-in-aid for scientific research (No.18300053) from the Japanese Ministry of Education, Culture, Sport, Science and Technology, and the Open Foundation of Key Laboratory of Multimedia and Intelligent Software Technology (Beijing University of Technology) Beijing.

References

1. Robert, L.: Limblic System. In: Encyclopedia of Life Sciences, vol. 10, pp. 1038–1076 (1982)
2. Craik, F.I.M., Moroz, T.M., Moscovitch, M.: In search of the self: a positron emission tomography study. Psychological Science 10, 26–34 (1999)
3. Ochsner, K.N., Beer, J.S., Robertson, E.R., Cooper, J.C., Gabrieli, J., Kihsltrom, J.F., D'Esposito, M.: The neural correlates of direct and reflected self-knowledge. Neuroimage 28, 797–814 (2005)
4. Vogt, B.A., Laureys, S.: Posterior cingulate, precuneal and retrosplenial cortices: cytology and components of the neural network correlates of consciousness. Prog. Brain Res. 150, 205–217 (2005)
5. Northoff, G., Bermpohl, F.: Cortical midline structures and the self. Trends Cogn. Sci. 8, 102–107 (2004)
6. Johnson, S.C., Baxter, L.C., Wilder, L.S., Pipe, J.G., Heiserman, J.E., Prigatano, G.P.: Neural correlates of self-reflection. Brain 125, 1808–1814 (2002)
7. Fossati, P., Hevenor, S.J., Graham, S.J., Grady, C., Keightley, M.L., Craik, F., Mayberg, H.: In search of the emotional self: An fMRI study using positive and negative emotional words. Am. J. Psychiat. 160, 1938–1945 (2003)
8. Macrae, C.N., Moran, J.M., Heatherton, T.F., Banfield, J.F., Kelley, W.M.: Medial prefrontal activity predicts memory for self. Cereb. Cortex 14, 647–654 (2004)
9. Frith, U., Frith, C.: The biological basis of social interaction. Current Directions in Psychological Science 10, 151–155 (2001)
10. Mitchell, J.P., Banaji, M.R., Macrae, C.N.: General and specific contributions of the medial prefrontal cortex to knowledge about mental states. Neuroimage 28, 757–762 (2005)
11. Mayberg, H.S.: Limbic-cortical dysregulation: A proposed model of depression. J. Neuropsych. Clin. N 9, 471–481 (1997)
12. Simpson, J.R., Drevets, W.C., Snyder, A.Z., Gusnard, D.A., Raichle, M.E.: Emotion-induced changes in human medial prefrontal cortex: II. During anticipatory anxiety. P. Natl. Acad. Sci. USA 98, 688–693 (2001)
13. Maddock, R.J.: The retrosplenial cortex and emotion: new insights from functional neuroimaging of the human brain. Trends Neurosci. 22, 310–316 (1999)
14. Maddock, R.J., Garrett, A.S., Buonocore, M.H.: Posterior cingulate cortex activation by emotional words: fMRI evidence from a valence decision task. Hum. Brain Mapp. 18, 30–41 (2003)
15. Mantani, T., Okamoto, Y., Shirao, N., Okada, G., Yamawaki, S.: Reduced activation of posterior cingulate cortex during imagery in subjects with high degrees of alexithymia: A functional magnetic resonance imaging study. Biol. Psychiat. 57, 982–990 (2005)
16. Bar, M., Aminoff, E., Mason, M., Fenske, M.: The units of thought. Hippocampus 17, 420–428 (2007)
17. Ferstl, E.C., Neumann, J., Bogler, C., Cramon, D.Y.: The extended language network: A meta-analysis of neuroimaging studies on text comprehension. Hum. Brain Mapp. 29, 581–593 (2008)

18. Bar, M., Aminoff, E.: Cortical analysis of visual context. Neuron. 38, 347–358 (2003)
19. Bar, M.: Visual objects in context. Nat. Rev. Neurosci. 5, 617–629 (2004)
20. Aminoff, E., Boshyan, J., Bar, M.: The division of labor within the cortical network mediating contextual associations of visual objects. In: Society for Neuroscience Annual Conference, Washington, DC (2005)
21. Aminoff, E., Gronau, N., Bar, M.: The parahippocampal cortex mediates spatial and nonspatial associations. Cereb. Cortex 17, 1493–1503 (2007)
22. Abdullaev, Y.G., Bechtereva, N.P., Melnichuk, K.V.: Neuronal activity of human caudate nucleus and prefrontal cortex in cognitive tasks. Behav. Brain Res. 97, 159–177 (1998)
23. Pickett, E.R., Kuniholm, E., Protopapas, A., Friedman, J., Lieberman, P.: Selective speech motor, syntax and cognitive deficits associated with bilateral damage to the putamen and the head of the caudate nucleus: a case study. Neuropsychologia 36, 173–188 (1998)
24. Verney, S.P., Brown, G.G., Frank, L., Paulus, M.P.: Error-rate-related caudate and parietal cortex activation during decision making. Neuroreport 14, 923–928 (2003)
25. Haruno, M., Kuroda, T., Doya, K., Toyama, K., Kimura, M., Samejima, K., Imamizu, H., Kawato, M.: A neural correlate of reward-based behavioral learning in caudate nucleus: A functional magnetic resonance Imaging study of a stochastic decision task. J. Neurosci. 24, 1660–1665 (2004)
26. Filoteo, J.V., Maddox, W.T., Simmons, A.N., Ing, A.D., Cagigas, X.E., Matthews, S., Paulus, M.P.: Cortical and subcortical brain regions involved in rule-based category learning. Neuroreport 16, 111–115 (2005)
27. Monchi, O., Petrides, M., Petre, V., Worsley, K., Dagher, A.: Wisconsin card sorting revisited: Distinct neural circuits participating in different stages of the task identified by event-related functional magnetic resonance imaging. J. Neurosci. 21, 7733–7741 (2001)
28. Rao, S.M., Bobholz, J.A., Hammeke, T.A., Rosen, A.C., Woodley, S.J., Cunningham, J.M., Cox, R.W., Stein, E.A., Binder, J.R.: Functional MRI evidence for subcortical participation in conceptual reasoning skills. Neuroreport 8, 1987–1993 (1997)
29. Seger, C.A., Cincotta, C.M.: Striatal activity in concept learning. Cogn. Affect Behav. Neurosci. 2, 149–161 (2002)
30. Shawn, W.E., Natalie, L.M., Richard, B.I.: Focal putamen lesions impair learning in rule-based, but not information-integration categorization tasks. Neuropsychologia 44, 1737–1751 (2006)
31. Gazzaniga, M., Ivry, R., Mangun, G.: Cognitive neuroscience: the biology of the mind, pp. 530–535. W.W. Norton & Company, NewYork (2002)
32. Bechara, A., Tranel, D., Damasio, H., Damasio, A.R.: Failure to respond autonomically to anticipated future outcomes following damage to prefrontal cortex. Cereb. Cortex 6, 215–225 (1996)
33. Devinsky, O., Morrell, M.J., Vogt, B.A.: Contributions of anterior cingulated cortex to behavior. Brain 118, 279–306 (1995)
34. Carter, C.S., Braver, T.S., Barch, D.M., Botvinick, M.M., Noll, D., Cohen, J.D.: Anterior cingulate cortex, error detection, and the online monitoring of performance. Science 280, 747–749 (1998)
35. Botvinick, M.M., Braver, T.S., Barch, D.M., Carter, C.S., Cohen, J.D.: Conflict monitoring and cognitive control. Psychol. Rev. 108, 624–652 (2001)

36. Kerns, J.G., Cohen, J.D., MacDonald, A.W., Cho, R.Y., Stenger, V.A., Carter, C.S.: Anterior Cingulate conflict monitoring and adjustments in control. Science 303, 1023–1026 (2004)
37. Hampton, A.N., O'Doherty, J.P.: Decoding the neural substrates of reward-related decision making with functional MRI. PNAS 104, 1377–1382 (2007)
38. Dehaene, S., Posner, M.I., Don, M.T.: Localization of a neural system for error detection and compensation. Psychological Science 5, 303–305 (1994)
39. Posner, M.I., Rothbart, M.K., Sheese, B.E., Tang, Y.: The anterior cingulate gyrus and the mechanism of self-regulation. Cognitive Affective & Behavioral Neuroscience 7, 391–395 (2007)
40. Rueda, M., Posner, M., Rothbart, M.: Attentional control and self-regulation, pp. 283–300. Guilford, New York (2004)
41. Maddock, R.F., Garrett, A.S., Buonocore, M.H.: Remembering familiar people: The posterior cingulate cortex and autobiographical memory retrieval. Neuroscience 104, 667–676 (2001)
42. Watanabe, K., Lauwereyns, J., Hikosaka, O.: Neural correlates of rewarded and unrewarded eye movements in the primate caudate nucleus. J. Neurosci. 23, 10052–10057 (2003)
43. Lauwereyns, J., Watanabe, K., Coe, B., Hikosaka, O.: A neural correlate of response bias in monkey caudate nucleus. Nature 418, 413–417 (2002)
44. Eleonore, S., Benno, K., Michael, S., Rolf, D., Irene, D.: The Role of the Thalamus in Recognition Memory. International Graduate School of Neuroscience (2005)
45. Volz, K.G., Schubotz, R.I., Cramon, D.Y.: Predicting events of varying probability: uncertainty investigated by fMRI. Neuroimage 19, 271–280 (2003)
46. Turner, R.S., Desmurget, M., Grethe, J., Crutcher, M.D., Grafton, S.T.: Motor subcircuits mediating the control of movement extent and speed. J. Neurophysiol. 90, 3958–3966 (2003)
47. DeLong, M.R., Wichmann, T.: Circuits and circuit disorders of the basal ganglia. Arch. Neurol.-Chicago 64, 20–24 (2007)
48. Francis, C.C., Christof, K.: What is the function of the claustrum? Phil. Trans. R. Soc. B 360, 1271–1279 (2005)

Knowledge Representation Meets Simulation to Investigate Memory Problems after Seizures

Youwei Zheng and Lars Schwabe

Universität Rostock, Dept. of Computer Science and Electrical Engineering, Adaptive and Regenerative Software Systems, 18051 Rostock, Germany
{youwei.zheng,lars.schwabe}@uni-rostock.de

Abstract. Despite much efforts in data and model sharing, the full potential of community-based and computer-aided research has not been unleashed in neuroscience. Here we argue that data and model sharing shall be complemented with machine-readable annotations of scientific publications similar to the semantic web, because this would allow for automated knowledge discovery as recently demonstrated using so-called "robot scientists". We consider a particular example, namely the potentially disruptive role of synaptic plasticity for memories during paroxysmal brain activity. A systematic simulation study is performed where we compare the combinations of different rules of spike-timing-dependent plasticity (STDP) and different kinds of paroxysmal activity in terms of how they affect memory retention. We translate the simulation results into a Bayesian network and show how new empirical evidence can be used in order to infer currently unknown model properties (the STDP mechanisms and the nature of paroxysmal brain activity).

1 Introduction

Recent years have seen an enormous interest in data and model sharing in neuroscience, which now also extends towards sharing formal models in machine-readable formats, such as NeuroML (neuroml.org), NineML (nineml.org), or yet to be developed model descriptions [1]. These efforts are ongoing and meet many challenges in practice, for example, convincing researchers to share their data, where major funding agencies and publishers certainly have to establish more rigid measures in the future. While standards for model exchange in systems biology and cellular computational neuroscience have been established [2], the sharing of network models in neuroscience is currently hindered by the lack of widely accepted standards for describing these models. However, even if both data and model sharing would be in place and supported by proper platforms like web-portals, here we ask: *In which way would such platforms support research in neurotheory and modeling?*

Data and model sharing is desperately needed as the data provides the yardstick for any model, and accurate quantitative models are needed for proper predictions as required in, for example, personalized medicine. Having both data

B. Hu et al. (Eds.): BI 2011, LNAI 6889, pp. 76–87, 2011.

and models available in machine-readable formats is also beneficial for computer-aided or fully automatic model generation from data using statistical and machine learning approaches. However, despite the inherent complexity of neuronal systems, we still believe that their understanding in terms of theories embodying simple principles is possible. Researchers in neurotheory, who work out such principles, will make use of such platforms as a source of inspiration to validate their theories which are usually developed without much informatics support and are largely informed by the available scientific literature. We hypothesize that even the development of theories, which go beyond plain model fitting, can be performed in a computer-aided or fully automatic manner [3] as demonstrated recently by so-called "robot scientists" [4].

We envision annotations of scientific publications using formal statements of the empirical findings (see Fig. 1). This is similar to the semantic web, which is still only a vision, *because it depends on the authors of web pages to annotate their content.* For the majority of content on the web, this may not even be worth the effort. However, from scientists, one shall expect the motivation and skills to formulate such annotations. Once such annotations are available, including references to proper domain ontologies, they could enter inference engines for automated knowledge discovery, which is a well-studied topic in classical artificial intelligence.

In this paper, we selected a challenging problem from computational neuroscience and show how to address it using a combination of knowledge representation and simulations. More specifically, we investigated how memories are affected by paroxysmal brain activity observed during seizures. This is a challenge for multiple reasons. First, despite decades of investigations on the mechanisms of synaptic plasticity and memory, we still have only a partial understanding of how the former underlies the network phenomena of encoding, maintenance, recall, and loss of memories. Second, after more than a decade of theoretical investigations of spike-timing-dependent plasticity (STDP), the modeling of STDP remains controversial, i.e. there is not even a census yet regarding phenomenological STDP models. Third, long-term memory retention via STDP has been studied only recently [5]. Consequently, to the best of our knowledge, the possibly perturbing role of STDP during paroxysmal brain activity as observed during epileptic seizures has not been studied.

Therefore, we performed a systematic simulation study of how transient paroxysmal activity may affect memories via STDP. We explicitly considered alternatives for the currently unknown STDP mechanisms and the nature of the paroxysmal activity. For different choices of these unknowns, the simulations make different predictions and we demonstrate how Bayesian networks, which are a prominent method for representing knowledge with uncertainty in expert systems, could be used in order to combine the simulation results with prior assumptions and new empirical evidence. In Sec. 2, we introduce our Bayesian network, connect it to the simulations, and we describe the simulated models. In Sec. 3, we present the simulation results and show how one could use them for reasoning within the Bayesian network. Finally, in Sec. 4, we discuss our findings

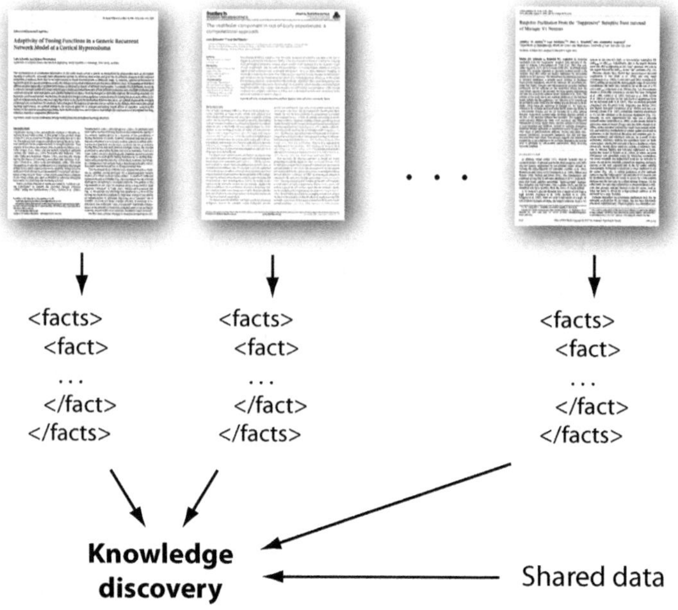

Fig. 1. Illustration of how to exploit semantic annotations of publications. Scientific publications will be annotated using formal statements of the empirical findings, similar to the semantic web and with reference to domain ontologies. Then, new knowledge could be inferred based on these qualitative findings, which are already interpreted by the experimentalists. Shared data can be used to validate existing and inferred theories.

from the simulations and what we can learn about the possibly disruptive role of STDP during epileptic seizures using our new method.

2 Methods

2.1 From Data-Model Comparison to Knowledge Representation

The integration of data and models has a long tradition in neuroscience, and the Bayesian approach is emerging as the *de facto* standard for that. Here, prior assumptions and a generative model for the data are combined with new observations in order to arrive at the posterior distribution over candidate models. It is widely used when the signal to noise ratio is low such as in, for example, functional brain imaging. Fig. 2a shows a graphical model for Bayesian model comparison and selection, where different models M can be parameterized with a parameter vector θ. Once prior distributions $P(\theta|M)$ are specified, observed data D can be used in order to compare different models M_1 and M_2 using the posterior odds $P(M_1|D)/P(M_2|D)$. This is certainly the method of choice once

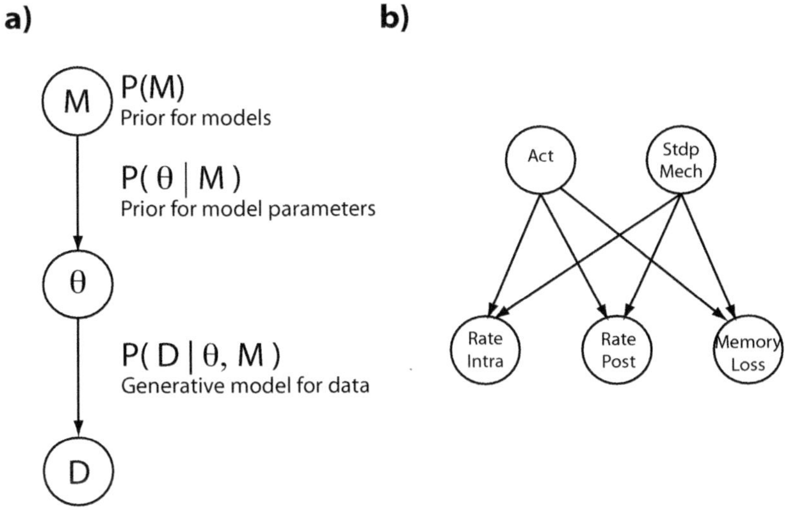

Fig. 2. Two Bayesian approaches to inference in neuroscience. **a)** The graphical model for Bayesian model comparison and selection, which depends on actual experimental data. **b)** The Bayesian network we use in this paper as an example of a representation of expert knowledge informed by simulation studies, which only needs qualitative observations (lower three nodes) in order to make inference about unknown model properties (upper two nodes) using Belief propagation.

the raw data is available, even though such a comparison is technically demanding because defining the prior distributions $P(\theta|M)$ and estimating the Bayes factor is non-trivial.

Here we focus on comparing models when only qualitative observations are available. We suggest to set up Bayesian networks for a particular domain and then perform inference given new experimental evidence. Fig. 2b shows the Bayesian network we set up for this study, where all nodes are binary. Paroxysmal brain activity such as seizures can be identified clearly using local field potentials and electroencephalography, but until today it is not clear if the individual neurons are synchronizing their discharges, or if the high-frequency population spikes are only a property at the level of neuronal populations without synchronicity of individual spikes. Therefore, we define two modes of paroxysmal activity, which correspond to two extreme scenarios in the population of neurons, namely changes in the mean firing rate and changes in the synchronicity with an unchanged mean firing rate, i.e. $Act \in \{\text{rate, sync}\}$. Another unknown is the nature of STDP, where we consider the "additive" and "mixed" rules (see Sec. 2.3), i.e. $StdpMech \in \{\text{add, mix}\}$. As observables, first, we consider changes in the postsynaptic firing rate of a neuron, which is driven by the paroxysmal activity via plastic synapses. The firing rate of this neuron could be transiently increased and then decay during the intra-ictal period, or be elevated throughout entire intra-ictal period, i.e. $RateIntra \in$

{transient, elevated}.Interestingly, recent experimental evidence suggests heterogeneous changes [5,6]; we return to this in the Discussion. Second, we consider activity in this neuron during the post-ictal period, where the firing rate can be lowered but recovers to the pre-ictal level, or be unchanged relative to the pre-ictal period, i.e. $RatePost \in$ {recovering, unchanged}. Third, we consider memory retention after a seizure, where we distinguish between mild and severe memory loss, i.e. $MemoryLoss \in$ {mild, severe}.

2.2 Leaky Integrate-and-Fire Neuron and Synapse Model

Following [7], we simulate a one-compartment conductance-based leaky integrate-and-fire neuron (see Fig. 3a) with membrane potential dynamics given by

$$\tau_m \frac{dV_m}{dt} = (V_{rest} - V_m) + \frac{G_{exc}(t)}{G_L}(E_{exc} - V_m) + \frac{G_{inh}(t)}{G_L}(E_{inh} - V_m), \quad (1)$$

where $\tau_m = 20\,\text{ms}$ is the membrane time constant and $G_L = 10\,\text{nS}$ is the membrane leak-conductance. $E_{exc} = 0\,\text{mV}$ and $E_{inh} = -70\,\text{mV}$ are the excitatory and inhibitory reversal potentials, respectively. When the membrane potential V_m reaches the threshold value $-54\,\text{mV}$, the neuron fires an action potential, and V_m is reset to $-60\,\text{mV}$. The model neuron has 1000 excitatory and 200 inhibitory synapses. Synaptic strengths of individual synapses are also conductance-based. Synaptic strengths $G_{exc}(t)$ and $G_{inh}(t)$ in Eq. 1 represent the summed contribution from excitatory and inhibitory synapses. On arrival of a presynaptic spike at the i-th excitatory synapse, the overall excitatory synaptic strength is increased instantaneously by g^i_{exc}, i.e. $G_{exc}(t) \leftarrow G_{exc}(t) + g^i_{exc}$ and then decays with a time constant $\tau_{syn} = 20\,\text{ms}$. The same applies to inhibitory synapses, where the synaptic strength $g^i_{inh} = 500\,\text{pS}$ is kept fix (no learning occurs at inhibitory synapses). All simulations were performed using Matlab with a forward Euler integration of 0.1 ms resolution.

2.3 Spike-Timing-Dependent Plasticity Models

The strengths of excitatory synapses, g^i_{exc}, are subject to learning modeled via spike-timing-dependent plasticity (STDP). Under STDP, the modification of synaptic strength of individual synapses depends on the relative timing of pre- and postsynaptic spikes [8]. The STDP learning rules encompass both synaptic potentiation *and* depression. This property will turn out to be important for our simulations, where we show how STDP rules adjust postsynaptic firing rate in response to changes in the presynaptic activity. More specifically, we use "additive" and "mixed" [9] update rules: In the "additive" rule, the modification is independent of the current synaptic strength but strengths are bounded, i. e. $0 \leq g^i_{exc} \leq \overline{g}_{max}$ with $\overline{g}_{max} = 150\,\text{pS}$. This update rule is given by

$$\Delta w = \begin{cases} \overline{g}_{max} \cdot A_+ \cdot \exp(-\Delta t/\tau_+) & \text{if } \Delta t < 0 \\ -\overline{g}_{max} \cdot A_- \cdot \exp(\Delta t/\tau_-) & \text{if } \Delta t > 0, \end{cases} \quad (2)$$

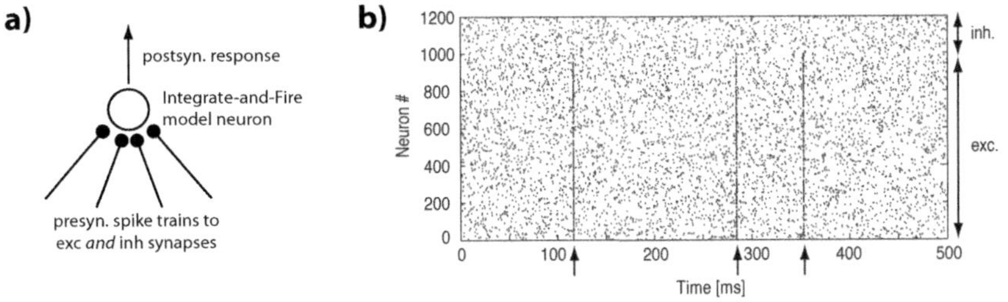

Fig. 3. Model setup and examples of synchronicity events. **(a)**Conductance-based single compartment leaky integrate-and-fire model neuron. The presynaptic activity for 1000 excitatory and 200 inhibitory neurons is sampled using statistical models (see Sec. 2.4), i.e. the presynaptic neurons are not modeled and simulated explicitly. Learning occurs only at excitatory, not inhibitory synapses.**(b)**Example rasterplot of presynaptic activity with three synchronicity events (see arrows), where for each synchronicity event 200 excitatory neurons are randomly selected. Dots indicate the time of presynaptic spikes for the excitatory $(1 \ldots 1000)$ and inhibitory $(1001 \ldots 1200)$ neurons.

where $\Delta t = t_{post} - t_{pre}$ is the time difference between post- and presynaptic spikes on an individual synapse. $A_+ = 0.005$ and $A_- = \alpha A_+$ are scaling factors, where $\alpha = 1.05$. One of the original experimental studies of STDP [10] showed a dependence of the magnitude of synaptic depression on initial synaptic strength. Such a dependence has been modeled using the "mixed" rule given by

$$\Delta w = \begin{cases} \overline{g}_{max} \cdot A_+ \cdot \exp\left(-\Delta t/\tau_+\right) & \text{if } \Delta t < 0 \\ -g^i_{exc} \cdot \tilde{A}_- \cdot \exp\left(\Delta t/\tau_-\right) & \text{if } \Delta t > 0, \end{cases} \tag{3}$$

with $\tilde{A}_- = 0.0114$.

2.4 Modeling Presynaptic Population Activity

All presynaptic spikes were generated via Poisson processes. During an initial phase of learning, the rate of presynaptic spike trains for both excitatory and inhibitory synapses was set to 10 sp/s. In order to mimic paroxysmal brain activity of an epileptic seizure, we employed two different transient modification schemes. First, the rate of Poisson processes is increased from 10 sp/s to 12 sp/s. Second, the synchronicity between presynaptic spikes is increased while the Poisson rate remains unchanged. This is done as follows. One synchronized "spike train" is sampled to determine a synchronicity event with Poisson rate of 10 Hz. Whenever such an event takes place, 5 % of *randomly* selected presynaptic excitatory neurons synchronize their discharges. Compared to the first scenario, the average activity could be regarded unchanged, but synchronous discharges of a subset of presynaptic neurons at each synchronicity event strongly drive the postsynaptic neuron to fire action potentials. Fig. 3b shows a rasterplot for the second scenario with 20 % synchronicity.

2.5 Quantification of Memory Loss/Memory Retention

A change in the firing rate of postsynaptic model neuron is an observable which can easily be measured. However, the "memory loss" is not straight-forward to quantify using single neuron models. It is generally assumed that the pattern of synaptic strengths is one important form of memory storage. Therefore, here we calculate the correlation between the strength-vectors of all excitatory synapses at two different times as an index of memory retention. We use the Pearson product-moment correlation coefficient [11]. A reference time t_{ref} is set before the simulated paroxysmal activity at which the distribution of synaptic weights reaches its equilibrium (see Fig. 4a). The strength-vector at t_{ref} is denoted as $\mathbf{W}\left(t_{ref}\right)$. Afterwards we let the model neuron continue to experience presynaptic activity and learn to adapt its synaptic strengths according to the two STDP rules. Then, the correlation coefficient $r\left(t,\, t_{ref}\right)$ between two strength-vectors $\mathbf{W}\left(t_{ref}\right)$ and $\mathbf{W}\left(t\right)$, where by default $t > t_{ref}$, is given by

$$\mathrm{r}(t,\ t_{ref}) = \frac{\sum\left(W_i(t_{ref}) - \overline{\mathbf{W}(t_{ref})}\right)\left(W_i(t) - \overline{\mathbf{W}(t)}\right)}{\left[\sum\left(W_i(t_{ref}) - \overline{\mathbf{W}(t_{ref})}\right)^2 \sum\left(W_i(t) - \overline{\mathbf{W}(t)}\right)^2\right]^{\frac{1}{2}}}, \tag{4}$$

where $\overline{\mathbf{W}\left(t\right)} = 1/N \cdot \sum W_i\left(t\right)$ and $\overline{\mathbf{W}\left(t_{ref}\right)} = 1/N \cdot \sum W_i\left(t_{ref}\right)$. The coefficient $r\left(t,\, t_{ref}\right)$ quantifies how much memory is retained.High values of r correspond to high memory retention whereas low values correspond to less memory retention, i. e. a stronger fading of memory. Note that even though the pattern may have reached equilibrium, individual synapses are still undergoing changes and this is most prominent for "additive" STDP rule (see Fig. 4b for an example). The ongoing changes of synaptic strengths are the main cause of memory fading, and this course of inevitable memory fading will be the baseline for our quantification of additional memory loss due to the paroxysmal activity. The baselines are shown for two STDP rules in Fig. 4c in terms of the coefficient $r\left(t,\, t_{ref}\right)$, where no paroxysmal activity was simulated.

3 Results

3.1 Simulation Results

The structure of the Bayesian network shown in Fig. 2b needs to be accompanied with the definition of conditional probability tables (CPTs), which embody the expert knowledge. This is where the simulation and analysis of the models enter. Thus, let us first interpret the simulation results, and then, in Sec. 3.2, we show how we translate these results into a CPT and perform inference.

Fig. 5 shows the simulation results for all combinations of $Act \in \{\text{rate, sync}\}$ and $StdpMech \in \{\text{add, mix}\}$. The top four panels show the predicted postsynaptic firing rate before (pre-ictal), during (intra-ictal) and after (post-ictal) a simulated seizure. The four lower panels show the memory retention during intra-ictal period in terms of the correlation coefficient of the strength-vectors (Fig. 5, thick red lines) in comparison with the memory retention predicted when

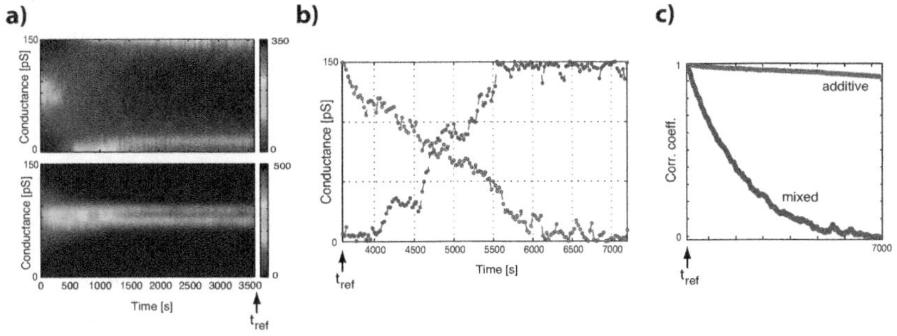

Fig. 4. Dynamics of the synaptic strengths. **a)** Evolving distribution (in terms of absolute numbers) of the excitatory synaptic strengths g^i_{exc} for "additive" (upper panel) and "mixed" (lower panel) STDP rules. **b)**Example synaptic strength traces of two selected excitatory synapses under "additive " STDP rule, where individual synapses are undergoing changes, for example, a weak synapse gets stronger and a strong synapse gets weaker. Note that these dynamics of individual synapses take place after the distribution reaches equilibrium (see $t_{ref} = 3600\,\text{s}$). **c)**baseline dynamics of memory retention in terms of the correlation coefficient for both STDP rules where no paroxysmal activity was employed.

no seizure is simulated (dashed blue lines). Interestingly, the postsynaptic firing rate remains elevated in three out of four scenarios. Only under "additive" STDP, an increase of presynaptic mean firing rate results in a transient increase of postsynaptic rate, which decays afterwards because the STDP rule weakens many strong synapses (see also Fig. 4b). The postsynaptic rate for the "additive" STDP with increased synchronicity remains elevated, because here many previously weak synapses are strengthened. The firing rates for the "mixed" STDP (Fig. 5, right column) during pre-ictal and post-ictal periods are low ($\approx 1\,\text{sp/s}$) and an increase in presynaptic firing rate is directly reflected in the postsynaptic response.

It has been shown before that "mixed" STDP leads to very poor memory retention [5] (compare dashed blue lines in Fig. 5e and f). Here we demonstrate that the memory loss due to the perturbing activity is even more severe for the "mixed" than for the "additive" rule (compare dashed blue with thick red lines in Fig. 5f and h). In contrast, the memory fading for the "additive" STDP during intra-ictal period is though obvious bigger caused by perturbing presynaptic activity than non-perturbing one, but much less pronounced than for the "mixed" STDP. It is particularly worth noting that synchronicity perturbation is more disruptive than rate perturbation, due to the fact that many previously weak synapses are strengthened, reshaping the distribution of synaptic strengths.

3.2 Inference with the Bayesian Network

The simulation results give valuable insights into the consequences of STDP for regulating neuronal responses and how paroxysmal activity may cause harm beyond the actual seizure, namely changing the network connectivity and hence disrupting long-term memory. Based on the simulation results, a human expert could resort to the scientific literature or laboratory in order to reason about the actual mechanisms. However, as we have considered only a small set of possible alternatives, it is likely that mechanisms we have not included are operating as well during a seizure, for example, an increase in both firing rate *and* synchronicity. In addition, the experimental literature shows that the changes in firing rates before, during, and after a seizure are diverse [12,6]. Thus, simply reading off the most likely combination of the unobserved model properties by having a human expert comparing the simulation results with the experimental literature is not even straight-forward in our very simple example.

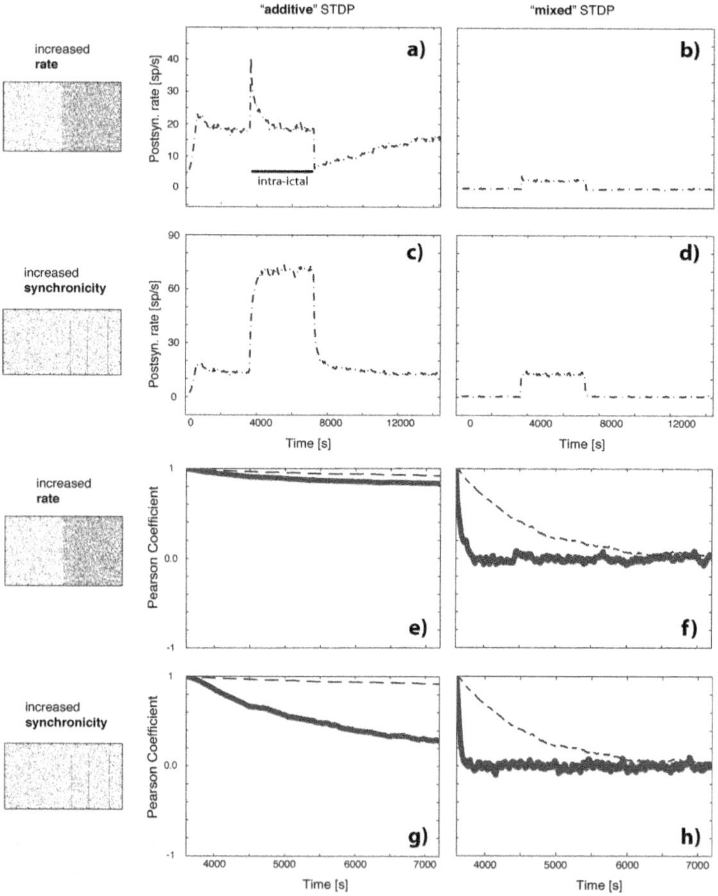

Fig. 5. Simulation results for all four combinations of paroxysmal activities (see icons, left) and STDP rules. See text for details

a)

	rate add	rate mix	sync add	sync mix
transient	0.9	0.1	0.1	0.1
elevated	0.1	0.9	0.9	0.9
recovering	0.9	0.1	0.1	0.1
unchanged	0.1	0.9	0.9	0.9
mild	0.9	0.1	0.6	0.1
severe	0.1	0.9	0.4	0.9

b)

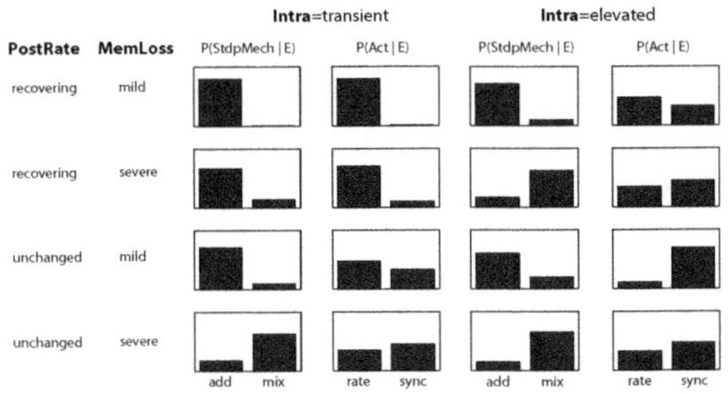

Fig. 6. Conditional probabilities for the Bayesian network and inferred posteriors. **a)** CPTs set up based on the simulation results. **b)**Inferred posterior distributions over the latent variables for all combinations of observable evidence at the three evidence nodes (leaf nodes in Fig. 2b).

Therefore, we first translated our simulation results from Fig. 5 into a CPT of the Bayesian network shown in Fig. 2b. This CPT is shown in Fig. 6a, where for all four combinations of the latent variables *Act* and *StdpMech*, the probability of the values at the evidence nodes *RateIntra*, *RatePost*, and *MemLoss* is given. Even though the simulations showed crisp results in the sense that some properties were only observed for a certain combination values of the latent variables, such as *RateIntr* = transient for rate increases under "additive" STDP, we decided to express this via probabilities 0.9 vs. 0.1 instead of 1.0 vs. 0. The prior probabilities for each of the latent variables were set to 0.5. Now we determine how new evidence changes our prior beliefs by setting evidence nodes to certain values and applying Pearl's belief propagation algorithm to update the marginal probabilities over the latent variables. We implemented this inference step using the Bayes Net Toolbox for Matlab [13]; the code is available at our site http://neurobench.org/publications/bi2011-bnet.m. The updated posteriors for all combination of evidence. are shown in Fig. 6b. Obviously, when the three observations correspond exactly to the simulation results, the corresponding latent variables have high posterior probabilities. For example, for observed transient decay of postsynaptic activity during the seizure (*RateIntra* = transient), a "recovering" post-ictal firing rate (*RatePost* = recovering) and "mild" memory loss (*MemLoss* = mild) are predictable only by "additive" STDP. However, it is conceivable that experimental evidence may yield results not compatible with any of the four combinations of latent variables such as *RateIntra* = elevated, *RatePost* = recovering, and *MemLoss* = severe, which leads to almost equal posterior probabilities for *Act* (second row, fourth column).

We argue that such a systematic comparison of different mechanisms, even without a full data-driven Bayesian model comparison, will yield valuable insights into the actually employed mechanisms. Most importantly, however, we believe that this approach of comparing alternative mechanisms is ideally suited as a basis for further refinement of the models and the domain knowledge expressed in terms of a Bayesian network.

4 Discussion

We propose that data and model sharing in neuroscience shall be accompanied with the sharing of knowledge via annotating scientific publications with formal statements of the qualitative empirical findings, similar to the semantic web. In this work, one particular knowledge representation is demonstrated where inferences generated from qualitative observations could easily be translated to machine-readably annotations. We have shown how to translate simulation results into a Bayesian network and how to perform such inferences using qualitative observations from the literature even without access to the raw quantitive data. Certainly, the annotation of scientific publications using semantic knowledge is desirable. But this, of course, leaves open the problem of how to get these annotations in the first place. Ideally, for new publications, the authors themselves formulate the findings and hypotheses in a machine-readable format. A prerequisite for that is the availability of proper ontologies and markup languages. Efforts for standardized ontologies in neuro- and brain science are under way, and research in semantic web technologies has produced methods and tools for formalizing knowledge. However, for already published works such annotations need to be made *post hoc*. We envision a web site with curated annotations, which would then be applicable for both new and older publications, where standards are enforced as part of the curation procedure.

The particular example we considered here is challenging, because as of now, it is not known in which way paroxysmal brain activity may affect memory via STDP. Directly measuring this will remain beyond the technical possibilities for the foreseeable future. Thus, making use of a variety of experimental observations both from animal and human studies will be most promising. The experimental literature shows a diverse picture: for example, the intra-ictal activity of some granule cells in the rat hippocampus was observed to be elevated while others remained unchanged [12]. In addition, the firing of some cells became more regular approx. 1 min before seizure onset, and some other cells showed a firing rate reduction for the seizure. Recent observations from human spike activity during seizures revealed that the single neuron activity is indeed "highly heterogeneous, not hypersynchronous" and showed clear termination of activity after a seizure [6]. Within the class of the mutually exclusive alternatives we considered, the latter findings are most compatible with an "additive" STDP rule, and an increased firing rate of the presynaptic neurons. Taken the poor performance of the "mixed" STDP in terms of memory retention, however, one could even rule it out as a candidate mechanism.

Future work will have to i) derive formal statements of these experimental findings using, for example, temporal logic expressions, ii) extend the space of models to more alternatives for the presynaptic spike activity to allow for increased rates, increased synchronicity and changes in the regularity of firing, iii) introduce more observables such as the Fano factor for the postsynaptic response, and iv) link all descriptions to neuro-ontologies.

Acknowledgements. YZ is funded by DFG GRK dIEM oSiRiS. YZ and LS developed the idea for this study and jointly wrote the manuscript. YZ conducted all simulations and analyses.

References

1. Ansorg, R., Schwabe, L.: Domain-specific modeling as a pragmatic approach to neuronal model descriptions. Brain Informatics, 168–179 (2010)
2. Le Novère, N.: Model storage, exchange and integration. BMC Neuroscience 7 (suppl.1), S11 (2006)
3. Langley, P., Simon, H.A., Bradshaw, G.L., Zytkow, J.M.: Scientific Discovery: Computational Explorations of the Creative Processes. The MIT Press, Cambridge (1987)
4. Sparkes, A., Aubrey, W., Byrne, E., Clare, A., Khan, M.N., Liakata, M., Markham, M., Rowland, J., Soldatova, L.N., Whelan, K.E., Young, M., King, R.D.: Towards Robot Scientists for autonomous scientific discovery. Automated Experimentation 2, 1 (2010)
5. Billings, G., van Rossum, M.C.W.: Memory Retention and Spike-Timing-Dependent Plasticity. J. Neurophysiol. 101(6), 2775 (2009)
6. Truccolo, W.J., Donoghue, J.A., Hochberg, L.R., Eskandar, E.N., Madsen, J.R., Anderson, W.S., Brown, E.N., Halgren, E., Cash, S.S.: Single-neuron dynamics in human focal epilepsy. Nat. Neurosci., 1–9 (2011)
7. Song, S., Miller, K.D., Abbott, L.F.: Competitive Hebbian learning through spike-timing-dependent synaptic plasticity. Nat. Neurosci. 3(9), 919–926 (2000)
8. Markram, H., Leubke, J., Frotscher, M., Sakmann, B.: Regulation of synaptic efficacy by coincidence of postsynaptic APs and EPSPs. Science 275(5297), 213 (1997)
9. Kepecs, A., van Rossum, M.C.W., Song, S., Tegner, J.: Spike-timing-dependent plasticity: common themes and divergent vistas. Biol. Cybern. 87(5-6), 446–458 (2002)
10. Bi, G.Q., Poo, M.M.: Synaptic modifications in cultured hippocampal neurons: dependence on spike timing, synaptic strength, and postsynaptic cell type. J. Neurosci. 18(24), 10464–10472 (1998)
11. Rodgers, J.L., Nicewander, W.A.: Thirteen ways to look at the correlation coefficient. American Statistician 42(1), 59–66 (1988)
12. Bower, M.R., Buckmaster, P.S.: Changes in granule cell firing rates precede locally recorded spontaneous seizures by minutes in an animal model of temporal lobe epilepsy. J. Neurophysiol. 99(5), 2431–2442 (2008)
13. Bayes Net Toolbox for Matlab: `http://code.google.com/p/bnt`

An Event-Response Model Inspired by Emotional Behaviors

S. Nirmal Kumar, M. Sakthi Balan, and S.V. Subrahmanya

E Commerce Research Labs, Education & Research,
Infosys Technologies Ltd., Bangalore, India
{nirmal_sivaraman,sakthi_muthiah,subrahmanyasv}@infosys.com

Abstract. In most attempts to define a system with emotions, researchers have tried to incorporate human emotions in them. In this paper, human emotional behavior is studied in a larger perspective of problem solving. The similarity among reflex action, emotional behavior and common sense behavior is observed. Based on these observations an event-response model for artificial system is introduced.

Keywords: Emotions, Emotional systems, Affective systems, Emotional intelligence, Common sense computing, Intelligent systems, Self adaptive systems.

1 Introduction

We propose a framework for an event-response model in an artificial system based on the human emotional behavior to various events that a human faces in his life. For achieving this we first focus on the study of human emotional behavior in a very fundamental way in the larger perspective of problem solving and we observe the similarities of it with the reflex actions and common sense. We see a common trait of reusing the solutions from the history in all the three behaviors. Also, from these observations, we infer that a problem is solved using all these three behaviors in an incremental fashion.

Emotional systems being a core part of any intelligent systems are being studied with much interest in this era. In the human-computer interaction perspective, we would feel more comfortable to use systems that understand and respond to our emotions. An example for such a system is emotional e-learning system. These systems use emotions for efficient human-machine interaction.

Even though communication is a very important goal of emotions, studies have shown that it is not the only goal of emotions in human beings. Recent studies on patients with frontal lobe disorders suggests that those who are unable to feel are unable to take decisions [32]. This shows that a decision cannot be the result of pure rational thinking alone. Of course, rational thinking or reasoning is important for decision making, but it results in good decisions in the presence of emotions. This shows the importance of imparting emotions in an artificial system.

It is now felt that emotions are an integral part of any intelligent systems, the exact role of emotions in human intelligence is still not clear. This is an important question to answer, in order to build a real intelligent system with emotions. It has been shown that emotions play a significant role in cognitive processing [9,26,31] perception [31],

B. Hu et al. (Eds.): BI 2011, LNAI 6889, pp. 88–97, 2011.

decision making, social interaction [8], behavior, beliefs [33], etc in humans. Also, emotional phenomenon has been correlated with effective decision-making processes, memory, learning and other high-level cognitive capabilities and skills [9]. In short, we can consider emotions as a problem solving tool as well.

Thus, if the aspect of emotion is incorporated in software systems, we will be able to empower them with better intelligence and problem solving capabilities. The intelligence aspect of emotions has been incorporated in some systems already. Some examples of various emotional agent models are presented in [1,2,10,11,13,17,27]. Studies on emotional coping and cognitive architectures are presented in [5,8,14,18].

The organization of our paper is described as follows. In Section 2 we study human emotional behaviors in a broader perspective of problem solving. In Section 3 we observe that reflex actions, emotions and common sense have the same problem solving strategy at different levels of complexities. In Section 4, an event-response model is proposed by extending these observations.

2 Understanding Emotional Behavior

If we have to impart emotions into a system with functionalities like decision making, strategizing, goal management, etc, we need to think more fundamentally on the human emotional behavior. That is, we need to understand what human emotions are and how does it help us.

In [23], Frijda defines emotions this way:

> Emotional Phenomena are non-instrumental behavior and non-instrumental features of behavior, physiological changes, and evaluative, subject related experiences, as evoked by external or mental events, and primarily by the significance of such events. An emotion is either an occurrence of phenomena of these three kinds or the inner determinant of such phenomena; the choice will be made later.

In the above definition, *the significance of such events* is stressed upon by the word *primarily*. Here, the *event* is the one that evokes the emotion. To understand the definition, the word *significance* has to be interpreted correctly. If we claim that an event is significant to us, that means, it is significant to our survival directly or indirectly, positively or negatively. Also, which event would be significant to us would depend on our definition of survival. The definition of survival depends on the problems that we encounter.

Even though there are many definitions for emotions and emotional behavior, there is no definition that is universally agreed upon. The definitions vary depending on the objectives of the studies. Ortony et al in [4] identifies three predominant approaches to studying emotions in the literature. We quote from [4]:

> Some theorists (e.g., [3,12,16]) focus on what one might call the input side of emotions by attending to the cognitive and perceptual aspects. Others (e.g., [23]) devote more attention to the output side by concentrating on action tendencies. Yet others (e.g., [25,6]) have undertaken extensive studies of the facial expressions of emotions.

Our objective is to use the technique of emotional behavior in intelligent system designs to make it better. When we study a behavior for this purpose, we need to observe and understand the inputs and outputs and how an input leads to an output. Emotional behaviors that we see and experience today cannot be explained completely in this simple way because of the complexities such as the continuous variation in the appraisal information [15], inter dependency of perception and action [28,30], occurrence of appraisals at different levels and different sequences in complex fashion [15], etc. With all these complexities on one side, let us try to understand emotional behavior at the very basic level.

Emotional behaviors are triggered by events [23]. Here, the event can be internal or external. An external event can be identified by the significance of any change in the environment [12,23]. An internal event can be some thoughts or mental activity [15,23]. The emotion depends on the interpretation of the event. So, we cannot say whether an event would elicit one particular emotion always. Different events may elicit same emotion, and same event may elicit different emotions [21]. For example, we can observe that one may get angry in all the following situations.

- When hurt physically by someone.
- When insulted by someone.
- When someone violates a social rule. E.g. A young person disrespects an elderly person.

A situation when one gets his dream job at a far place shows that different emotions can occur because of the same event. The person who got the job will be feeling both happy and sad – happy, because he got his dream job and sad, because he has to go away from his dear ones. This shows how different kinds of appraisal of the same event can end up in different emotions. Here, getting the dream job is an example for external event and being aware of the fact that he needs to go away from his dear ones is an example for internal event.

Emotional behaviors are some actions or action tendencies to some events [12]. We call them reactions. It is important to know what reactions are to be given at what situation. This can be observed from how emotions are elicited in some cases like the one given below.

> Conditioned electro dermal response persisted indefinitely after shock, in the same way that a smell of burning evokes a sense of panic in anyone who has ever been in a conflagration [24].

This suggests that emotional responses are learned. Phobia is also a good example that suggests that emotional responses are learned. In [7] it is mentioned that 60 percentage of people who suffer from phobia remember when the fear crisis occurred for the first time.

Even though these suggests that emotional reactions can be learned, we cannot conclude that all emotional reactions are learned. According to Frijda, feeling means more than knowing. He gives an example to illustrate that in [24] – we get angry when someone steps on our toes even if we know that he is not to be blamed. This suggests that not all these reactions are based on explicitly learned knowledge. Studies on infants also suggest the same. The infant reactions like crying and smiling are their emotional reactions [29]. They did not learn it from their experience, but these are instinctive reactions.

So, emotional reactions are some reactions that are either learned or instinctive. In other words, we have a knowledge repository about what all reactions are to be given in what all situations. This repository consists of knowledge that is passed on to us through our genes and that is acquired by us. The problem that is caused by the event may not be completely solved by these reactions. These reactions are action readiness [24] that would help solving the problem. Since the reactions are action readiness, they can be used to help to solve a variety of problems that are similar. This helps the system to adapt to different environments by providing some solution to the problems that are similar in some sense, but different in some other sense. In short, these reactions make the system ready to face the problem and adapt to the situations.

3 Extending the Traits of Problem Solving found in Emotional Behaviors

Let us consider three behaviors, reflex action, emotional behavior and common sense behavior.

The difference between emotional behavior and reflex action is that reflexes are stereotyped reactions whereas emotions are flexible and generic reactions [22].

According to Minsky [20], common sense is defined as below.

> it is an immense society of hard earned practical ideas of multitudes of life-learned rules and exceptions, dispositions and tendencies, balances and checks.

Of course common sense is more than just some reactions that are learned, but the above quote suggests that common sense behaviors are also reactions that are learned. One difference between common sense behavior and emotions is that emotions can be instinctive. Another difference is that the process of acquiring knowledge is less obvious to us, in case of emotions.

Let us consider the following scenario.

A girl wants to cross the road. When she is near the zebra lines, she hears a sound. She turns her head and sees a car speeding from a distance. She gets afraid to cross the road. She thinks if she crosses the road now, the car may hit her. But, she is on the zebra lines and the driver would stop the car for her to cross. So, she crosses the road.

In the above scenario, when she heard the sound, she turned her head. This is a reflex action. She got afraid to cross the road. This is emotional behavior. She understood that if she crosses the road when the car is speeding, it may hit her. This is common sense. She thought that when she is on the zebra lines, the driver is supposed to stop the car. This is thought behavior.

In all these three behaviors, we observe that there is one thing in common. All three can be seen as mechanisms to invoke predefined reactions to events that we face repeatedly in our life. These reactions may have been acquired through genes, learned through one's own experiences or from other fellow beings. There are many learning theories like classical conditioning (also known as Stimulus-Response theory), operant conditioning, etc, but our focus in this paper is on the mechanism of problem solving and hence learning approaches are not dealt with in more detail.

Each reflex action solves different purposes using the same strategy of reusing the known reactions. These reactions are different and specific to the problem that is solved. Since they act almost at the same level of complexity, we tend to group them and represent using a single name *Reflex actions*. Similarly, each phenomenon that we are able to identify as an emotion solves different purposes using the same strategy of reusing the learned reactions. They also act nearly at the same level of complexity but different from the level of reflex actions. So, we represent this group of phenomena using a different word *Emotions*. We can observe the same with the term *Common sense* as well.

Identifying how many such levels of complexities are to be considered is a tough task. The more intelligence we need to give to the system, the more are the number of levels of complexities that are to be incorporated in it.

We look up to human mind as the ultimate intelligent system and we can see that the complexities involved in it are enormous. Though research has been carried out in this direction, we are still not able to understand how it works. Minsky proposed a six-level model of mind [19] as shown in Fig. 1.

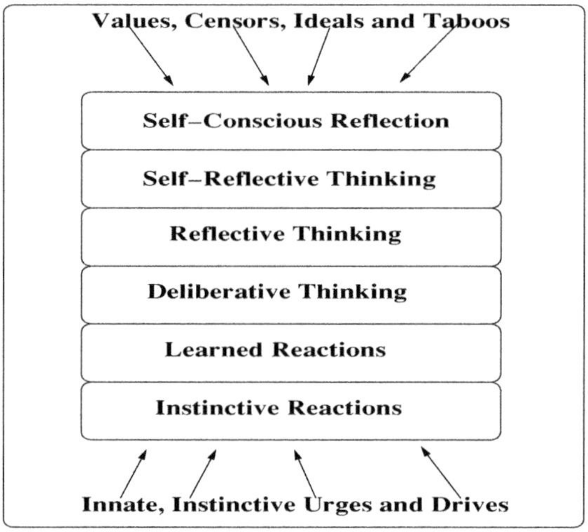

Fig. 1. The six-level model of mind proposed by Minsky

In this model, the six levels of mental activities are *Instinctive Reactions, Learned Reactions, Deliberative Thinking, Reflective Thinking, Self Reflective Thinking* and *Self Conscious Reflection*. However, there is no rigid boundary for any of the labeled levels.

According to the discussions at the beginning of this section, reflex actions are instinctive reactions and are not behaviors that are learned explicitly. Emotional behaviors are instinctive or learned and common sense behaviors are learned. So these three behaviors - *Reflex action, Emotional behavior and Common sense behavior* can be mapped into the first two levels of mental activity in Minsky's mind model as shown in Fig. 2.

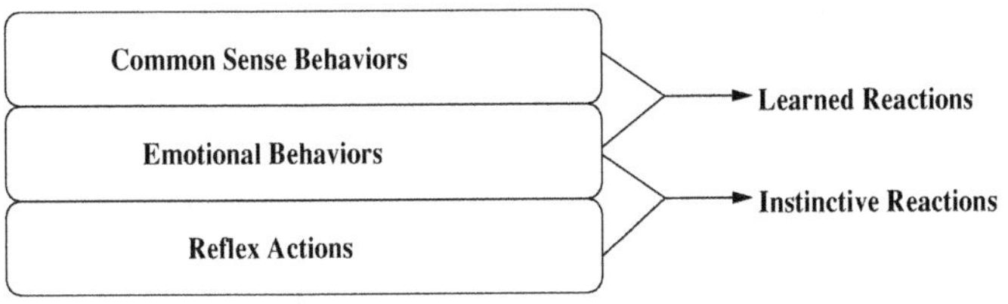

Fig. 2. Three behaviors mapped to two levels of mental activity

The fact that the three behaviors we observed are mapped to only two levels in the mind model suggests that there may be many more levels of complexities if we consider all the six levels of mental activity. Also, we cannot discard the fact that it may be possible to observe and group the behaviors further and label them within each level of mental activity itself. So, it may not be a good idea to conclude that there are only a fixed number of levels of complexity. Instead, we can imagine it to have many more levels of complexity. In all these levels, we use the same strategy of reusing the reactions that are instinctive or learned. We can keep on finding the reactions at each level of complexity till we find that the environment is favorable. So, the solution to the problem that is caused by an event will be a series of reactions each at different level of complexity, collectively called as the response to the event. This is shown in Fig. 3.

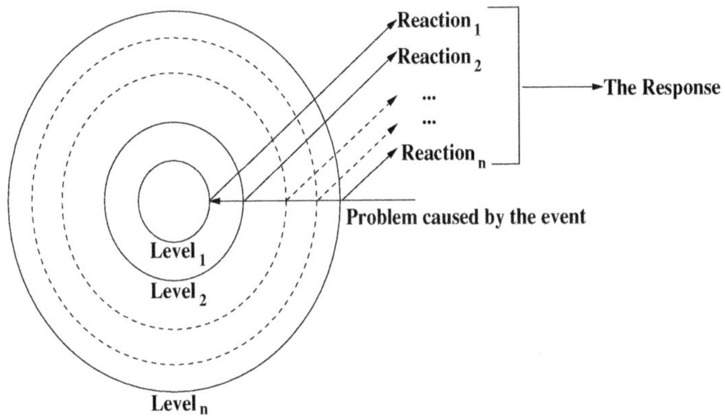

Fig. 3. The response

Here, the circles shows part of the problem that can be handled in each level of complexity. For example, the inner-most circle represents part of the problem that can be solved at $Level_1$. Here, that part of the problem is solved and the solution is given as $Reaction_1$. It leaves the part that cannot be addressed by $Level_1$ to $Level_2$. Similarly, many reactions are generated till the environment becomes favorable. All these reactions put together forms the response to the event. As we observed in the road crossing scenario, even though this response does not solve the problems that are caused by the event completely, it enhances the chances of survival of the system.

4 An Event-Response Model

In the previous section, we saw that the response to events is a collection of many reactions. From this it is logical to formulate a model to find the reactions in an incremental fashion to form the response. Here, we suggest a model to find the response to events. The model is shown in Fig. 4.

The first step is to identify that there is an event. This is done by analyzing the change in the environment. Once the event is identified, the change in the environment and the impact that it brings to the state of the system is examined. If the changes impact the system negatively, then it is identified as a problem. To solve the problem, first the complexity level is fixed to the least one. The history of solutions is checked to find an analogous problem and solution. If an analogous problem is not found in the history at that level of complexity, the history at the next level of complexity is checked. Once an analogous problem is found, its solution is used to find an appropriate reaction. This is $Reaction_1$ as mentioned in the previous section. This reaction and the problem description are updated in the history. The environment is analyzed to know whether it is favorable or not. If the environment is favorable, it is assumed that the problem is solved and the process is stopped. If the environment is not favorable, it means that there is still some problem. This situation is identified as a new problem and the same strategy of checking the history and giving the reaction is continued till the environment is found to be favorable.

In the road crossing scenario that is given in the previous section, the girl identified the goal as *to cross the road* when she decided that she needs to cross the road. When she heard the sound, she identified a potential problem that may stop her from achieving her goal or may affect her survival in a negative way. Turning the head is an instinctive reaction that is already there in the history as a solution to similar problems. This solution is executed and the environment is observed to check whether it is favorable or not. Since the environment is still not favorable, the problem is redefined. Now, the history is checked again to find a solution for this problem. Since no solution is found, the level of complexity of her mental activity is increased and the history of the new complexity level is checked to find a solution. She finds a solution as *Switch to a particular mode in which the mental and physical activities happen only in a particular pattern.* This particular pattern of activities or mode is commonly referred to as *fear*. Now she gets afraid to cross the road. But the problem is not solved yet. So, the level of complexity is increased again. Now, she considers more facts and arrives at a new problem definition that she may get hit by the car if she crosses the road. So, this leads to the next solution - *refrain from crossing the road*. Still, the problem is not solved completely since her goal is not achieved. So, the level of complexity is increased again. Now she considers more details about the environment like what the zebra lines signify, how a driver would respond if he see someone crossing the road through the zebra lines, etc and concludes that it is safe to cross at that time.

Here, the response consists of four reactions. Turning the head when hearing the sound is $Reaction_1$. Identifying a possible threat produces $Reaction_2$ - being afraid. Understanding the possibility of the car hitting her produces $Reaction_3$ - not crossing the road. Anticipating the driver to stop the car because she is on the zebra lines produces $Reaction_4$ - to cross the road. These reactions are obtained from the history.

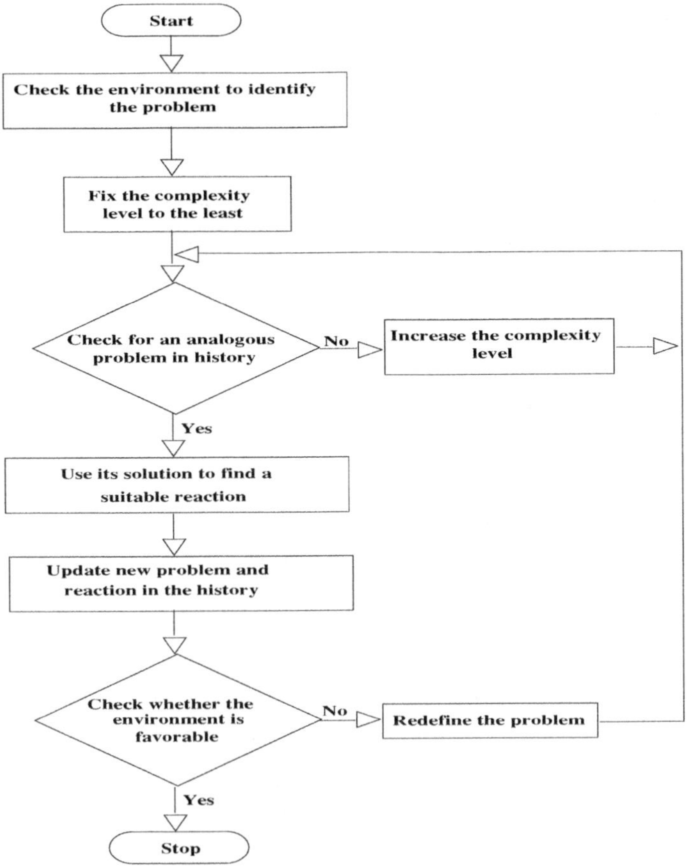

Fig. 4. The event-response model

Each time when a reaction is given, the event-reaction pair is updated in the history for future reference.

This system will keep on improving as it acquires more knowledge. This framework does not identify different emotions of the system and use them for communication. This work is the first step towards making such an emotionally intelligent system. Even though this model is not a complete intelligent system that can solve problems that are completely new to it, this is an essential part that helps the system to adapt to new situations.

5 Conclusion

We studied the emotional behavior in problem solving perspective. We observed similarity among reflex action, emotional behavior and common sense behavior and introduced an event-response model based on these observations. This model responds to events in an incremental fashion and is a self-adaptive one.

This work is the first step towards imparting emotional behaviors in artificial systems and we feel that this will lead to a better model for a self-adaptive system. The framework presented in this paper needs implementation and needs to be studied further. In consequent to that, work needs to be done to enhance this models adaptability and towards building formal models for the environment and the system itself. Moreover, the future models can also include knowledge representation structures for representing history, and defining and modeling of different levels of complexity.

References

1. Rhalibi, A.E., Baker, N., Merabti, M.: Emotional agent model and architecture for NPCs group control and interaction to facilitate leadership roles in computer entertainment. In: Proceedings of the 2005 ACM SIGCHI International Conference on Advances in Computer Entertainment Technology, ACM 2005, pp. 156–163 (2005)
2. Campos, A.M.C., Santos, E.B., Canuto, A.M.P., Soares, R.G., Alchieri, J.C.: A flexible framework for representing personality in agents. In: Proceedings of the Fifth International Joint Conference on Autonomous Agents and Multi Agent Systems, ACM 2006, pp. 97–104 (2006)
3. Ortony, A., Clore, G.L., Collins, A.: The cognitive structure of emotions. Cambridge University Press, New York (1988)
4. Ortony, A., Revelle, W., Zinbarg, R.: Why Emotional Intelligence Needs a Fluid Component. In: Matthews, G., Zeidner, M., Roberts, R.D. (eds.) The Science of Emotional Intelligence. Oxford University Press, New York (2007)
5. Smith, C.A., Lazarus, R.S.: Emotion and adaptation. In: Pervin, L.A. (ed.) Handbook of Personality: Theory and Research, pp. 609–637. Guilford, New York (1990)
6. Izard, C.E.: The face of emotion. Appleton Century-Crofts, New York (1971)
7. Masci, C.: Phobias: When Fear is a Disease, `http://www.cerebromente.org.br/n05/doencas/fobias_i.htm` (last accessed date: June 24, 2011)
8. Hudlicka, E.: Beyond cognition: modeling emotion in cognitive architectures. In: Proceedings of the Sixth International Conference on Cognitive Modeling, CMU, Pittsburgh, pp. 118–123 (2004)
9. Oliveira, E., Sarmento, L.: Emotional advantage for adaptability and autonomy. In: Proceedings Of The Second International Joint Conference on Autonomous Agents and Multiagent Systems, ACM 2003, pp. 305–312 (2003)
10. Sklar, E., Richards, D.: The use of agents in human learning systems. In: Proceedings of the Fifth International Joint Conference on Autonomous Agents and Multiagent Systems, ACM 2006, pp. 767–774 (2006)
11. Wang, H., Chignell, M., Ishizuka, M.: Empathic tutoring software agents using real-time eye tracking. In: Proceedings of the 2006 Symposium on Eye Tracking Research and Applications, ACM 2006, pp. 73–78 (2006)
12. Roseman, I.J.: Cognitive Determinants of Emotion: A Structural Theory. In: Shaver, P. (ed.) Review of Personality & Social Psychology, Emotions, Relationships, and Health, pp. 11–36. Sage, Beverly Hills (1984)
13. Bates, J., Loyall, A.B., Reilly, W.S.: An architecture for action, emotion, and social behavior. LNCS, pp. 55–68. Springer, Heidelberg (1994)
14. Mahboub, K., Clement, E., Bertelle, C., Jay, V.: Emotion: appraisal coping model for the cascades problem, from system complexity to emergent properties. Springer, Berlin

15. Scherer, K.R., Shorr, A., Johnstone, T. (eds.): Appraisal processes in emotion: theory, methods, research. Oxford University Press, Canary (2001)
16. Scherer, K.R.: On the nature and function of emotion: A component process approach. In: Scherer, K.R., Ekman, P. (eds.) Approaches to Emotion, pp. 293–317. Erlbaum, Hillsdale (1984)
17. Morgado, L., Gaspar, G.: Emotion based adaptive reasoning for resource bounded agents. In: Proceedings of the Fourth International Joint Conference on Autonomous Agents and Multiagent Systems, ACM 2005, pp. 921–928 (2005)
18. Eckschlager, M., Bernhaupt, R., Tscheligi, M.: NEmESys neural emotion eliciting system. In: Chi 2005 Extended Abstracts on Human Factors in Computing Systems, ACM 2005, pp. 1347–1350 (2005)
19. Minsky, M.: The Emotion Machine. Simon & Schuster paperbacks (2006)
20. Minsky, M.: The society of mind. Simon & Schuster paperbacks (1988)
21. Siemer, M., Mauss, I., Gross, J.J.: Same Situation Different Emotions: How Appraisals Shape Our Emotions. Emotion 7(3), 592–600 (2007)
22. Frijda, N.H.: Flexibility, `http://home.medewerker.uva.nl/n.h.frijda/bestanden/flexibility.100y.pdf` (last accessed date: June 24, 2011)
23. Frijda, N.H.: The emotions, p. 4. Cambridge University Press, Cambridge (1986)
24. Frijda, N.H.: The laws of emotion. American Psychologist 43(5), 349–358 (1988)
25. Ekman, P. (ed.): Emotion in the human face. Cambridge University Press, New York (1982)
26. Ekman, P.: Basic emotions. In: Dalgleish, T., Power, M. (eds.) Handbook of cognition and emotion, ch. 3, John Wiley & Sons, Ltd., Sussex (1999)
27. Gmytrasiewicz, P.J., Lisetti, C.L.: Emotions and personality in agent design. In: Proceedings of the First International Joint Conference on Autonomous Agents and Multiagent Systems: part 1, ACM 2002, pp. 360–361 (2002)
28. Lowe, R., Herrera, C., Morse, A., Ziemke, T.: The Embodied Dynamics of Emotion, Appraisal and Attention, Attention in Cognitive Systems. In: Theories And Systems From an Interdisciplinary Viewpoint. Springer, Heidelberg (2008)
29. Restak, R.M.: The Infant Mind. Doubleday & Company Inc., Garden City (1986)
30. Lazarus, R.S.: Emotion and adaptation. Oxford University Press, New York (1991)
31. Picard, R.W.: Affective computing, M.I.T Media Laboratory Perceptual Computing Section Technical Report No. 321
32. DMello, S., Graesser, A., Picard, R.W.: Toward an affect- sensitive autotutor. IEEE Intelligent Systems 22(4), 53–61 (2007)
33. Marsella, S., Gratch, J.: A step toward irrationality: using emotion to change belief. In: Proceedings of the First International Joint Conference on Autonomous Agents and Multiagent Systems: part 1, ACM 2002, pp. 334–341 (2002)

Generating Decision Makers' Preferences, from their Goals, Constraints, Priorities and Emotions

Majed Al-Shawa

Electrical and Computer Engineering, University of Waterloo,
200 University Avenue West, Waterloo, Ontario, Canada N2L 3G1
mmalshawa@uwaterloo.ca

Abstract. The Constrained Rationality framework, a formal qualitative goals and constraints reasoning framework for single and multi agents to analyze and rationalize about strategic decisions/conflicts, is extended in this paper by adding: 1) modeling mechanisms to include the agent's priorities, emotions and attitudes within the context of the conflict; and 2) eliciting the agent's cardinal and ordinal preferences over his alternatives using the amount of achievement the strategic goals of the agent can harness from each alternative, given the collective goals, constraints, priorities, emotions and attitudes, the agent has. An illustrative example and some experimental results are given to demonstrate the effectiveness of the framework and the proposed modeling and reasoning mechanisms in the context of a strategic decision making case.

Keywords: Strategic Decision Analysis, Conflict Analysis, Decision Support, Formal Reasoning Methods, Agents Modeling and Reasoning.

1 Introduction

Strategic decision making conflicts are mostly ill-structured decision making situations, with outcomes that rely on the rich contextual knowledge that each has. Despite the fact that agents' preferences are usually not clear, or hard to validate, and that agents' options/moves are hard to completely capture in such conflicts, we find that dominant modeling and analysis tools, such as decision and game theoretic methods, assume predetermined agents' preferences, or utility functions, and predetermined set of alternatives to evaluate. This leads to a lack of applicability of such models to represent and analyze real-life strategic conflicts [1,2].

Because of the many limitation of the decision theory and game theory approaches, in general [1,2], and for agent systems [3], a new direction starts to emerge within the research community, namely within the decision analysis [1], the AI multi-agent BDI [4,5] and the software requirements engineering [6] communities: Modeling Goals and Reasoning about them. But the current frameworks lack the representation mechanisms to support modeling goals (interrelationships, constraints, prioritization, etc.), and therefore reason about them. Recently, in [7,8], we talked about the short comings of the current frameworks,

B. Hu et al. (Eds.): BI 2011, LNAI 6889, pp. 98–110, 2011.

and the need to extend them at different levels to make them well suited for multi-agent knowledge-based systems to support strategic decision making.

Constrained Rationality is a formal qualitative value-driven enterprise knowledge management modeling and analysis framework [9,8], with a robust methodological approach, that addresses such challenge by bringing back the decision and conflicts analysis to its roots: reasoning about goals and plans to achieve the strategic goals the agent has. The framework: 1) uses each agent's individual contextual knowledge about his goals and constraints to suggest the set of options the agent has; 2) takes in consideration the agent's priorities, emotions and attitudes; and 3) elicits accordingly the agent's preferences over his alternatives. The framework allows decision makers, especially at the strategic level, model their goals, model their internal and external constraints (realities which limit or open opportunities to their goals - from this the name of the framework came), model the interrelations among these goals and constraints and how they affect each other, and then finally evaluate their plans based on the collective overall goals-constraints model they have.

In this paper, we extend our previous work, the viewpoint-based value-driven conceptual modeling [7] and the Constrained Rationality's basic goal and constraint modeling and reasoning [9], and propose new modeling facilities to capture the agent's priorities (importance), emotions (likeness) and attitudes (towards acting rationally or emotionally); and propose a method to generate the agent's cardinal and ordinal preferences over his alternatives (options or plans). First, Section 2 provides an overview of the agent's Goal and Constraints Model (GCM) and its constructs (goal and constraint nodes and interrelationships). Section 3 discusses how the agent's priorities, emotions and attitudes will be modeled; and Section 4 shows how the cardinal and ordinal preferences of an agent, over his alternatives, will be calculated and represented. Finally, Section 5 and 6 conclude with an illustrative application of the concepts and methods proposed in this paper, preliminary experimental results, and some discussion around limitations and future work.

2 Agent's Goals and Constraints Model

In [9], we presented the Goals and Constraints Model (GCM), a sub-model of each agent's Viewpoint model. GCM captures the agent's goals and constraints with regard to the specific situation/conflict his viewpoint model is concerned with. *GCM* is a graph like structure $\langle \mathcal{G}, \mathcal{C}, \mathcal{R} \rangle$ where $\mathcal{G}$ is a set of goal nodes, $\mathcal{C}$ is a set of constraint nodes, and $\mathcal{R}$ is a set of interrelationships over the nodes of $\mathcal{G}$ and $\mathcal{C}$. Figure 1 shows an illustration of a simple one goals-tree GCM model.

The goal nodes in GCM represent the motivation the agent has. Goal nodes are modeled by first inserting the ultimate strategic goals the agent has. Then go through a reduction process, by using reduction relations, refining these big goals, called *Desires*, to a set of smaller Desires, and so on until a set of primitive very-refined goals, called *Intentions*, are produced. Intentions are goals that could be operationalized by means of Plans, whilst Desires are goals that could be operationalized by other Desires or Intentions. The end result of the goals reduction process is a goal tree, or a set of goal trees, where ultimate strategic Desires form the roots of these trees, and with Intentions at the bottom of each goal tree. In addition, *Constraint* nodes form an an important component of each GCM. Constraints represent not only limitations on goals, i.e. affecting goals negatively, but also they could represent opportunities. Representing constraints as nodes, instead of variables within goal nodes, allow for complex and realistic constraint representation, as discussed in [7,8]. We discussed there also how goal nodes are interconnected through a set of goal-to-goal (G-G) reduction and lateral relations, and constraint nodes affect goal nodes through a set lateral constraint-to-goal (C-G) relations.

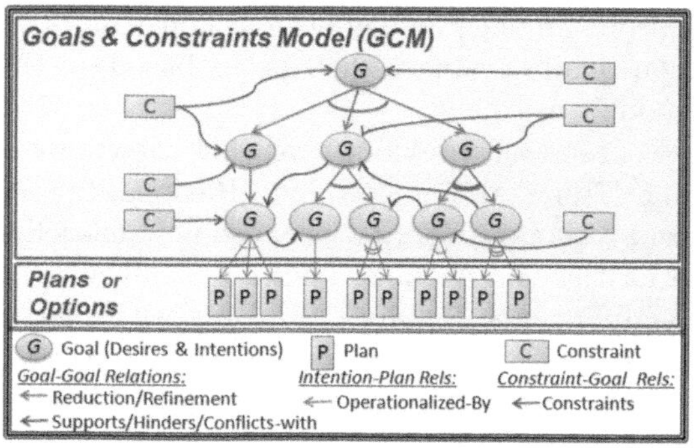

Fig. 1. Goals & Constraints Model (GCM), with simple one goals-tree

Each goal node $G \in \mathcal{G}$ has three value properties, as discussed in [9]. First, *Goal Achievement* provides a measure of the achievement level of G, and denoted as $Achv(G)$. Goals' achievement levels propagates up the goals reduction tree from the intentions at the bottom (based on results from the plans attached to those intentions) and up the goals tree until a value is assigned to the achievement level of the goal, or through the G-G lateral relations. Second, *Goal Prevention* describes the hindering (negative) effect that other goal's achievement has on G, and denoted as $Prvn(G)$. The Prevention property is especially important to track conflicting/hindering effect that may be hidden otherwise (if we have only achievement level indicators for goals). Third, *Goal Operationalization* describes the operationalization level of G, and denoted as $Opr(G)$. This property will state whether the agent has committed itself to a set of plans that will ensure a degree of operationalization for the goal, or not. Higher goals in the trees have operationalization levels that reflect the degree of operationalization that is provided to each by the lower level goals, mainly the Intentions. It is important to track Operationalization, separate from Achievement, because the maximum level of achievability possible for any goal depends on the level of operationalization the agent commits to it. For each constraint node $C \in \mathcal{C}$, there are two value properties: First, *Constraint Achievement* value attached to C to reflect the true reality/strength of the constraint C as imposed by the enforcer, or as believed to be enforced/exist, and denoted as $Achv(C)$. Second, *Constraint Prevention* value attached to C to reflect the prevention the constraint suffers from, stopping it fully or partially from having its effect on the goals it affects, and denoted as $Prvn(C)$.

For the purpose of the Constraint Rationality's qualitative reasoning framework [9,8], let us consider a limited number of satisfaction levels (instead of considering all the levels between 0-100%) for these value properties' variables. And let these levels be defined as fuzzy sets, each is given a name which represent a meaningful linguistic label such as Full or Some. Each fuzzy sets to be defined by a fuzzy membership function mapping the actual satisfaction level of the property (0-100%) to a set membership degree $[0, 1]$. While the fuzzy domain of any value property's satisfaction-levels can be divided into any number of fuzzy sets, as deemed beneficial to the framework user, we introduce a simple but sufficient scheme to divide the fuzzy satisfaction level domain of each value property to seven sets: *Full*, *Big*, *Much*, *Moderate*, *Some*, *Little*, and *None*. These fuzzy sets cover all the value properties (Operationalization, Achievement or Prevention) for goals/constraints, as shown in Figure 2. The figure shows the membership functions to be trapezoidal in shape, for simplicity only (not as a restriction). In practice, the fuzzy sets should be defined as per the user needs.

Now, let us introduce $\mathcal{L}$ as a set of labels. $\mathcal{L}$'s elements match in number and names the fuzzy sets chosen to divide the satisfaction levels of the operationalization, achievement, and prevention value properties. In our case, $\mathcal{L} = \{Full, Big, Much, Moderate, Some, Little, None\} = \{F, B, M, Mo, S, L, N\}$. And let $F>B>M>Mo>S>L>N$, matching the order of the fuzzy sets coverage over the satisfaction levels domain, with the meaning that the *Full* label represents a higher satisfaction level than *Big*, and so on. Let the *Achievement* value property of a goal G_i is represented as $Achv(G_i) = L_{achv}$, where $L_{achv} \in \mathcal{L}$, and L_{achv} is a label that matches the name of the fuzzy set which the achievement level of G_i has the highest membership of. The same is assumed for both $Opr(G_i)$ and $Prvn(G_i)$. We also use the proposition $Null$ to represent the Null trivially true statement that the status of the satisfaction level of the value property for a goal/constraint is unknown or negative. We also add the $Null$ label to $\mathcal{L}$, making $\mathcal{L} = \{F, B, M, Mo, S, L, N, Null\}$, where $F>B>M>Mo>S>L>N>Null$.

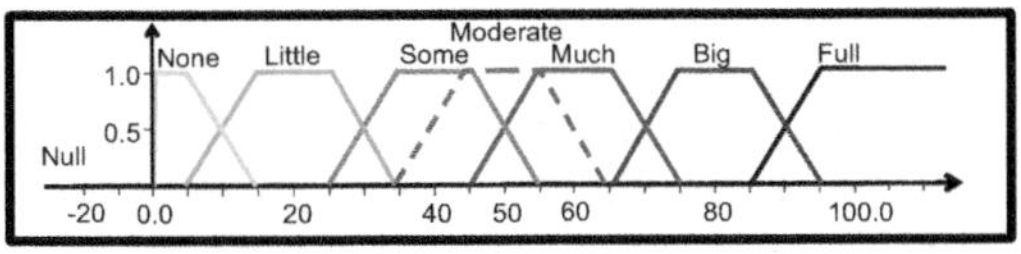

Fig. 2. Fuzzy Sets dividing the satisfaction levels of the goals' value properties

In [9,8], we proposed a comprehensive, but flexible and extendable, set of G-G and C-G interrelationships that includes: 1) Goal Reduction/Refinement *AND/OR* Relations responsible for generating the tree like structures found in goal-tree/s; and 2) Goal-Goal Lateral Relations, to represent: *Supports*,

Hinders and *Conflicts-with* among goal nodes in GCMs. The G-G lateral relations are named based on whether the cause/effect is positive (achievement or operationalization) or negative (prevention) of the goal at that end of the relation. For example, if G_1 is achieved fully and this will cause G to be fully achieved as well, then we call the relation: a "++" relation; and if having G_1 fully achieve will cause G to be fully prevented, then the relation is called: a "+−" relation. Each G-G lateral relation has a *Modifier*. For example, the lateral relation of "+(*Some*+)" represents a relation in which a full or partial satisfaction of the source node will make the satisfaction level of the target node be partial. This relation's *Modifier* is "*Some*". The relation's *Modifier* M is a label that belongs to the same set of labels $\mathcal{L}$ used for value properties, i.e. $M \in \mathcal{L}$. Note that an assignment of $Null$ as a label to a relation's *Modifier* makes the relation has no effect on the target node, i.e. as if the relation does not exist.

Constraints are connected to goal nodes through Constraint-Goal (C-G) Lateral Relations, which are similar to the G-G Lateral ones, with similar propagation rules for value labels, with two exception: constraints do not have operationalization value and do not affect the target goal-nodes' operationalization; and constraints set the upper and lower limits of the $Achv(G_i)$ not actual achievement level s for G_i to harness through the C-G lateral relations.

Table 1. The Propagation Rules of Value Labels using Goal-to-Goal Relations

G-G AND Reduction Relations	*G-G OR Reduction Relations:*
$(G_1, G_2) \xrightarrow{and} G$:	$(G_1, G_2) \xrightarrow{or} G$:
$Opr(G) = \min\{Opr(G_1), Opr(G_2)\}$ (1)	$Opr(G) = \max\{Opr(G_1), Opr(G_2)\}$ (4)
$Achv(G) = \min\{Achv(G_1), Achv(G_2)\}$ (2)	$Achv(G) = \max\{Achv(G_1), Achv(G_2)\}$ (5)
$Prvn(G) = \max\{Prvn(G_1), Prvn(G_2)\}$ (3)	$Prvn(G) = \min\{Prvn(G_1), Prvn(G_2)\}$ (6)
G-G Symmetric Consistent Lateral Rels	*G-G Symmetric Conflicting Lateral Rels:*
$G_1 \xrightarrow{(M=)} G$:	$G_1 \xrightarrow{(M\times)} G$:
$Opr(G) = \min\{Opr(G_1), M\}$ (7)	$Opr(G) = Null$ (10)
$Achv(G) = \min\{Achv(G_1), M\}$ (8)	$Achv(G) = \min\{Prvn(G_1), M\}$ (11)
$Prvn(G) = \min\{Prvn(G_1), M\}$ (9)	$Prvn(G) = \min\{Achv(G_1), M\}$ (12)
G-G Asymmetric Consistent Lateral Rels:	*G-G Asymmetric Conflicting Lateral Rels:*
$G_1 \xrightarrow{+(M+)} G$:	$G_1 \xrightarrow{+(M-)} G$:
$Opr(G) = \min\{Opr(G_1), M\}$ (13)	$Opr(G) = Achv(G) = Null$ (18)
$Achv(G) = \min\{Achv(G_1), M\}$ (14)	$Prvn(G) = \min\{Achv(G_1), M\}$ (19)
$Prvn(G) = Null$ (15)	
$G_1 \xrightarrow{-(M-)} G$:	$G_1 \xrightarrow{-(M+)} G$:
$Opr(G) = Achv(G) = Null$ (16)	$Achv(G) = \min\{Prvn(G_1), M\}$ (20)
$Prvn(G) = \min\{Prvn(G_1), M\}$ (17)	$Prvn(G) = Opr(G) = Null$ (21)

In [9,8] a complete set of propagation rules for the goals' fuzzy value property labels, to propagate through the G-G relations (reduction and lateral) and C-G lateral relations, was proposed. We list here the G-G relations' propagation rules, and leave out the C-G ones (because of the space constraint and their similarity to the G-G lateral ones –with minor differences–, [8] lists them all). The final values labels of G_i at any time t are concluded by the following propagation rules (an algorithm to calculate the final value property labels for each G_i the agent has in his GCM model is provided in [9,8]):

$$Opr(G_i) = \left(Opr(G_i) \vee \bigvee_{r_j \in \mathcal{R}_{G-G_i}} Opr_{r_j}(G_i) \right) \tag{22}$$

$$Achv(G_i) = \left(Achv(G_i) \vee \bigvee_{r_j \in \mathcal{R}_{G-G_i}} Achv_{r_j}(G_i) \right) \wedge \left(\bigwedge_{r_k \in \mathcal{R}_{C-G_i}} Achv_{r_k}(G_i) \right) \tag{23}$$

$$Prvn(G_i) = \left(Prvn(G_i) \wedge \bigwedge_{r_j \in \mathcal{R}_{G-G_i}} Prvn_{r_j}(G_i) \right) \vee \left(\bigvee_{r_k \in \mathcal{R}_{C-G_i}} Prvn_{r_k}(G_i) \right) \tag{24}$$

3 Modeling Agent's Priorities, Emotions and Attitudes

3.1 Identifying the Agent's Strategic Goals and Alternatives

Let, decision maker $DM_i \in \mathcal{DM}$, at time t of the decision making situation, has a set of strategic goals $\mathcal{SG}_{DM_i,t}$, and $\mathcal{SG}_{DM_i,t} \subseteq \mathcal{G}_{DM_i,t}$, where $\mathcal{G}_{DM_i,t}$ is the set of all goals part of DM_i's GCM model $GCM\_Graph_{DM_i,t}\ \langle \mathcal{G}_{DM_i,t}, \mathcal{C}_{DM_i,t}, \mathcal{R}_{DM_i,t} \rangle$. What differentiate the goals in $\mathcal{SG}_{DM_i,t}$ from the rest of goals in $\mathcal{G}_{DM_i,t}$ is that the strategic goals are the aims, or the ends, DM_i is ultimately looking to achieve while the rest of the goals form the means. Also, the strategic goals in $\mathcal{SG}_{DM_i,t}$ are usually, but not necessarily, the top/root goals of the GCM's goal-trees.

Let $\mathcal{A}_{DM_i,t}$ be the set of alternatives (plans, options, moves) that the decision maker $DM_i \in \mathcal{DM}$ is considering at time t in his decision making situation. Each alternative $A \in \mathcal{A}_{DM_i,t}$ produces certain level of operationalization, achievement or prevention to each strategic goal $SG \in \mathcal{SG}_{DM_i,t}$, by propagating value labels for such value properties through the goal-trees and up to the strategic goals.

3.2 Modeling Final Achievement Levels of Agent's Strategic Goals

The Constrained Rationality forward propagation reasoning algorithm which uses the above propagation rules to finalize the value labels for each goal node in GCM (proposed in [9,8]) purposely keeps track of the achievement, operationalization and prevention values of the goal nodes, within the agent's GCM model, all separate from each other. The algorithm will not try to consolidate the value properties for each goal node to a single achievement value for the node. The idea is to highlight these values, and allow the DM, or the analyst modeling the decision making situation, to track what caused these values for each goal node in the model. But for the purpose of evaluating each alternative, a consolidated achievement level value property is adopted to measure how good the alternative in helping the agent getting closer to his ultimate goals.

For a strategic goal SG, its Final Achievement value property will be denoted as $FAchv(SG)$. Understandably, $FAchv(SG)$ should receive a value that represent the result of subtracting its final prevention value ($Prvn(SG)$) from its final achievement one ($Achv(SG)$), taking in consideration the achievement upper limit that is set by both the constraints targeting SG and the level of operationalization SG managed to gain from the alternative the agent adopts. At time t of the decision making situation and for a strategic goal $SG \in \mathcal{SG}_{DM_i,t}$, let the three final value labels that value propagation algorithm produces for SG's operationalization, achievement and prevention are denoted as $Opr(SG)$, $Achv(SG)$ and $Prvn(SG)$, respectively. The *Final Achievement* value of SG, denoted as $FAchv(SG)$, is defined as follows:

$$FAchv(SG)=\begin{cases} Achv(SG)\ominus Prvn(SG) & \text{if } Achv(SG)\geq Opr(SG) \\ Opr(SG)\ominus Prvn(SG) & \text{if } Achv(SG)<Opr(SG). \end{cases} \tag{25}$$

Let the fuzzy linguistic value label given to $FAchv(SG)$ based on the definition above is denoted as L_{FAchv} and is assigned by applying the "$\ominus$" operator's table shown in Figure 3b (implemented as reasoning rules). In other words, $FAchv(SG)=L_{FAchv}$, where $L_{FAchv}\in\mathcal{L}=\{$*Full, Big, Much, Moderate, Some, Little, None, -Little, -Some, -Moderate, -Much, -Big, -Full, Null*$\}$ $= \{F,B,M,Mo,S,L,N,-L,-S,-Mo,-M,-B,-F,Null\}$. And, with the complete order of $F>B>M>Mo>L>N>-L>-S>-Mo>-M>-B>-F>Null$, where the labels range from representing *Full* goal achievement to *Full* goal prevention, covering the Final Achievement satisfaction level of 100% to -100% or -1 to 1, and that the *Null* label represents an unknown achievement/prevention of the goal. The fuzzy membership functions defining these linguistic value labels are given in Figure 3a. The number of fuzzy sets and their membership functions (shown in the figure to be trapezoidal in shape) should be defined based on the user needs and requirements, as discussed in [9,8].

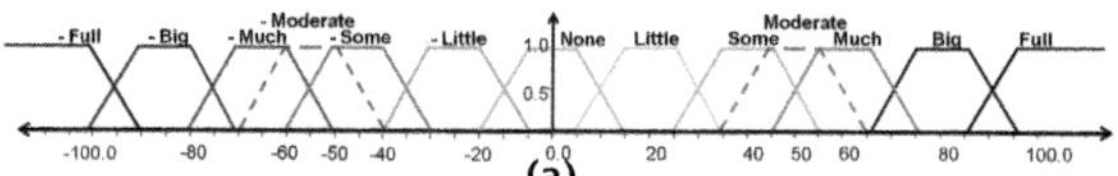

(a)

⊖	N	L	S	Mo	M	B	F	Null
N	N	-L	-S	-Mo	-M	-B	-F	Null
L	L	N	-L	-S	-S	-M	-B	Null
S	S	L	N	-L	-L	-S	-M	Null
Mo	Mo	S	L	N	-L	-S	-Mo	Null
M	M	S	L	L	N	-L	-S	Null
B	B	M	S	S	L	N	-L	Null
F	F	B	M	Mo	S	L	N	Null
Null	Null	Null	Null	Null	Null	Null	Null	Null

(b)

Fig. 3. (a) fuzzy sets dividing the satisfaction levels of $FAchv$ value property; and (b) definition of $\ominus$ showing the resultant linguistic value label from the operation

3.3 Modeling the Strategic Importance of Agent's Goals

To model the priorities a DM might give to his strategic goals, we introduce here the *Strategic Importance* value property. A value property that will be attached to each strategic goal node, the DM has, and given a fuzzy linguistic value label that represents qualitatively the importance/priority given to this strategic goal. For $DM_i \in \mathcal{DM}$, and at time t of the decision making situation, let the *Strategic Importance* value property for a strategic goal $SG \in \mathcal{SG}_{DM_i,t}$ be denoted as $SImprt(SG)$. And, let $SImprt(SG_i) = L_{SImprt}$, where L_{SImprt} is a fuzzy linguistic value label that represents the name of the fuzzy set which the strategic

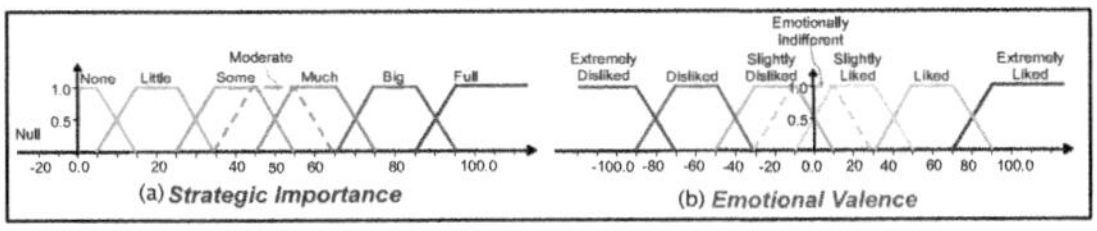

Fig. 4. The membership functions of the fuzzy sets dividing: (a) the importance levels of $SImprt(G)$; and (b) the emotionally likeness/dislike levels of $EVlnc(G)$

importance of SG, as assigned to it by DM_i, has the highest membership of. Let us assume $L_{SImprt} \in \mathcal{L}$, where $\mathcal{L}$ is shown in Figure 4a and the same value labels set used before with the same fuzzy membership functions –shown in Figure 2. In practice, the fuzzy sets (number and functions) should be defined as per the user needs. the total of all strategic importance values given to all goals do not have to add up to be 1, or *Full*, as other frameworks demand (e.g. priorities in AHP must add up to 1 [10]).

3.4 Modeling Agent's Emotional Likes and Dislikes

Following the steps of many researchers who introduced emotions into cognitive models by adding valences or affective tags (e.g [11]), we propose here to represent the effect of emotions on concepts in our models by adding emotional valences. These numerical valences can indicate likability, desirability, or other positive or negative attitudes towards the concept by the agent. [11] discussed experimental evidence that shows evaluation on the good/bad (positive/negative) dimension is a ubiquitous component of human thinking. But, assigning precise numeric value for emotional valence is not practical, or even real. In this paper, we propose to attach an *Emotional Valence* value property, to each strategic goal the agent has. Each assigned a qualitative linguistic value label based on fuzzy membership functions. This value property will capture a different, but real, importance level than the importance level given by the Strategic-Importance.

For $DM_i \in \mathcal{DM}$, and at time t of the decision making situation, let the *Emotional Valence* value property for a strategic goal $SG \in \mathcal{SG}_{DM_i,t}$ be denoted as $EVlnc(SG)$. And, let $EVlnc(SG) = L_{EVlnc}$, where L_{EVlnc} is a fuzzy linguistic value label that represents the name of the fuzzy set which the degree of like or dislike, that DM_i feels toward working and achieving SG, has the highest membership of. And, let $L_{EVlnc} \in \mathcal{L}_{\mathcal{EV}} = \{$*ExtremelyLiked*, *Liked*, *SlightlyLiked*, *EmotionallyIndifferent*, *SlightlyDisliked*, *Disliked*, *ExtremelyDisliked*, *Null*$\} = \{EL, L, SL, EI, SD, D, ED, Null\}$, with the complete order of $EL > L > SL > EI > SD > D > ED > Null$. The suggested membership functions for the fuzzy linguistic labels in $\mathcal{L}_{\mathcal{EV}}$ are given in Figure 4b. The actual fuzzy sets should be defined as per the user needs. Similarly here, the total of all emotional valence values given to an agent's strategic goals do not have to add up to 1, or 100%.

3.5 Modeling Agent's Overall Rationality or Emotionality Attitudes

To account for situations in which a decision maker decides to act completely rational even when having strong emotional likes/dislikes (i.e. act emotionless or in an extremely disciplined manner) or act completely emotional (i.e. give no regard to the strategic importance of goals), we offer two weighting factors: the *Rationality Factor* and *Emotionality Factor*. The two factors are intended to show the overall agent's attitude toward acting rationally and/or emotionally in general, and at times when there are conflicts among the strategic order versus the emotional order of goals. For $DM_i \in \mathcal{DM}$, and at time t of the decision making situation, let the *Rationality Factor* of DM_i be denoted as RF_{DM_i}, and let his *Emotionality Factor* be denoted as EF_{DM_i}. And, let $RF_{DM_i} = L_{RF}$ and $EF_{DM_i} = L_{EF}$, where L_{RF} and L_{EF} are fuzzy linguistic value labels that represent the name of the fuzzy sets which the rationality weighting factor and the emotionality weighting factor, respectively (that DM_i holds or expected to hold at time t of the decision making situation) have the highest memberships of. Let $L_{RF} \in \mathcal{L}$ and $L_{EF} \in \mathcal{L}$, where $\mathcal{L}$, here too, is the same value labels set used before (Figure 2). We will show in the next subsection, how these factors will be used. We will also show the flexibility this representation scheme provide to the modeling of decision makers' preferences.

4 Eliciting Agents' Preferences over Alternatives

Now, for the purpose of calculating the effectiveness of adopting an alternative over another, for DM_i, we calculate how much each alternative contributes to the final achievement of the strategic goals in $\mathcal{SG}_{DM_i}$. We introduce here the *Weighted Final Achievement* value property. A property that will be attached to each of strategic goals in $\mathcal{SG}_{DM_i}$, and provide a weight-adjusted Final Achievement value based on the importance given to the strategic goal, the emotional valence given to the goal, in addition to DM_i's overall attitudes towards rationality and emotionality. This value property will be represented as a numerical value, not a qualitative fuzzy linguistic value label, that captures the relationship between value properties all of which are represented by fuzzy linguistic value labels. Therefore, we adopt the simple but effective Centroid defuzzification scheme. For DM_i, at time t, let the Weighted Final Achievement of a strategic goal $SG \in \mathcal{SG}_{DM_i}$, as a result of having alternative $A \in \mathcal{A}$ been adopted, to be denoted as $WFAchv(SG, DM_i, A, t)$, and calculated algebraically as follows:

$$WFAchv(SG, DM_i, A, t) = \begin{cases} W(SG, DM_i, t) \cdot FAchv(SG, A, t) & \text{if } W(SG, DM_i, t) \geq 0 \\ 0 & \text{if } W(SG, DM_i, t) < 0. \end{cases} \quad (26)$$

where:

$$W(SG, DM_i, t) = (RF^*_{DM_i} \cdot SImprt^*(SG)) + (EF^*_{DM_i} \cdot EVlnc^*(SG)) \quad (27)$$

where $SImprt^*(SG)$, $EVlnc^*(SG)$, $RF^*_{DM_i}$ and $EF^*_{DM_i}$ represent the defuzzified values of their respective fuzzy values, and where none of the original fuzzy values is *Null*, and all reflect the state of mind and beliefs of DM_i at time t

$$FAchv(SG, A, t) = [FAchv^*(SG)]_{\text{if } A \text{ was fully applied to GCM at } t-1} \quad (28)$$

where $FAchv^*(SG)$ represents the defuzzified values of $FAchv(SG)$, and $FAchv(SG) \neq Null$; and where "A was fully applied at time $t-1$" means that the intention to apply A was fully achieved, i.e. $Achv(A) = F$, at $t-1$

The way the weighting factor $W(SG, DM_i, t)$ is calculated suggests that if DM_i has a $RF_{DM_i} = F$ and $EF_{DM_i} = N$ (i.e. DM_i will act completely rational with no regard to his emotions); and if DM_i has a $RF_{DM_i} = N$ and $EF_{DM_i} = F$ (i.e. DM_i will act completely emotional with no regard to his goals importance). But, the weighted final achievement value, $WFAchv(SG, DM_i, A, t)$ calculated in Equation 26, shows only the affect of adopting an alternative A to one specific strategic goal SG that DM_i has. For a DM_i, at time t, let the effect of the full application of alternative $A \in \mathcal{A}$ into DM_i's strategic goals in the none-empty $\mathcal{SG}_{DM_i}$ collectively be represented by a Total Weighted Final Achievement value property; and let this value property be denoted as $TWFAchv(DM_i, A, t)$, and calculated algebraically as follows:

$$TWFAchv(DM_i, A, t) = \frac{1}{|\mathcal{SG}_{DM_i}|} \sum_{SG \in \mathcal{SG}_{DM_i}} WFAchv(SG, DM_i, A, t) \tag{29}$$

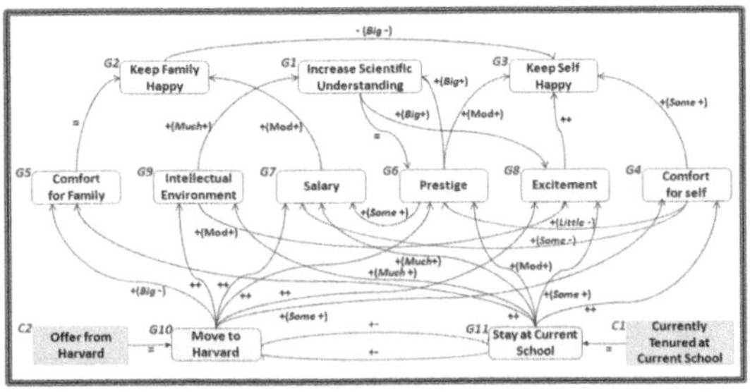

Fig. 5. Goal & Constraints Model of the Howard's Dilemma example

Howard at his Current School, and has no offer from Harvard

	Initial		run 1		run 2		run 3		run 4		run 5	
	Achv	Prvn	Achv	Prvn	Achv	Prvn	Achv	Prvn	Achv	Prvn	Achv	Prvn
G1					M		M		M		M	
G2					F		F		F		F	
G3					O		O		M		M	
G4			F		F		F		F		F	
G5			F		F		F		F		F	
G6			O		O	L	M	L	M	L	M	L
G7			M		M	S	M	S	M	S	M	S
G8			S		O		M		M		M	
G9			M		M		M		M		M	
G10				F		F		F		F		F
G11	F		F		F		F		F		F	
C1	F											
C2		F										

Howard, if he accepts Harvard's offer

	Initial		run 1		run 2		run 3		run 4	
	Achv	Prvn	Achv	Prvn	Achv	Prvn	Achv	Prvn	Achv	Prvn
G1					B		B		B	
G2					O	B	O	B	O	B
G3					F		F	B	F	B
G4			S		S		S		S	
G5				B		B		B		B
G6			F		F	L	F	L	F	L
G7			F		F	S	F	S	F	S
G8			F		F		F		F	
G9			F		F		F		F	
G10	F		F		F		F		F	
G11				F		F		F		F
C1		F								
C2	F									

Labels: Full "F" | Big "B" | Much "M" | Moderate "O" | Some "S" | Little "L" | None "N" | Null " "

Fig. 6. Algorithm Runs for the Howard Dilemma Example

For a single DM_i, in a single-agent decision making situation, at time t, let the *Cardinal Preference* that DM_i has over alternative $A \in \mathcal{A}_{DM_i}$ be represented as a *Weighted Payoff* value property attached to A, and be denoted as $WP(A, DM_i, t)$. Let $WP(A, DM_i, t) = TWFAchv(DM_i, A, t)$. Based on the cardinal preferences, or weighted payoffs, calculated for DM_i over each of his alternatives $A \in \mathcal{A}_{DM_i}$, there will be a *Preference Vector*, denoted as $Pref(DM_i, \mathcal{A}_{DM_i})$, showing the order of the alternatives in $\mathcal{A}_{DM_i}$ from the *most preferred* to the *least preferred*. The preference order of a specific alternative $A \in \mathcal{A}_{DM_i}$, to DM_i

at time t, is given as an *Ordinal Preference* value property attached to A, and is denoted by $OP(A, DM_i, t)$. Let $OP(A, DM_i, t)$ be given an integer number that reflects A's position in DM_i's preference vector $Pref(DM_i, \mathcal{A}_{DM_i})$ at t.

5 Example: Howard's Personal Dilemma

An interesting real-life "personal dilemma" was presented by [12]. As per the dilemma, Howard, a professor in a good university, receives an offer to move to Harvard. Howard has many personal goals that range from research-related to family-related goals. The goals conflict with each other. Satisfaction of some will lead to dissatisfaction of others. Figure 5 shows Howard Dilemma modeled using the Constrained Rationality framework. Howard goals' final value labels, as finalized by the reasoning algorithm discussed earlier are shown in Figure 6, for the two scenarios: 1) Howard continues at current school ($G11$) with no offer received from Harvard ($C1$); and 2) Howard activates the "move to Harvard" intention ($G10$) after the "Offer from Harvard" constraint ($C2$) changed from

(a) Achv & Prvn values for Goals within the decision making situation

Strategic Goals of DMs	SGs:	Howard SGHoward SGH 1	SGH 2	SGH 3
Alternative AH 0	Achv(SGk)	S	M	Mo
Status Quo (Howard	Prvn(SGk)	N	N	N
Stays at Current School)	FAchv(SGk)	S	M	Mo
{ Achv(AH 0)=F }	FAchv*(SGk)	0.40	0.60	0.50
Alternative AH 1	Achv(SGk)	B	M	F
Howard Moves	Prvn(SGk)	N	L	B
to Harvard	FAchv(SGk)	B	S	L
{ Achv(AH 1)=F }	FAchv*(SGk)	0.80	0.40	0.20

(b)

	Strategic Goals of DMs	SGs:	decision making situation # 1 Howard SGHoward SGH 1	SGH 2	SGH 3	decision making situation # 2 Howard SGHoward SGH 1	SGH 2	SGH 3
	Strategic Importance	SImprt(SGi)	F	B	Mo	F	B	Mo
	Emotional Valence	EVlnc(SGi)	L	EL	SL	El	EL	SL
Extremely Rational; Rationality Factor = 1.0; Emotionality Factor = 0.0	Alternative AH 0	FAchv(SGk, AH 0,t)	0.40	0.60	0.50	0.40	0.60	0.50
		W(SGk,H,t)	1.00	0.80	0.50	1.00	0.80	0.50
	Status Quo (Howard Stays at Current School)	WFAchv(SGk,H,AH 0,t)	0.40	0.48	0.25	0.40	0.48	0.25
		WP(AH 0, H, t)		0.38			0.38	
	{ Achv(AH 0)=F }	OP(AH 0, H, t)		2 (Worst)			2 (Worst)	
	Alternative AH 1	FAchv(SGk, AH 1,t)	0.80	0.40	0.20	0.80	0.40	0.20
		W(SGk,H,t)	1.00	0.80	0.50	1.00	0.80	0.50
	Howard Moves to Harvard	WFAchv(SGk,H,AH 1,t)	0.80	0.32	0.10	0.80	0.32	0.10
		WP(AH 1, H, t)		0.41			0.41	
	{ Achv(AH 1)=F }	OP(AH 1, H, t)		1 (Best)			1 (Best)	
Extremely Emotional; Rationality Factor = 0.0; Emotionality Factor = 1.0	Alternative AH 0	FAchv(SGk, AH 0,t)	0.40	0.60	0.50	0.40	0.60	0.50
		W(SGk,H,t)	0.60	1.00	0.20	0.00	1.00	0.20
	Status Quo (Howard Stays at Current School)	WFAchv(SGk,H,AH 0,t)	0.24	0.60	0.10	0.00	0.60	0.10
		WP(AH 0, H, t)		0.31			0.23	
	{ Achv(AH 0)=F }	OP(AH 0, H, t)		Same			1 (Best)	
	Alternative AH 1	FAchv(SGk, AH 1,t)	0.80	0.40	0.20	0.80	0.40	0.20
		W(SGk,H,t)	0.60	1.00	0.20	0.00	1.00	0.20
	Howard Moves to Harvard	WFAchv(SGk,H,AH 1,t)	0.48	0.40	0.04	0.00	0.40	0.04
		WP(AH 1, H, t)		0.31			0.15	
	{ Achv(AH 1)=F }	OP(AH 1, H, t)		Same			2 (Worst)	
Fully Rational & Emotions are Considered Fully; Rationality Factor = 1.0; Emotionality Factor = 1.0	Alternative AH 0	FAchv(SGk, AH 0,t)	0.40	0.60	0.50	0.40	0.60	0.50
		W(SGk,H,t)	1.60	1.80	0.70	1.00	1.80	0.70
	Status Quo (Howard Stays at Current School)	WFAchv(SGk,H,AH 0,t)	0.64	1.08	0.35	0.40	1.08	0.35
		WP(AH 0, H, t)		0.69			0.61	
	{ Achv(AH 0)=F }	OP(AH 0, H, t)		2 (Worst)			1 (Best)	
	Alternative AH 1	FAchv(SGk, AH 1,t)	0.80	0.40	0.20	0.80	0.40	0.20
		W(SGk,H,t)	1.60	1.80	0.70	1.00	1.80	0.70
	Howard Moves to Harvard	WFAchv(SGk,H,AH 1,t)	1.28	0.72	0.14	0.80	0.72	0.14
		WP(AH 1, H, t)		0.71			0.55	
	{ Achv(AH 1)=F }	OP(AH 1, H, t)		1 (Best)			2 (Worst)	
Mostly Rational & Slightly Emotional; Rationality Factor = 0.8; Emotionality Factor = 0.2	Alternative AH 0	FAchv(SGk, AH 0,t)	0.40	0.60	0.50	0.40	0.60	0.50
		W(SGk,H,t)	0.92	0.84	0.44	0.80	0.84	0.44
	Status Quo (Howard Stays at Current School)	WFAchv(SGk,H,AH 0,t)	0.37	0.50	0.22	0.32	0.50	0.22
		WP(AH 0, H, t)		0.36			0.35	
	{ Achv(AH 0)=F }	OP(AH 0, H, t)		2 (Worst)			Same	
	Alternative AH 1	FAchv(SGk, AH 1,t)	0.80	0.40	0.20	0.80	0.40	0.20
		W(SGk,H,t)	0.92	0.84	0.44	0.80	0.84	0.44
	Howard Moves to Harvard	WFAchv(SGk,H,AH 1,t)	0.74	0.34	0.09	0.64	0.34	0.09
		WP(AH 1, H, t)		0.39			0.35	
	{ Achv(AH 1)=F }	OP(AH 1, H, t)		1 (Best)			Same	

Fig. 7. (a) Value Labels of Howard's Strategic Goals; and (b) Calculating Howard's Preferences using different Rationality/Emotionality Factors, and Emotional Valences

full prevention (no offer) to full achievement (offer received). For the first scenario, the figure shows that while Howard's goal of keeping his family happy ($G2$) is fully achieved, Howard's goals of "increase scientific understanding"($G1$) and "keep self happy" ($G3$) are moderately achieved. For the second scenario, the figure shows the effect of moving to Harvard on all Howard's goals. While he managed to satisfy fully $G1$, his and his family's happiness goals received prevention. Changing some of the lateral relation types, or their modifiers, provide more insight on Howard's thinking, beliefs and values.

Now, we use the same dilemma, with Howard having the same alternatives: A_{H0}: stay at current school (shown in Figure 5 as intention node G_{11}); and A_{H1}: move to Harvard (intention node G_{10}). But, let the GCM model, presented in Figure 5 be modified to generate, for each of the alternatives, a set of different final achievement and prevention value labels for Howard's ultimate strategic goals: SG_{H1}; SG_{H2}; and SG_{H3}. And, let the final achievement and prevention labels of these strategic goals be the ones given in the table shown in Figure 7a. Final Achievement value for each goal is given as fuzzy linguistic label, and as a defuzzified real number. We analyze Howard's dilemma to generate his cardinal and ordinal preferences over his two alternatives. But, we assume different scenarios where different strategic importance, emotional valences, rationality and emotionality factor values are employed. This is done to show how the preferences change as these values change, as in the analysis results in Figure 7b.

6 Conclusion

In this paper, we extended Constrained Rationality's basic goal and constraint modeling and reasoning [9], and proposed new modeling facilities to capture agents' priorities (importance), emotions (likeness) and attitudes (towards acting rationally or emotionally); and an effective method to generate the agents' cardinal and ordinal preferences over their alternatives (options or plans), from their goals, constraints, priorities, emotions and attitudes. Preferences, that other decision and game theoretic approaches assume to be well known in advance. An illustrative application is used to demonstrate how effective and flexible the modeling and reasoning methods to represent different scenarios of a strategic personal decision making situation. As future work, we are looking to expand the representation of: priorities and emotions to cover all goals, not only strategic goals; and attitudes to include attitudes towards the alternatives not just goals.

References

1. Keeney, R.: Value-focused thinking: A path to creative decisionmaking. Harvard University Press, Cambridge (1992)
2. Raiffa, H., Richardson, J., Metcalfe, D.: Negotiation Analysis: The Science and Art of Collaborative Decision Making. Harvard University Press, Cambridge (2002)
3. Wooldridge, M.: Reasoning About Rational Agents. MIT Press, Cambridge (2000)

4. Winikoff, M., Harland, J., Padgham, L.: Linking Agent Concepts and Methodology with CAN. In: Submitted to the First International Joint Conference on Autonomous Agents and Multi-Agent Systems (2002)
5. Shaw, P.H., Bordini, R.H.: Towards Alternative Approaches to Reasoning About Goals. In: Baldoni, M., Son, T.C., van Riemsdijk, M.B., Winikoff, M. (eds.) DALT 2007. LNCS (LNAI), vol. 4897, pp. 104–121. Springer, Heidelberg (2008)
6. Dardenne, A., van Lamsweerde, A., Fickas, S.: Goal-directed Requirements Acquisition. Science of Computer Programming 20, 3–50 (1993)
7. Al-Shawa, M.: Viewpoints-based Value-Driven - Enterprise Knowledge Management (ViVD-EKM). MASc thesis, Electrical and Computer Engineering. University of Waterloo (2006)
8. Al-Shawa, M.: Constrained Rationality: Formal Value-Driven Enterprise Knowledge Management Modelling and Analysis Framework for Strategic Business, Technology and Public Policy Decision Making & Conflict Resolutio. Ph.D. dissertation, Electrical and Computer Engineering, University of Waterloo (2011)
9. Al-Shawa, M., Basir, O.: Constrained Rationality: Formal Goals-Reasoning Approach to Strategic Decision & Conflict Analysis. In: Proceedings of the 2009 IEEE International Conference on Systems, Man, and Cybernetics (2009)
10. Saaty, T.L.: The Analytic Hierarchy Process: Planning, Priority Setting, Resource Allocation. McGrawHill, New York (1980)
11. Thagard, P.: Hot Thought: Mechanisms and Applications of Emotional Cognition. The MIT Press, Cambridge (2006)
12. Thagard, P., Millgram, E.: Inference to the best plan: A coherence theory of decision. In: Ram, A., Leake, D. (eds.) Goal-Driven Learning, pp. 439–454 (1995)

Modeling and Analyzing Agents' Collective Options in Collaborative Decision Making

Majed Al-Shawa

Electrical and Computer Engineering, University of Waterloo,
200 University Avenue West, Waterloo, Ontario, Canada N2L 3G1
mmalshawa@uwaterloo.ca

Abstract. Despite the cooperation and collaboration in Multi-Agent Collaborative Decision Making Situations, such as Requirements Engineering, System Design, and Product Development, the involved agents still have to satisfy different and conflicting strategic goals and constraints (internal and external) that they have. In most cases, agents adopt an option that considers only the needs and realities of few, while ignoring or suppressing the others' needs and realities. Constrained Rationality is a formal qualitative framework, with a robust methodological approach, to model and analyze ill-structured strategic multi-agent collaborative decision making situations and conflicts. In this paper, we show how the framework is used to: 1) model the collective and individual goals, constraints and priorities of the agents; 2) analyze each of the proposed collective options; and 3) elicit the agents' collective ordinal and cardinal preferences over their options. We illustrate the framework usage and benefits by modeling and analyzing a multi-stakeholder requirements engineering collaborative decision making case.

Keywords: Collaborative Decision Making, Conceptual Decision Making Models, Decision Analysis, Multi-Agent Decision Making.

1 Introduction

Collaborative Strategic decision making situations, such as Requirements Engineering, System Design, and Product Development, are mostly ill-structured situations, with outcomes that rely on the rich contextual knowledge that each has. Despite the cooperation and collaboration among the involved agents, the agents still have to satisfy different and most likely conflicting strategic goals and constraints (internal and external) that they have. In most cases, agents adopt an option (set of requirements, design, product or plan) that considers only the needs and realities of few, while ignoring or suppressing others' needs and realities. This leaves many collaborative decision making initiatives, such as software implementation initiatives, with high ratio of failure (see the CHAOS reports by the Standish group, for example). In such initiatives, the agents' preferences are usually not clear, or hard to validate, and that agents' options/moves are hard to completely capture. Nevertheless, we find that most dominant modeling and analysis tools, such as decision and game theoretic methods, assume

B. Hu et al. (Eds.): BI 2011, LNAI 6889, pp. 111–123, 2011.

predetermined agents' preferences, or utility functions, and predetermined set of alternatives to evaluate. This leads to a lack of applicability of such methods to model and analyze real-life strategic conflicts [1,2].

Because of the many limitation of the decision theory and game theory approaches, in general [1,2], and for agent systems [3], a new direction starts to emerge within the research community, namely within the decision analysis [1], the AI multi-agent BDI [4,5] and the software requirements engineering [6] communities: Modeling Goals and Reasoning about them. But the current frameworks lack the representation mechanisms to support modeling goals (interrelationships, constraints, prioritization, etc.), and therefore reason about them. Recently, in [7,8], we talked about the short comings of the current frameworks, and the need to extend them at different levels to make them well suited for multi-agent knowledge-based systems to support strategic decision making.

Constrained Rationality is a formal qualitative value-driven enterprise knowledge management modeling and analysis framework [9,8], with a robust methodological approach, that addresses such challenge by bringing back the decision and conflicts analysis to its roots: reasoning about goals and plans to achieve the strategic goals the agents has. The framework: 1) uses the agents' individual and collective contextual knowledge about their goals and constraints to suggest set of options; 2) takes in consideration the agent's priorities; and 3) elicits accordingly the agent's preferences over their collective alternatives. The framework allows decision makers, especially at the strategic level, to model their goals, their internal and external constraints, and the interrelations among these goals and constraints and how they affect each other. It, then, allow them to evaluate their plans/options based on their collective overall goals-constraints model.

In this paper, we extend our previous work, the viewpoint-based value-driven conceptual modeling [7] and the Constrained Rationality's basic goal and constraint modeling and reasoning [9], and propose new modeling and reasoning facilities, for collaborative decision making situations, to help generate the agents' collective cardinal and ordinal preferences over their shared alternatives. First, Section 2 provides an overview of the agent's Goal and Constraints Model (GCM) and its constructs (goal and constraint nodes and interrelationships). Section 3 discusses how the agent's GCMs will be integrated, and how their priorities, over their individual strategic goals, are added and modeled. Section 4 shows how the collective cardinal and ordinal preferences of the agents, over the alternatives, will be calculated. Finally, Section 5 and 6 conclude with an illustrative application of the concepts and methods proposed in this paper, focusing primarily on the process, the decision makers will use, to model their collaborative decision making situation and evaluate their alternatives.

2 Agent's Goals and Constraints Model

The Goals and Constraints Model (GCM), presented in [9], is a sub-model of each agent's Viewpoint model. GCM captures the agent's goals and constraints with regard to the specific situation/conflict his viewpoint model is concerned with. *GCM* is a graph like structure $\langle \mathcal{G}, \mathcal{C}, \mathcal{R} \rangle$ where $\mathcal{G}$ is a set of goal nodes, $\mathcal{C}$

is a set of constraint nodes, and $\mathcal{R}$ is a set of interrelationships over the nodes of $\mathcal{G}$ and $\mathcal{C}$. Figure 1 shows an illustration of a simple one goals-tree GCM model.

Goal nodes in GCM represent the motivation the agent has, and are modeled by first inserting the ultimate strategic goals the agent has. Then go through a reduction process, by using reduction relations, refining these big goals, called *Desires*, to a set of smaller Desires, and so on until a set of primitive very-refined goals, called *Intentions*, are produced. Intentions are goals that could be operationalized by means of Plans, whilst Desires are goals that could be operationalized by other Desires or Intentions. The end result of the goals reduction process is a goal tree, or a set of goal trees, where ultimate strategic Desires form the roots of these trees, and with Intentions at the bottom of each goal tree. In addition, *Constraint* nodes form an an important component of each GCM. Constraints represent not only limitations on goals, i.e. affecting goals negatively, but also they could represent opportunities. Representing constraints as nodes, instead of variables within goal nodes, allow for complex and realistic constraint representation, as discussed in [7,8]. We discussed there also how goal nodes are interconnected through a set of goal-to-goal (G-G) reduction and lateral relations, and constraint nodes affect goal nodes through a set lateral constraint-to-goal (C-G) relations.

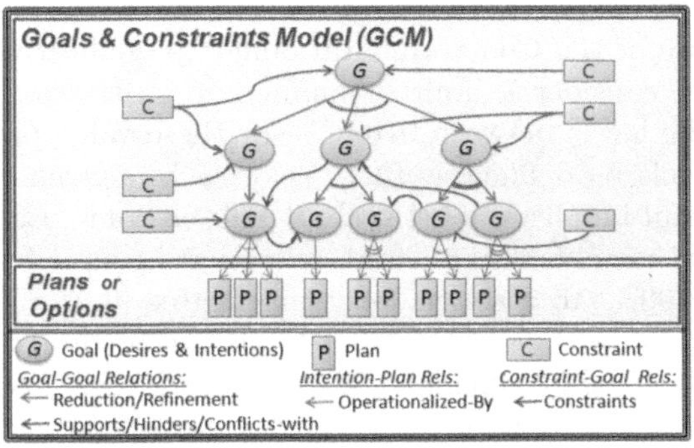

Fig. 1. Goals & Constraints Model (GCM), with simple one goals-tree

Within the GCM, each goal node $G \in \mathcal{G}$ has three value properties, as discussed in [9]. First, *Goal Achievement* provides a measure of the achievement level of G, and denoted as $Achv(G)$. Goals' achievement levels propagates up the goals reduction tree from the intentions at the bottom (based on results from the plans attached to those intentions) and up the goals tree until a value is assigned to the achievement level of the goal, or through the G-G lateral relations. Second, *Goal Prevention* describes the hindering (negative) effect that other goal's achievement has on G, and denoted as $Prvn(G)$. The Prevention property is especially important to track conflicting/hindering effect that may be hidden otherwise (if we have only achievement level indicators for goals). Third, *Goal Operationalization* describes the operationalization level of G, and denoted as $Opr(G)$. This property will state whether the agent has committed itself to a set of plans that will ensure a degree of operationalization for the goal, or not. Higher goals in the trees have operationalization levels that reflect the degree of operationalization that is provided to each by the lower level goals, mainly the Intentions. It is important to track Operationalization, separate from Achievement, because the maximum level of achievability possible for any goal depends on the level of operationalization the agent commits to it. For each constraint node $C \in \mathcal{C}$, there are two value properties: First, *Constraint Achievement* value attached to C to reflect the true reality/strength of the constraint C as imposed by the enforcer, or as believed to be enforced/exist, and denoted as $Achv(C)$. Second, *Constraint Prevention* value attached to C, denoted as $Prvn(C)$, to reflect the prevention the constraint suffers from, stopping it fully or partially from having its effect on the goals it affects.

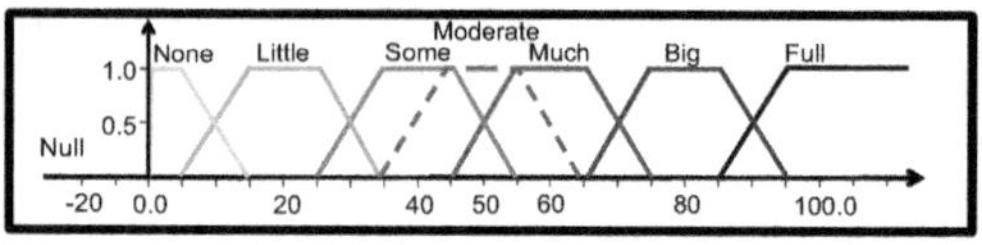

Fig. 2. Fuzzy Sets dividing the satisfaction levels domain of the different Goals' Value Properties (operationalization, achievement, and prevention)

For the purpose of the Constraint Rationality's qualitative reasoning framework [9,8], let us consider a limited number of satisfaction levels (instead of considering all the levels between 0-100%) for these value properties' variables. And let these levels be defined as fuzzy sets, each is given a name which represent a meaningful linguistic label such as Full or Some. Each fuzzy sets to be defined by a fuzzy membership function mapping the actual satisfaction level of the property (0-100%) to a set membership degree $[0, 1]$. While the fuzzy domain of any value property's satisfaction-levels can be divided into any number of fuzzy sets, as deemed beneficial to the framework user, we introduce a simple but sufficient scheme to divide the satisfaction level of each value property to seven fuzzy sets: *Full*, *Big*, *Much*, *Moderate*, *Some*, *Little*, and *None*. These fuzzy sets cover all the value properties (Operationalization, Achievement or Prevention) for goals/constraints, as shown in Figure 2. In practice, the membership functions should be defined as per the user needs.

Let us introduce $\mathcal{L}$ as a set of labels. $\mathcal{L}$'s elements match in number and names the fuzzy sets chosen to divide the satisfaction levels of the operationalization, achievement, and prevention value properties. In our case, $\mathcal{L} = \{Full, Big, Much, Moderate, Some, Little, None\} = \{F, B, M, Mo, S, L, N\}$. And let $F > B > M > Mo > S > L > N$, matching the order of the fuzzy sets coverage over the satisfaction levels domain. Let the *Achievement* value property of a goal G_i is represented as $Achv(G_i) = L_{achv}$, where $L_{achv} \in \mathcal{L}$, and L_{achv} is a label that matches the name of the fuzzy set which the achievement level of G_i has the highest membership of. The same is assumed for both $Opr(G_i)$ and $Prvn(G_i)$. We also use the proposition

$Null$ to represent the Null trivially true statement that the status of the satisfaction level of the value property for a goal/constraint is unknown or negative. We also add the $Null$ label to $\mathcal{L}$, making $\mathcal{L} = \{F, B, M, Mo, S, L, N, Null\}$, where $F>B>M>Mo>S>L>N>Null$.

A comprehensive, flexible and extendable, set of G-G and C-G interrelationships was proposed in [9,8] to include: 1) Goal Reduction/Refinement *AND/OR* Relations responsible for generating the tree like structures found in goal-tree/s; and 2) Goal-Goal Lateral Relations, to represent: *Supports*, *Hinders* and *Conflicts-with* among goal nodes in GCMs. The G-G lateral relations are named based on whether the cause/effect is positive (achievement or operationalization) or negative (prevention) on the goal at that end of the relation. For example, if G_1 is achieved fully and this will cause G to be fully achieved as well, then we call the relation: a "++" relation; and if having G_1 fully achieve will cause G to be fully prevented, then the relation is called: a "+−" relation. On the other hand, constraints are connected to goal nodes through Constraint-Goal (C-G) Lateral Relations, which are similar to the G-G Lateral ones, with similar propagation rules for value labels, with two exception: constraints do not have operationalization value and do not affect the target goal-nodes' operationalization; and constraints set the upper and lower limits of the $Achv(G_i)$ not actual achievement level s for G_i to harness through the C-G lateral relations. Each G-G, or C-G, lateral relation has a *Modifier*. For example, the lateral relation of "+(*Some*+)" represents a relation in which a full or partial satisfaction of the source node will make the satisfaction level of the target node be partial. This relation's *Modifier* is "*Some*". The relation's *Modifier* M is a label that belongs to the same set of labels $\mathcal{L}$ used for value properties, i.e. $M \in \mathcal{L}$. Note that an assignment of $Null$ as a label to a relation's *Modifier* makes the relation has no effect on the target node, i.e. as if the relation does not exist.

Table 1. The Propagation Rules of Value Labels using Goal-to-Goal Relations

G-G AND Reduction Relations	*G-G OR Reduction Relations:*
$(G_1, G_2) \xrightarrow{and} G$: $Opr(G) = \min\{Opr(G_1), Opr(G_2)\}$ (1) $Achv(G) = \min\{Achv(G_1), Achv(G_2)\}$ (2) $Prvn(G) = \max\{Prvn(G_1), Prvn(G_2)\}$ (3)	$(G_1, G_2) \xrightarrow{or} G$: $Opr(G) = \max\{Opr(G_1), Opr(G_2)\}$ (4) $Achv(G) = \max\{Achv(G_1), Achv(G_2)\}$ (5) $Prvn(G) = \min\{Prvn(G_1), Prvn(G_2)\}$ (6)
G-G Symmetric Consistent Lateral Rels	*G-G Symmetric Conflicting Lateral Rels:*
$G_1 \xrightarrow{(M=)} G$: $Opr(G) = \min\{Opr(G_1), M\}$ (7) $Achv(G) = \min\{Achv(G_1), M\}$ (8) $Prvn(G) = \min\{Prvn(G_1), M\}$ (9)	$G_1 \xrightarrow{(M\times)} G$: $Opr(G) = Null$ (10) $Achv(G) = \min\{Prvn(G_1), M\}$ (11) $Prvn(G) = \min\{Achv(G_1), M\}$ (12)
G-G Asymmetric Consistent Lateral Rels:	*G-G Asymmetric Conflicting Lateral Rels:*
$G_1 \xrightarrow{+(M+)} G$: $Opr(G) = \min\{Opr(G_1), M\}$ (13) $Achv(G) = \min\{Achv(G_1), M\}$ (14) $Prvn(G) = Null$ (15) $G_1 \xrightarrow{-(M-)} G$: $Opr(G) = Achv(G) = Null$ (16) $Prvn(G) = \min\{Prvn(G_1), M\}$ (17)	$G_1 \xrightarrow{+(M-)} G$: $Opr(G) = Achv(G) = Null$ (18) $Prvn(G) = \min\{Achv(G_1), M\}$ (19) $G_1 \xrightarrow{-(M+)} G$: $Achv(G) = \min\{Prvn(G_1), M\}$ (20) $Prvn(G) = Opr(G) = Null$ (21)

[9,8] proposed a complete set of propagation rules for the goals' fuzzy value property labels to propagate through the G-G relations (reduction and lateral) and C-G lateral relations. We list here the G-G relations' propagation rules, and leave out the C-G ones (because of the space constraint and their similarity to the G-G lateral ones –with minor differences–, [8] lists them all). The final values labels of G_i at any time t are concluded by the following propagation rules (an algorithm to calculate the final value property labels for each G_i the agent has in his GCM model is provided in [9,8]):

$$Opr(G_i) = \left(Opr(G_i) \vee \bigvee_{r_j \in \mathcal{R}_{G-G_i}} Opr_{r_j}(G_i) \right) \quad (22)$$

$$Achv(G_i) = \left(Achv(G_i) \vee \bigvee_{r_j \in \mathcal{R}_{G-G_i}} Achv_{r_j}(G_i) \right) \wedge \left(\bigwedge_{r_k \in \mathcal{R}_{C-G_i}} Achv_{r_k}(G_i) \right) \quad (23)$$

$$Prvn(G_i) = \left(Prvn(G_i) \wedge \bigwedge_{r_j \in \mathcal{R}_{G-G_i}} Prvn_{r_j}(G_i) \right) \vee \left(\bigvee_{r_k \in \mathcal{R}_{C-G_i}} Prvn_{r_k}(G_i) \right) \quad (24)$$

3 Integrating Agents' GCMs and Modeling their Strategic Priorities

3.1 Integrating the Agents' GCMs, and Identifying their Strategic Goals and Shared Alternatives

After the agents are identified, a GCM for each is built, comes the step of capturing the agents' alternatives. The alternatives, which they will be modeled as intention nodes as we said earlier, could be reduced from the refined desire-type goals at the agent's goals-tree/s, elicited directly from the agents themselves, or identified through a process of brainstorming or creative thinking. The alternatives are then connected to the goals and constraints in the agent's GCM. Then, comes the step of integrating all the agents' GCMs. This is done by capturing the the positive and negative effects that the different agents' goals and constraints have on each other's goals. The integration process is intended mainly to test and highlight the effect of each agent's GCM on the others' GCMs. Figure 3 (and the one for the example at the end of this paper –Figure 5–) provides an illustration of how an end product of this integration process looks like.

Let each $DM_i \in \mathcal{DM}$, individually at time t of the decision making situation, has a set of strategic goals $\mathcal{SG}_{DM_i,t}$, and $\mathcal{SG}_{DM_i,t} \subseteq \mathcal{G}_{DM_i,t}$, where $\mathcal{G}_{DM_i,t}$ is the set of all goals part of DM_i's GCM model $GCM\_Graph_{DM_i,t} \langle \mathcal{G}_{DM_i,t}, \mathcal{C}_{DM_i,t}, \mathcal{R}_{DM_i,t} \rangle$. What differentiate the goals in $\mathcal{SG}_{DM_i,t}$ from the rest of goals in $\mathcal{G}_{DM_i,t}$ is that the strategic goals are the aims/ends, DM_i is ultimately looking to achieve while the rest of the goals form the means. Also, the strategic goals in $\mathcal{SG}_{DM_i,t}$ are usually, but not necessarily, the top goals or root goals of the goal-trees part of the GCM. And let for each $DM_i \in \mathcal{DM}$, where $\mathcal{DM}$ is the set of all decision makers in the collaborative decision making situation, at time t, let their be a set of strategic goals $\mathcal{SG}_{DM_i}$ (chosen by DM_i). Let, the set of all strategic goals by all decision makers in $\mathcal{DM}$ is called the strategic

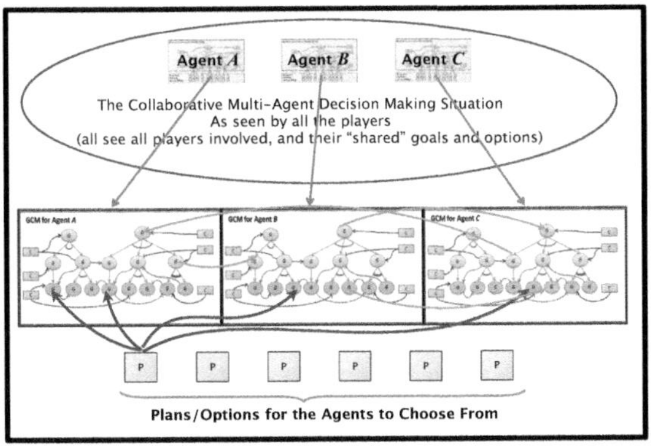

Fig. 3. Each Shared Alternative, the involved agents have in a Multi-Agent Collaborative Decision Making Situation, contribute positively/negatively to the agents' goals

goals of the collaborative decision making situation, and is denoted as $\mathcal{SG}$, where $\mathcal{SG} = \bigcup_{DM_i \in \mathcal{DM}} \mathcal{SG}_{DM_i}$. And, let the decision makers in $\mathcal{DM}$ collectively decided on a set of shared alternatives $\mathcal{A}$ to choose one from, based on how much each alternative contributes to the achievement of all strategic goals in $\mathcal{SG}$.

For each collaborative decision making situation, there are two important sets to be set up-front: 1) $\mathcal{SG}$: the set of all strategic goals, of all involved DMs; and 2) $\mathcal{A}$: the set of all shared alternatives that DMs have.

3.2 Modeling Final Achievement of Each Agent's Strategic Goals

Constrained Rationality forward propagation reasoning algorithm which uses the above propagation rules to finalize the value labels for each goal node in GCM (proposed in [9,8]) purposely keeps track of the achievement, operationalization and prevention values of the goal nodes all separate from each other. The algorithm will not try to consolidate the value properties for each goal node to a single achievement value for the node. The idea is to highlight these values, and allow the DM, or the analyst modeling the situation, to track what caused the values for each goal node in the model. But for the purpose of evaluating each alternative, a consolidated achievement level value is adopted to measure how good the alternative in helping the agent getting closer to his ultimate goals.

Understandably, the Final Achievement value property for a strategic goal SG, denoted as $FAchv(SG)$, should receive a value that represent the result of subtracting its final prevention value ($Prvn(SG)$) from its final achievement one ($Achv(SG)$), taking in consideration the achievement upper limit that is set by both the constraints targeting SG and the level of operationalization SG managed to gain from the alternative the agent adopts. At time t and for a strategic goal $SG \in \mathcal{SG}_{DM_i,t}$, let the three final value labels that value propagation algorithm produces for SG's operationalization, achievement and prevention are denoted as $Opr(SG)$, $Achv(SG)$ and $Prvn(SG)$, respectively. The *Final Achievement* value of SG, denoted as $FAchv(SG)$, is defined as follows:

$$FAchv(SG) = \begin{cases} Achv(SG) \ominus Prvn(SG) & \text{if } Achv(SG) \geq Opr(SG) \\ Opr(SG) \ominus Prvn(SG) & \text{if } Achv(SG) < Opr(SG). \end{cases} \tag{25}$$

Let the fuzzy linguistic value label given to $FAchv(SG)$ based on the definition above is denoted as L_{FAchv} and is assigned by applying the "$\ominus$" operator's table shown in Figure 4b (implemented as reasoning rules). In other words, $FAchv(SG) = L_{FAchv}$, where $L_{FAchv} \in \mathcal{L} = \{$*Full, Big, Much, Moderate, Some, Little, None, -Little, -Some, -Moderate, -Much, -Big, -Full, Null*$\} = \{F, B, M, Mo, S, L, N, -L, -S, -Mo, -M, -B, -F, Null\}$. And, with the complete order of $F > B > M > Mo > L > N > -L > -S > -Mo > -M > -B > -F > Null$, where the labels range from representing *Full* goal achievement to *Full* goal prevention, covering the Final Achievement satisfaction level of 100% to -100% and that the *Null* label represents an unknown achievement/prevention of the goal. The fuzzy membership functions defining these linguistic labels are given in Figure 4a. As discussed in [9,8], the fuzzy sets, shown in the figure to be trapezoidal in shape, should be defined based on the user needs.

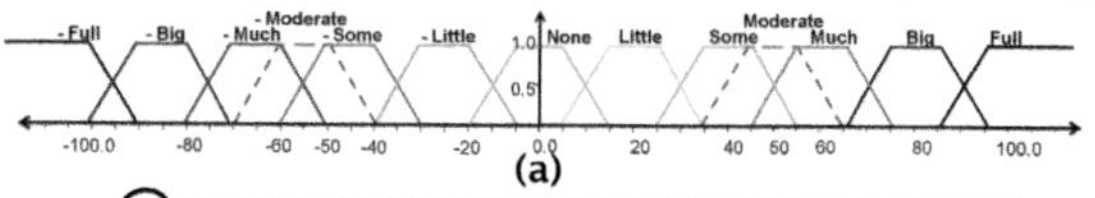

$\ominus$	N	L	S	Mo	M	B	F	Null
N	N	-L	-S	-Mo	-M	-B	-F	Null
L	L	N	-L	-S	-S	-M	-B	Null
S	S	L	N	-L	-L	-S	-M	Null
Mo	Mo	S	L	N	-L	-S	-Mo	Null
M	M	S	L	L	N	-L	-S	Null
B	B	M	S	S	L	N	-L	Null
F	F	B	M	Mo	S	L	N	Null
Null	Null	Null	Null	Null	Null	Null	Null	Null

(b)

Fig. 4. (a) fuzzy sets dividing the satisfaction levels of $FAchv$ value property; and (b) definition of $\ominus$ showing the resultant linguistic value label from the operation

3.3 Modeling Strategic Importance of Each Agent's Goals

To model the priorities a DM might give to his strategic goals, we introduce here the *Strategic Importance* value property. A value property attached to each strategic goal node and given a fuzzy linguistic value label that represents qualitatively the importance/priority of the strategic goal. For $DM_i \in \mathcal{DM}$, and at time t of the decision making situation, let the *Strategic Importance* value property for a strategic goal $SG \in \mathcal{SG}_{DM_i,t}$ be denoted as $SImprt(SG)$. And, let $SImprt(SG_i) = L_{SImprt}$, where L_{SImprt} is a fuzzy linguistic value label that represents the name of the fuzzy set which the strategic importance of SG, as assigned to it by DM_i, has the highest membership of. Let us assume $L_{SImprt} \in \mathcal{L}$, where $\mathcal{L}$ is the same value labels set used before with the same fuzzy membership functions (Figure 2). Note that the fuzzy sets should be defined based on the user needs; and the total of all goals' strategic importance values do not have to addup to be 1, or *Full*, as AHP requires [10].

4 Eliciting Agents' Collective Preferences over Shared Alternatives

For DM_i, to calculate the effectiveness of adopting an alternative over another, we calculate how much each alternative contributes to the final achievement of the strategic goals in $\mathcal{SG}_{DM_i}$. We introduce here the *Weighted Final Achievement* value property, attached to each strategic goals in $\mathcal{SG}_{DM_i}$, and provide a weight-adjusted Final Achievement value based on the importance given to the strategic goal. This value property will be represented as a numerical value, capturing the relationship between value properties represented by fuzzy labels. Therefore, we adopt the simple but effective Centroid defuzzification scheme. For DM_i, at time t, let the Weighted Final Achievement of a strategic goal $SG \in \mathcal{SG}_{DM_i}$, as a result of having alternative $A \in \mathcal{A}$ been adopted, to be denoted as $WFAchv(SG, DM_i, A, t)$, and calculated algebraically as follows:

$$WFAchv(SG, DM_i, A, t) = \begin{cases} SImprt^*(SG) \cdot FAchv^*(SG) & \text{if } SImprt^*(SG) \geq 0 \\ 0 & \text{if } SImprt^*(SG) < 0. \end{cases} \tag{26}$$

where $SImprt^*(SG)$ represent the defuzzified values of $SImprt(SG)$, and where $SImprt(SG) \neq Null$, and it reflects the state of mind and beliefs of DM_i at time t. And where $FAchv^*(SG)$ represents the defuzzified values of $FAchv(SG)$, and $FAchv(SG) \neq Null$; and where "A was fully applied at time $t-1$" means that the intention to apply A was fully achieved, i.e. $Achv(A) = F$, at $t-1$.

For all the decision maker in $\mathcal{DM}$ collectively, at time t of the situation, let the effect of the full joint application of alternative $A \in \mathcal{A}$ on all strategic goals in the none-empty $\mathcal{SG}$ is represented by a *Total Weighted Final Achievement* value property; and let this property value be denoted as $TWFAchv(\mathcal{DM}, A, t)$, and calculated algebraically as follows:

$$TWFAchv(\mathcal{DM}, A, t) = \frac{1}{|\mathcal{SG}|} \sum_{\substack{SG \in \mathcal{SG}_{DM_i} \\ DM_i \in \mathcal{DM}}} WFAchv(SG, DM_i, A, t) \tag{27}$$

Equation 27 requires that the set of strategic goals that decision maker DM_i have must not be empty, i.e. it requires that $|\mathcal{SG}_{DM_i}| \neq 0$. For the *Total Weighted Final Achievement* $TWFAchv(\mathcal{DM}, A, t)$ value to reflect the effect of alternative A, and only A, on all DMs in $\mathcal{DM}$, then the situation's integrated viewpoint with all its constructs and value properties' values must stay the same, and only A is applied fully. The achievement value of the intention node representing the intention to implement/apply alternative A changes from $Achv(A) = N$ to $Achv(A) = F$. All other alternatives have their respective intentions' achievement values stay the same unchanged, preferably unselected and stay at the *None* level, i.e. $(\forall A_k \in \mathcal{A} : A_k \neq A) \;\; Achv(A_k) = N$. Then, after the values forward propagation algorithm finalized the value labels for all goals, at t, we calculate $TWFAchv(\mathcal{DM}, A, t)$. The value of $TWFAchv(\mathcal{DM}, A, t)$, now, reflects the effect of applying alternative A, and only A, on all collaborating DMs in $\mathcal{DM}$.

Now, for all DMs in $\mathcal{DM}$, collectively, in a multi-agent collaborative decision making situation, at time t, let the *Cardinal Preference* that $\mathcal{DM}$ has over alternative $A \in \mathcal{A}$ be represented as a *Weighted Payoff* value property attached to A, and be denoted as $WP(A, \mathcal{DM}, t)$. Let $WP(A, \mathcal{DM}, t) = TWFAchv(\mathcal{DM}, A, t)$. Based on the cardinal preferences, weighted payoffs, calculated for $\mathcal{DM}$ over each shared alternatives in $\mathcal{A}$, $\mathcal{DM}$ will have a *Preference Vector* $Pref(\mathcal{DM}, \mathcal{A})$ showing the order of the alternatives in $\mathcal{A}$ from the *most preferred* to the *least preferred*. The preference order of a specific shared alternative $A \in \mathcal{A}$, collectively, to $\mathcal{DM}$ at time t, is given as an *Ordinal Preference* value property attached to A, and is denoted by $OP(A, \mathcal{DM}, t)$. Let $OP(A, \mathcal{DM}, t)$ be given an integer number that reflects A's position in $\mathcal{DM}$'s *Preference Vector*$Pref(\mathcal{DM}, \mathcal{A})$ at t.

5 Example: Modeling a System Requirements Collaborative Multi-agent Decision Making

In an effort to validate the Constrained Rationality framework and its suitability for the collaborative type of multi-agent decision making situations, we have used the framework to model and analyze two complex industrial collaborative multi-agent decision making situations: a strategic product development initiative and a strategic software requirements engineering initiative. The two initiatives were very successful, but contractually confidential to discuss here. Instead, we will use a simpler and heavily scaled-downed version of the software requirements engineering case to illustrate how the Constrained Rationality framework can be used to model and analyze a collaborative multi-agent decision making.

First, Define the Context: The purpose is to decide on the best architecture for a software system. There are three architectures to be reviewed for best fit (most accommodating to all the stakeholders' needs). Second, Relevant Decision Makers: The software architecture for such small system will be decided on by four agents: two represent the system's business users; one system architect/designer (also represents the rest of the technical team); and one project manager (responsible for the contractual obligations, delivery timing and reporting requirements). Third, Build a Viewpoint Model for each Decision Maker: The analyst will acquire the knowledge needed to build a viewpoint model for each agent. For collaborative decision making situations, the agents' individual viewpoint models include mainly the GCMs of the respective agents.

Fourth, Integrate All Viewpoint Models and Finalize the Base Mode: The analyst will integrate the individual agents' viewpoints (GCMs), adding cause-effect qualified fuzzy-labeled lateral relationships between the different goal and constraint nodes reside in different GCM models.The result will be similar to Figure 5. Note that the figure shows an integration of very simple GCMs, for a very simple system requirements example, with each agent has a GCM model with a two-layers goal-tree, and that goals in some GCMs conflict with each other. In real-life requirements engineering initiatives, there are usually many more stakeholders, each with a complex GCM model that has multiple goal-trees with goals conflict with others across the individual GCM boundaries. Also,

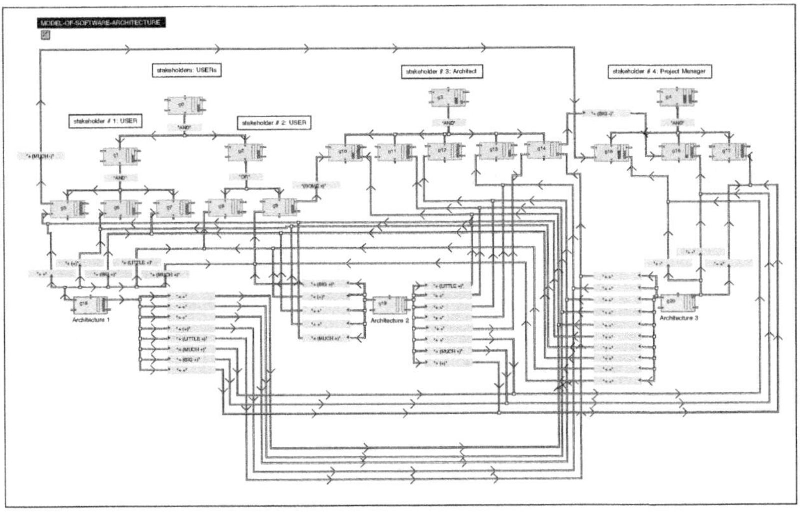

Fig. 5. Model of a Collaborative Multi-Stakeholder System Requirements Decision Making. Mobilizing an intention to implement Architecture 1 will provide different achievement levels to the agents' goals.

Figure 5 shows the three alternative architectures at the bottom, with each alternative connected to the agents' goals through lateral relations to show the positive/negative achievement/contribution that implementation of these alternatives have on the goals. In real-life requirements engineering initiatives though, there are many more alternatives (each has many variations/configurations).

Fifth, Add Priorities then Generate Agents' Preferences over Alternatives: In this step, the analyst will follow the same process used above to: 1) capture the agents' individual strategic importance over each of their respective strategic goals; and 2) elicit the agents' collective preferences over the shared alternatives. Figures 5 shows the effect (the achievement and prevention values) of implementing Architecture 1 on the agents' goals. Similar ones should be completed for the integrated model with each of alternatives 2 and 3 applied (Figures for alternatives 2 and 3 are not included for space constraint). After calculating the final achievement values for each strategic goal, for each architecture, the analyst can add the importance values for each of the agents' strategic goals, and generate the group's preferences over these alternatives, as shown in Figure 6. Finally, Sensitivity and What-If Analysis: The analyst will test variations to the value properties, the individual GCMs, or the integrated decision making situation as a whole. In this simple example, one can notice that all three alternatives show some serious weakness. In such case, which is not far from what real-life requirements projects face, the group has to rethink their alternatives, come up with other creative alternatives, break the system/project to smaller systems/projects, ask for a bigger budget and/or more resources.

(a)

Strategic Goals of DMs	SGs:	Collaborative $SG_{Collaborative}$ SG_{USERs}	$SG_{Architect}$	$SG_{ProjMangr}$
Architecture $A_{Arch\ 1}$	Achv(SG_k)	Mo	L	M
	Prvn(SG_k)	N	S	M
	FAchv(SG_k)	Mo	-L	N
{ Achv($A_{Arch\ 1}$)=F }	FAchv*(SG_k)	0.50	-0.20	0.00
Architecture $A_{Arch\ 2}$	Achv(SG_k)	M	L	Mo
	Prvn(SG_k)	N	S	B
	FAchv(SG_k)	M	-L	-S
{ Achv($A_{Arch\ 2}$)=F }	FAchv*(SG_k)	0.60	-0.20	-0.40
Architecture $A_{Arch\ 3}$	Achv(SG_k)	F	F	N
	Prvn(SG_k)	N	S	B
	FAchv(SG_k)	F	M	-B
{ Achv($A_{Arch\ 3}$)=F }	FAchv*(SG_k)	1.00	0.60	-0.80

(b)

Strategic Goals of DMs	SGs:	decision making situation # 1 Collaborative $SG_{Collaborative}$ SG_{USERs}	$SG_{Architect}$	$SG_{ProjMangr}$	decision making situation # 2 Collaborative $SG_{Collaborative}$ SG_{USERs}	$SG_{Architect}$	$SG_{ProjMangr}$	decision making situation # 3 Collaborative $SG_{Collaborative}$ SG_{USERs}	$SG_{Architect}$	$SG_{ProjMangr}$
Strategic Importance	SImprt(SG_k)	F	F	F	F	L	F	F	Mo	L
Architecture $A_{Arch\ 1}$	FAchv(SG_k, $A_{Arch\ 1}$, t)	0.50	−0.20	0.00	0.50	−0.20	0.00	0.50	−0.20	0.00
	W(SGk,DM,t)	1.00	1.00	1.00	1.00	0.20	1.00	1.00	0.50	0.20
	WFAchv(SGk,DM,$A_{Arch\ 1}$,t)	0.50	−0.20	0.00	0.50	−0.04	0.00	0.50	−0.10	0.00
	WP($A_{Arch\ 1}$, DM, t)		0.10			0.15			0.13	
{ Achv($A_{Arch\ 1}$)=F }	OP($A_{Arch\ 1}$, DM, t)		2			1 (Best)			3(Worst)	
Architecture $A_{Arch\ 2}$	FAchv(SG_k, $A_{Arch\ 2}$, t)	0.60	−0.20	−0.40	0.60	−0.20	−0.40	0.60	−0.20	−0.40
	W(SGk,DM,t)	1.00	1.00	1.00	1.00	0.20	1.00	1.00	0.50	0.20
	WFAchv(SGk,DM,$A_{Arch\ 2}$,t)	0.60	−0.20	−0.40	0.60	−0.04	−0.40	0.60	−0.10	−0.08
	WP($A_{Arch\ 2}$, DM, t)		−0.00			0.05			0.14	
{ Achv($A_{Arch\ 2}$)=F }	OP($A_{Arch\ 2}$, DM, t)		3(Worst)			3(Worst)			2	
Architecture $A_{Arch\ 3}$	FAchv(SG_k, $A_{Arch\ 3}$, t)	1.00	0.60	−0.80	1.00	0.60	−0.80	1.00	0.60	−0.80
	W(SGk,DM,t)	1.00	1.00	1.00	1.00	0.20	1.00	1.00	0.50	0.20
	WFAchv(SGk,DM,$A_{Arch\ 3}$,t)	1.00	0.60	−0.80	1.00	0.12	−0.80	1.00	0.30	−0.16
	WP($A_{Arch\ 3}$, DM, t)		0.27			0.11			0.38	
{ Achv($A_{Arch\ 3}$)=F }	OP($A_{Arch\ 3}$, DM, t)		1 (Best)			2			1 (Best)	

Fig. 6. Results (a) Final Achievement Levels for all Architectures; and (b) Generating the Preferences for the Group

6 Conclusion

Constrained Rationality's basic goal and constraint modeling and reasoning introduced in [9] has been extended by proposing new modeling and reasoning facilities to effectively generate the agents' collective cardinal and ordinal preferences (from their goals, constraints and priorities) over their collective shared alternatives in collaborative decision making situations. A simplified version of a systems requirements industrial case study is used to demonstrate: the process to model a collaborative decision making initiative; and to show how effective and flexible the extended framework is in modeling and reasoning about such situation. As a future work, we intend to solve some of the model management challenges we faced when used the framework in real-life cases, as the models increase in their size and details as the number of agents increase; and establish tools, templates and metrics to help the decision makers and analysts to be more effective in using the framework in complex initiatives.

References

1. Keeney, R.: Value-focused thinking: A path to creative decisionmaking. Harvard University Press, Cambridge (1992)
2. Raiffa, H., Richardson, J., Metcalfe, D.: Negotiation Analysis: The Science and Art of Collaborative Decision Making. Harvard University Press, Cambridge (2002)
3. Wooldridge, M.: Reasoning About Rational Agents. MIT Press, Cambridge (2000)

4. Winikoff, M., Harland, J., Padgham, L.: Linking Agent Concepts and Methodology with CAN. In: Submitted to the First International Joint Conference on Autonomous Agents and Multi-Agent Systems (2002)
5. Shaw, P.H., Bordini, R.H.: Towards alternative approaches to reasoning about goals. In: Baldoni, M., Son, T.C., van Riemsdijk, M.B., Winikoff, M. (eds.) DALT 2007. LNCS (LNAI), vol. 4897, pp. 104–121. Springer, Heidelberg (2008)
6. Dardenne, A., van Lamsweerde, A., Fickas, S.: Goal-directed Requirements Acquisition. Science of Computer Programming 20, 3–50 (1993)
7. Al-Shawa, M.: Viewpoints-based Value-Driven - Enterprise Knowledge Management (ViVD-EKM). MASc thesis, Electrical and Computer Engineering. University of Waterloo (2006)
8. Al-Shawa, M.: Constrained Rationality: Formal Value-Driven Enterprise Knowledge Management Modelling and Analysis Framework for Strategic Business, Technology and Public Policy Decision Making & Conflict Resolution. Ph.D. dissertation, Electrical and Computer Engineering. University of Waterloo (2011)
9. Al-Shawa, M., Basir, O.: Constrained Rationality: Formal Goals-Reasoning Approach to Strategic Decision & Conflict Analysis. In: Proceedings of the 2009 IEEE International Conference on Systems, Man, and Cybernetics (2009)
10. Saaty, T.L.: The Analytic Hierarchy Process: Planning, Priority Setting, Resource Allocation. Mc GrawHil, New York (1980)

Effects of Reaction Time on the Kinetic Visual Field

Xiaoya Yu[1,2], Jinglong Wu[1,3], Shuhei Miyamoto[4], and Shengfu Lu[1]

[1] International WIC Institute, Beijing University of Technology, Beijing, 100124, P.R. China
[2] Department of Computer Science, Beijing Institute of Education, Beijing, 100120, P.R. China
[3] Biomedical Engineering Laboratory, Division of Industrial Innovation Sciences, The Graduate School of Natural Science and Technology, Okayama University Okayama, Japan
[4] Department of Design Fukushima Branch, NOK Corporation, Fukushima, Japan

yuxiaoya@mails.bjut.edu.cn, wu@mech.okayama-u.ac.jp, lusf@bjut.edu.cn

Abstract. Kinetic visual field refers to the visual range in which a moving target can be seen. The reaction time in traditional Kinetic Perimetry was the time from the target was identified to the subject responded, without taking into account individual simple reaction time (SRT). This is problematic in that it mixes the evaluations of human visual performance with behavior performance. We redefined kinetic visual field by analyzed the components of the RT, and then measured SRT and kinetic visual field of six normal subjects, using a modified Goldman kinetic perimeter. The results showed that the newly defined kinetic visual field was wider than traditional defined, because the newly defined kinetic visual field without including SRT. Thus, Kinetic Perimetry using the newly defined method eliminates individual SRT differences to produce what we believe to be a more accurate evaluation indicator of human visual functions.

1 Introduction

Visual field is the entire area that can be seen when the eye is directed forward, including that which is seen with peripheral vision [1]. Kinetic visual field refers to the visual range in which a moving target can be seen [2][3], mapping of the visual field by using a moving rather than a static test object. It plays an important role in our daily life. Previous studies [4][5][6][7] on Kinetic Perimetry have reported such findings as the larger the target size and the greater the brightness, the wider the kinetic visual field[8][9], and in single-eye Kinetic Perimetry there are no differences between the left eye and the right eye [10][11][12], etc. However, previous studies neglected the simple reaction time (SRT) of subjects; it mixed the evaluations of human visual performance with behavior performance.

Psychologists have named three basic kinds of reaction time experiments [13][14]: In SRT experiments, there is only one stimulus and one response. In recognition reaction time experiments, there are some stimuli that should be responded to, and

B. Hu et al. (Eds.): BI 2011, LNAI 6889, pp. 124–135, 2011.

others that should get no response. There is still only one correct response. In choice reaction time experiments, the user must give a response that corresponds to the stimulus, such as pressing a key corresponding to a letter if the letter appears on the screen. We think humans make decisions and take appropriate action upon seeing external stimuli. The time required to make a decision is referred to as judgment time, while reaction time refers to the time it takes to begin acting after a stimulus is presented. As in Figure 1, judgment times are very short when reacting to simple stimuli, so reaction time in these situations is referred to as SRT. SRT do not rely on recognition and judgment differences, and can be thought of as human behavioral traits [15].

In the traditional kinetic visual field evaluation method, kinetic visual field was calculated by the time it took to press the reaction button after identifying the target. The target continued to move during the time from when it was perceived to the time the reaction button was pressed. Hence, the traditional definition of kinetic visual field was a mixed result of visual traits and behavioral traits. Thus, strictly speaking, it was not exactly kinetic visual field as a perceptual function of vision.

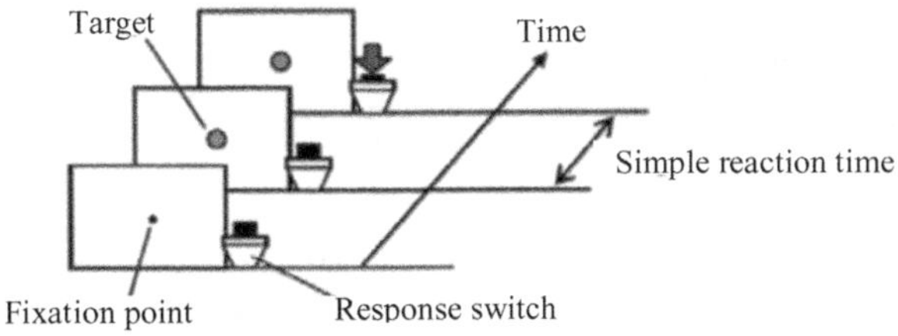

Fig. 1. Simple reaction time (SRT) measurement schematic diagram

This study compares the results obtained between measurements that employ the traditional kinetic field definition method, and those that employ this study's newly defined method. We used a modified kinetic perimeter system measured the SRT and visual field of six normal subjects, the results of the newly defined kinetic visual field was wider than traditional defined, because the newly defined kinetic visual field without including SRT. Thus, Kinetic Perimetry using the newly defined method eliminates individual differences in human behavioral traits to produce what we believe to be a more accurate evaluation indicator of human visual functions.

2 Methods

2.1 Apparatus

As seen in Figure 2, the kinetic perimeter apparatus used to measure kinetic visual field in this study employs an electric slider to replace the target movement operation of the manually operated Goldman perimeter, making it automatic.

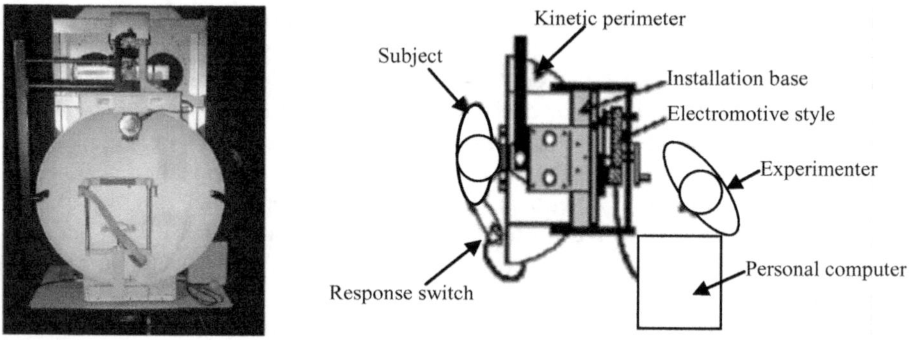

Fig. 2. The system of the kinetic perimeter. The left is the photo of Goldman perimeter, with an automatic target movement operation. The right is the kinetic perimeter system schematic diagram.

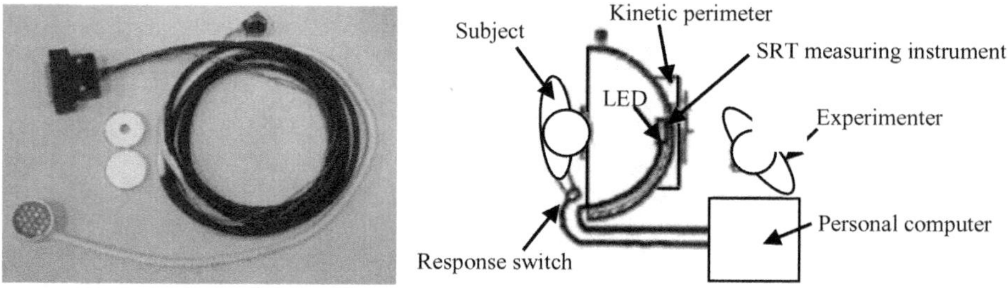

Fig. 3. This shows a figure of system of the SRT measuring instrument. The left is the photo of apparatus developed by the authors in past research; the right is the measurement system of the SRT schematic diagram.

The SRT measuring instrument system is shown in Figure 3. The apparatus developed by the authors in past research was used in this experiment [11]. It has the same experimental environment with Kinetic Perimety. We recorded the time between presentation of the LED light stimulus and subsequent pressing of a response switch, on the personal computer.

2.2 Subjects and Target Conditions

Six normal subjects aged 18-24, three males and three females, each with static visual acuities ranging from 0.6 – 2.0, with no eye disorders. There are seven target conditions, the details shown in Table 1.

Table 1. Target conditions

Condition number	Size (mm^2)	Luminance (cd/m^2)	Color
I	64	318	White
II	1	318	White
III	1	100	White
W	64	36	White
R	64	36	Red
G	64	36	Green
B	64	36	Blue

2.3 Procedure

Kinetic visual field measurements are conducted in a dark room with only the right eye, covering the subjects' left eyes with sterile gauze so they cannot see from that eye. The subjects' head fixed during Kinetic Perimetry. The background screen is 10 (cd/m^2) and white. The Goldman perimeter is used to measure SRT and kinetic visual field, a spot of light moves at a fixed rate of speed from the periphery of the visual field to its center. When the subjects see the target they press the reaction button, thereby measuring their kinetic visual fields.

As shown in Figure 4, the meridian directions are shown at angles centered on the fixation point, with the temple-side horizontal direction at 0 (deg), the counterclockwise upward vertical direction at 90 (deg), the nose side at 180 (deg), and the visual field's downward vertical direction at 270 (deg).

Target meridians are in 12 different directions, separated at 30º angles. In order to avoid blind spots, in horizontal direction making a 5 degree offset along a particular meridian. Take four measurements at each meridian and record the mean values.

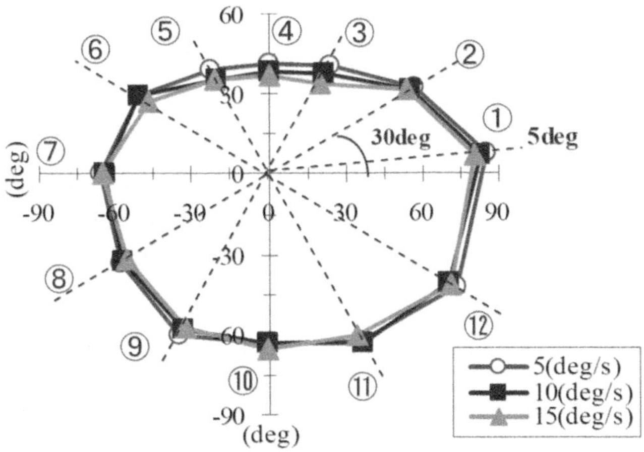

Fig. 4. The target movement speeds and meridians. Here show a sample of the kinetic visual fields of three movement speeds under target condition I

Take measurements using the three target movement speeds of 5, 10 and 15 (deg/s) for target conditions I, II, III, and the two target movement speeds of 5 and 15 (deg/s) for target condition W, R, G and B. Take four measurements for each target condition/meridian and use the mean values as results.

3 Results

3.1 Simple Reaction Time

The experimental environment is same with Kinetic Perimetry. Subjects sat in front of the Goldman perimeter, after 3 minutes of light adaptation, began by monocular fixating on the LED of the SRT measurement system located at the center of the background screen. When the LED lights the subject push the response switch, and the LED light turns off. After a randomly interval between 200ms and 600ms, the LED lights again. Repeat 30 times and record the SRT, use the mean values as the subject's SRT.

The average SRT time of the six subjects is shown in Table 2 respectively. The target condition in this experiment isφ9, visual angle is 1.7 (deg), luminance is 117 (cd/m^2).

Table 2. The individual experiment results of the SRT measurement

Initial	Age	SRT (ms)
MY	18	225.3
SN	18	212.9
AU	22	228.5
TM	22	235.2
AH	23	217.8
SM	24	211.0

3.2 Kinetic Visual Field

Kinetic visual field measurement results are shown by target conditions group in Figure 5. These were compiled by mean values of angles of eccentricity, measured by each meridian. Vertical and horizontal axes show a visual angle with a fixation point of 0 (deg).

From (a) to (g) in Figure 5 illustrate the average result of six subjects' kinetic visual field by seven target conditions group (I, II, III, W, R, G and B). The three/two polygonal lines in each of the graphs are the target movement speed. The three target movement speeds of 5 (deg/s), 10 (deg/s) and 15 (deg/s) for target conditions of I, II, III, and the two target movement speeds of 5 (deg/s) and 10 (deg/s) for target conditions W, R, G and B. These kinetic visual fields illustrated by each target condition are the results that reflect the individual SRT of the subjects.

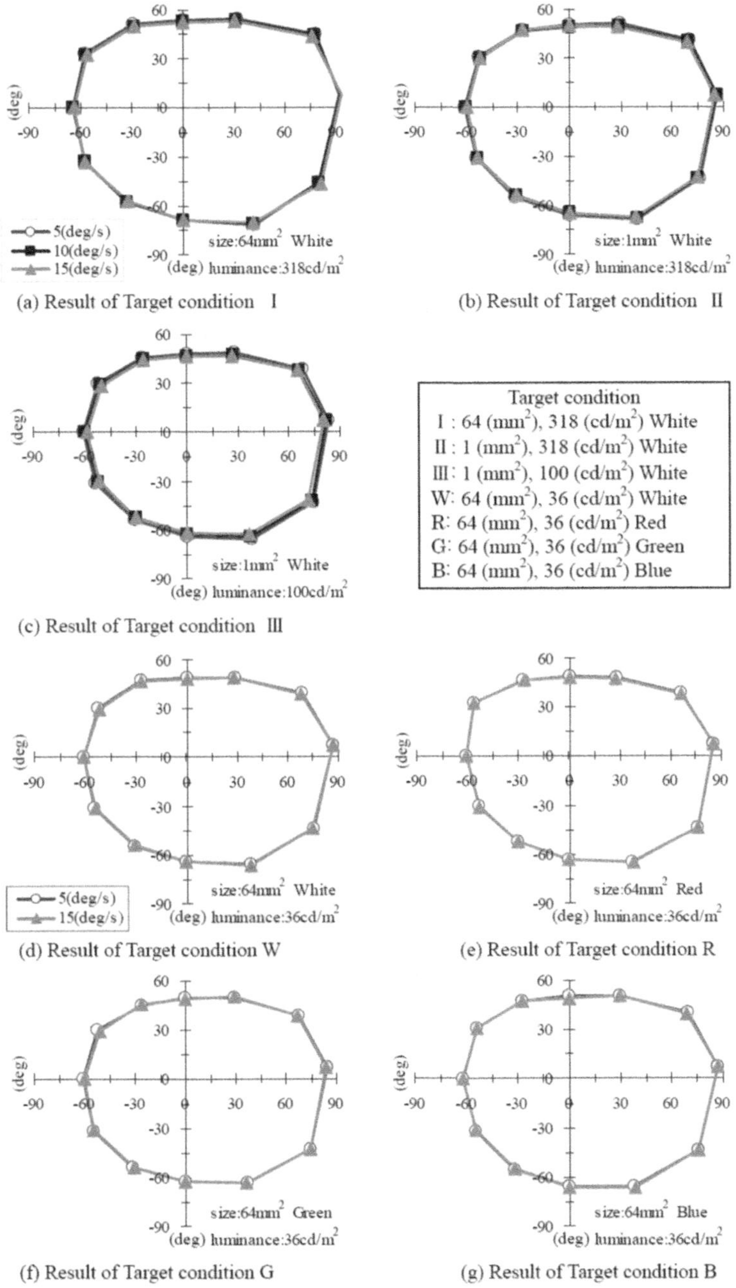

Fig. 5. Six subjects' kinetic visual fields by seven target conditions group. Target movement speed: 5 (deg/s), 10 (deg/s) and 15 (deg/s) for target condition I, II and II, 5 (deg/s) and 10 (deg/s) for target condition W, R, G and B.

3.3 Kinetic Visual Field Area

The kinetic visual field area is found by calculating the areas inside subject isopters. The reason for this is so that the amount of the visual field can be quantitatively described.

In this study, setting the fixation point as the eccentric angle of 0 (deg), subjects isopters are shown in polygons, so the area inside the polygons is calculated as the kinetic visual field area.

First we will describe the method to calculate the kinetic visual field area without taking into account the SRT of subjects.

As shown in Figure 6, the two response points a_i (deg), b_i (deg) and the single fixation point O determined the area of the section (A_i (deg2)), $A_i = (1/2) \times a_i \times b_i \times \sin\theta_i$. So we determine the areas of all the sections within isopter A, and total the sums to arrive at the kinetic visual field area without taking into account SRT.

Next, we will describe the method to calculate the kinetic visual field area while taking into account SRT. As shown in Figure 6, the eccentric angle R (deg), which is the response point of isopter A, obtained in the kinetic visual field measurement shown in Figure 6, is reduced by the amount of SRT it took for subjects to respond after seeing the target.

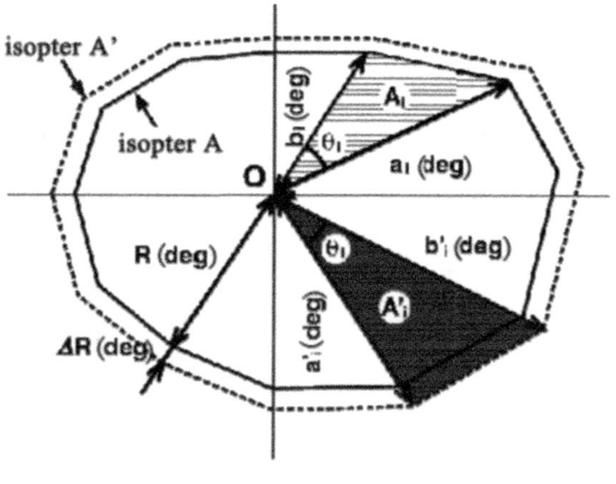

Fig. 6. The calculation method of kinetic visual field

In other words, the eccentric angles of subjects essentially have are larger than R (deg) by SRT (s) × target movement speed (deg/s) (= Δ R (deg)).

Thus, isopter A', which is the kinetic visual field taking into account SRT, is determined by adding Δ R (deg) to each of the response points in isopter A. The area of isopter A' is calculated the same way as the area for isopter A, determining the area of a section of isopter A' (A'_i (deg2)) from the two response points a'_i (deg) and b'_i (deg) and the single fixation point O. The kinetic visual field area, compensating for SRT, is then reached by $A'_i = (1/2) \times a'_i \times b'_i \times \sin\theta_i$ to calculate all the sections of isopter A' and adding them together.

We used the kinetic visual field testing measurement the subjects' kinetic visual field, used method above calculated the areas. Then we contrasted the target size and luminance effects on the kinetic visual field areas.

The averages of kinetic visual field areas under the same luminance (318 (cd/m^2) of target condition I (64mm^2) and II (1mm^2) in Figure 7. The results obtained by comparing the area showed the smaller target, the narrower kinetic visual field. Regarding the target size, the t test, revealed a significant difference in areas with respect to the kinetic visual field.

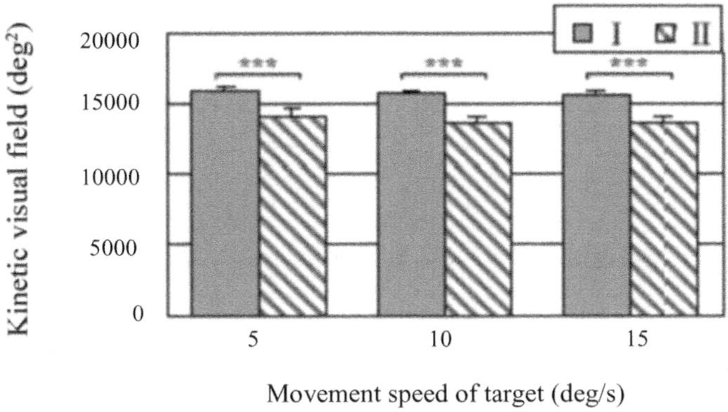

Fig. 7. Comparison size of kinetic visual field (*: $p<0.05$. **$p<0.01$, ***$p<0.001$.paired t-test)

In Figure 8, the targets size are same (1mm^2), the targets luminance are condition II (318(cd/m^2)) and III (100(cd/m^2)) respectively.

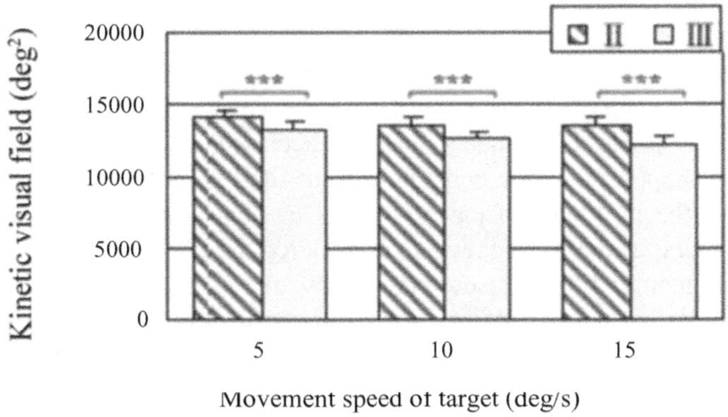

Fig. 8. Comparison luminance of kinetic visual field (*: $p<0.05$. **$p<0.01$, ***$p<0.001$.paired t-test)

From the contrast results in Figure 8, we know the higher of the target luminance, the broader the kinetic visual field area. With the paired t test, a significant difference was observed between the target condition II and III.

However, traditional Kinetic Perimetry defined SRT as the time from the target was identified to the time subjects responded. As shown in Figure 9, suppose t_s, t_c and t_r represent the time the target begins to be shown, the time it is perceived, and the reaction time, respectively. CT (consciousness time) is the time the target is perceived ($CT=t_c-t_s$), SRT (simple reaction time) is the time it takes to react to the target upon perception ($SRT=t_r-t_c$), and RT (reaction time) is the total time it takes to react to the target ($RT=t_r-t_s$). Traditional Kinetic Perimetry recorded the response time t_r, when moving the target at a fixed speed from a distant location, the location at which the subject accurately recognizes the moving target is designated as t_c, which is the subject's true kinetic visual field. However, by the time the subject reacts the target moves to the t_r location, the result are inaccurate. SRT is a behavioral trait occurring once the target is perceived, not a visual perception trait. Thus, the inclusion of SRT in the definition of kinetic visual field as a visual trait is problematic.

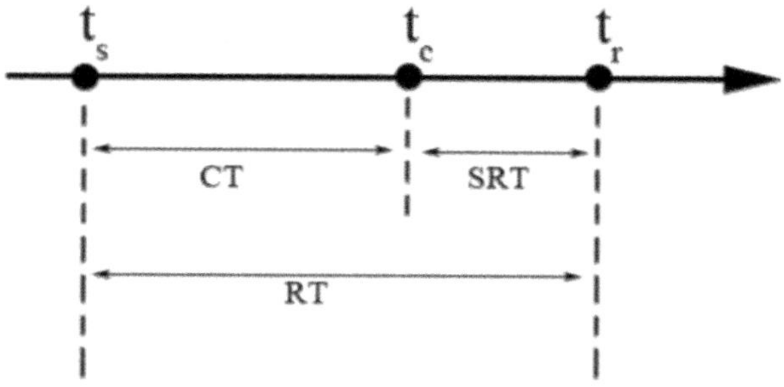

Fig. 9. The relationship among SRT and traditional reaction time, new defined kinetic visual field consciousness time. t_s, t_c and t_r represent the time the target begins to be shown, the time it is perceived, and the reaction time, respectively

Kinetic visual field, acting as indicator that assesses human visual perception functions, include behavioral traits, leaving the issue of inaccuracy unresolved.

In order to evaluate the human visual trait accurately, we define the more accurate reaction time, hope to exclude behavioral traits, and then gain the real kinetic visual field to solve the problems of past studies. Our next experiments will analysis and comparison of experimental data which considered the SRT or not.

Figure 10 illustrated the measurement results of six subjects' average kinetic visual field areas under considered SRT or not. From the results, when we take into account the SRT of the subjects, the kinetic visual field area increased. Since the new defined method can eliminate individual differences in human behavioral traits. Moreover, for combination of target conditions, seven target condition, three movement speed, on the basis of whether take into account the individual SRT differences or not, the results of paired sample t-test for comparing kinetic visual field areas demonstrate that the differences were significant. This trend was seen in all target conditions.

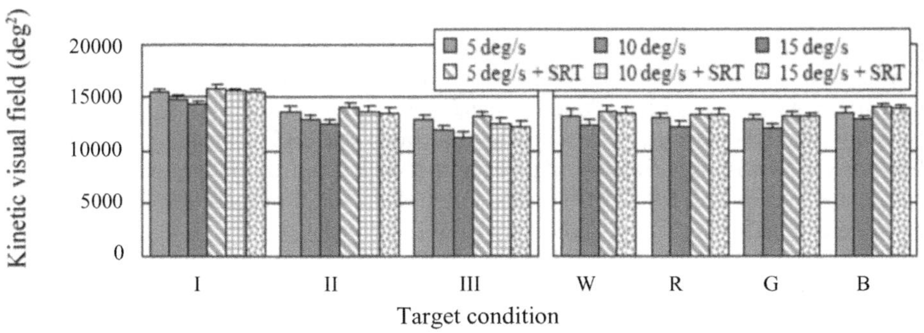

Fig. 10. This figure illustrated the average kinetic visual field areas of six subjects under considered SRT or not

From the above, the SRT affects the kinetic visual field measurement significantly. Kinetic Perimetry using the newly defined method eliminates individual SRT differences to produce what we believe to be a more accurate evaluation indicator of human visual functions.

4 Discussion

This study analyzed the components of the RT during traditional Kinetic Perimetry, pointed out the problem that mixed behavior traits into visual traits evaluation [16][17]made the Kinetic Perimetry inaccuracy. In order to solve the problem, this study redefined the kinetic visual field taking into account the individual SRT; propose a kinetic visual field evaluate method. Further, it experimentally investigated SRT, tested subjects to measure the relation of target size, luminance and speed to kinetic visual fields, quantitatively investigating the effects of the SRT on kinetic visual field. The appropriateness of the kinetic visual field eliminated SRT was proven by results of tests.

Traditional reaction time, as Figure 9 shown, includes consciousness time (CT) and SRT. From this study know, SRT includes the time from the target was been perceived to the time the reaction finished. So we think the SRT was a behavioral trait, not a vision trait. Past research did not take into account the above individual differences in the reaction time of subjects. Hence, kinetic visual field, acting as indicators that assess human visual perception functions, include behavioral traits, leaving the issue of inaccuracy unresolved. For example, your reaction time tends to slow with age, but your kinetic visual field maybe has not changed[18][19][20][21]. Under the traditional Kinetic Perimetry, the results would give you that the kinetic visual field narrowed evaluation. For another example, if one's brain was damaged lead to his behavioral reaction slow, the traditional Kinetic Perimetry maybe infer that your kinetic visual field was damaged. In fact, your kinetic visual field still perfected. So in this study, we defined the kinetic visual field only include visual trait's consciousness time (t_c), excluding SRT. We do some evaluative experiment to compare the results obtained between measurements that employ the traditional kinetic visual field definition method and those that employ this study's newly defined method. The experiment results show that the apparatus of Kinetic Perimetry is good, demonstrate the numbers of subjects meet the requirements, and we can estimate the overall trend on the basis of the experimental results. And then, we measurement the six subjects kinetic visual field under combination target conditions (seven types three speed), the results demonstrated the SRT affects the kinetic visual field measurement significantly. Kinetic Perimetry using the newly defined method eliminates individual SRT differences to produce what we believe to be a more accurate evaluation indicator of human visual functions.

Acknowledgments. This work is partially supported by Beijing Natural Science Foundation (4102007). The authors also would like to thank Mi Li and Linchan Qin in the International WIC Institute for their advices.

References

1. Webster's New World™ Medical Dictionary, 3rd edn. Wiley Publishing, Inc., Chichester (May 2008)
2. Ikeda, M., Uchikawa, K., Saida, S.: Static and dynamic functional visual fields. Optica Acta 26, 1103–1113 (1979)
3. Wu, J., Lu, S., Miyamoto, S., Hayashi, Y.: New definitions of kinetic visual acuity and kinetic visual field and their aging effects. IATSS Research 33(1), 27–34 (2009)
4. Spahr, J.: Optimization of the presentation pattern in automated static perimetry. Vision Res. 15, 1275–1281 (1975)
5. Johnson, C.A., Keltner, J.L., Lewis, R.A.: Automated kinetic perimetry: an efficient method of evaluating peripheral visual field loss. Appl. Opt. 26, 1409–1414 (1987)
6. Shigaki, H., Miyao, M.: Implications for Dynamic Visual Acuity with Changes in Age and Sex. Percept. Mot. Skills 77, 835–839 (1993)
7. Mashimo, I.: Sports Vision: Vision for Sports, 2nd edn. NAP Ltd. (1997) (in Japanese)
8. Hasjimoto, S.: Development of a Kinetic Visual Field Measuring Program Using an Automatic Perimeter. Medical Journal of Kinki University 28, 207–221 (2003)
9. Understanding Visual Fields, Part I; Goldman Perimetry. Journal of Ophthalmic Medical Technology 2(2) (2006)
10. Hasegawa, T., Yamashita, M., Suzuki, T., et al.: Active linear head motion improves dynamic visual acuity in pursuing a high-speed moving object. Exp. Brain Res. 194, 505–516 (2009)
11. Wu, J., Lu, S., Hayashi, Y.: Study and Development of a Visual Acuity Equipment with Multifunction for Three Subjects at Once. The Japan Society of Mechanical Engineers – Collected Papers. Group C 74-737, 83–89 (2008)
12. Ramirez, A.M., Chaya, C.J., Gordon, L.K., Giaconi, J.A.: A comparison of semiautomated versus manual Goldman kinetic perimetry in patients with visually significant glaucoma. J. Glaucoma 17(2), 111–117 (2008)
13. Luce, R.D.: Response times: Their role in inferring elementary mental organization. Oxford Univ. Press, New York (1986)
14. Whelan, R.: Effective Analysis of Reaction Time Data. The Psychological Record 58, 475–482 (2008)
15. Schiefer, U., Strasburger, H., Becker, S.T., et al.: Reaction time in automated kinetic perimetry: effects of stimulus luminance, eccentricity, and movement direction. Vision Res. 41, 2157–2164 (2001)

16. Johnson, C.A., Keltner, J.L., Balestrerya, F.: Effects of target size and eccentricity on visual detection and resolution. Vision Research 18, 1217–1222 (1978)
17. Parrish, R.K., Shiffman, J., Anderson, D.R.: Static and kinetic visual field testing, reproducibility in normal volunteers. Archives of Ophthalmology 102, 1497–1502 (1984)
18. Poulain, I., Giraudet, G., Dobrescu, N.: Age-related changes in perception of verticality with a static or kinetic visual-field disturbance. Perception 33 ECVP (2004)
19. Jaffe, G.J., Alvarado, J.A., Juster, R.P.: Age-related changes of the normal visual field. Arch. Ophthalmol. 104(7), 1021–1025 (1986)
20. Haas, A., Flammer, J., Schneider, U.: Influence of age on the visual fields of normal subjects. Am. J. Ophthalmol. 101(2), 199–203 (1986)
21. Drance, S.M., Berry, V., Hughes, A.: Studies on the effects of age on the central and peripheral isopters of the visual field in normal subjects. Am. J. Ophthalmol. 63(6), 1667–1672 (1967)

Robust and Stable Small-World Topology of Brain Intrinsic Organization during Pre- and Post-Task Resting States

Zhijiang Wang[1,2], Jiming Liu[1,2,3], Ning Zhong[1,2,4], Yulin Qin[1,2,5], Haiyan Zhou[1,2], and Kuncheng Li[6,2]

[1] International WIC Institute, Beijing University of Technology, China
[2] Beijing Municipal Lab of Brain Informatics, China
[3] Dept. of Computer Science, Hong Kong Baptist University, China
[4] Dept. of Life Science and Informatics, Maebashi Institute of Technology, Japan
[5] Dept. of Psychology, Carnegie Mellon University, USA
[6] Dept. of Radiology, Xuanwu Hospital, Capital Medical University, China
zhong@maebashi-it.ac.jp

Abstract. Brain functional network studies have demonstrated the small-world topology as the nature of large-scale spontaneous brain activity. Studies have also revealed that the temporal coherence of spontaneous activity could be reshaped during task-dependent (or post-task) resting states within local spatial patterns such as task-related and the default-mode networks. However, to our best knowledge, it is still a lack of rigorous investigations that whether the small-world topology of spontaneous intrinsic organization remains robust and stable during different resting states. To address the problem, we recorded blood oxygen level-dependent (BOLD) signals from two rests (namely, pre- and post-task resting states) before and after a simple semantic-matching task, and investigated the preceding task influences on the topology of the large-scale spontaneous intrinsic organization during the post-task resting state. The major findings are that the small-world configuration of spontaneous intrinsic organization remains robust and stable during resting states regardless of preceding task influences.

1 Introduction

Spontaneous brain activity, which is intrinsically generated in the absence of any explicit inputs or outputs (see the review [1]), consumes more than 80% of brain energy [1, 2]. But task-related increases in neuronal metabolism are usually less than 5% of the large resting energy consumption [1, 2]. These facts may suggest that spontaneous brain activity should develop the fundamental activity pattern in human brains either during rest or task-on conditions. Furthermore, topological investigations of brain intrinsic architecture could provide deep insights into the working mechanisms of spontaneous brain activity.

B. Hu et al. (Eds.): BI 2011, LNAI 6889, pp. 136–147, 2011.

With graph theories in complex networks, brain functional network studies have explored the nature of large-scale spontaneous brain activity. The small-world topology (high clustering coefficient and short characteristic path distance) has been demonstrated (for review, see [3–5]) in the large-scale spontaneous intrinsic organization using functional magnetic resonance imaging (fMRI) [6–10] as well as macaque cortex neurophysiological data [11], electroencephalograph (EEG) [12], magnetoencephalograph (MEG) [13, 14]. These global topological properties have also been demonstrated in anatomical networks [15–21]. According to discussions in some reviews, small-world topology can support parallel information processing of functional segregation and integration [3, 4, 22], which are two fundamental organizational principles of the cerebral cortex [23, 24]. Moreover, small-world topology can facilitate rapid adaptive reconfigurations of neuronal assemblies in support of cognitive states changing [4].

However, does the small-world topology of brain intrinsic organization remain robust and stable during pre- and post-task resting states? Studies have revealed temporal coherence modulations of spontaneous correlated activity within some local spatial patterns, such as task-related networks [25–27] and the default mode network (DMN) [25], during a post-task resting state. For the variability of large-scale coherent spatial patterns, a pioneer work using MEG found that the global topological properties of brain functional networks were not sensitive to a simple motor task during the task-on state by a two-sample contrast analysis [14]. In our previous work [28], two model perspectives of positively- and negatively-correlated brain functional networks (PCBFN and NCBFN) were proposed to investigate the topological modulation mechanisms of the large-scale spontaneous intrinsic organization during a post-task resting state. Both the PCBFN and NCBFN were determined by a series of group-level statistical significances. The between-state statistical comparisons in topological properties were not performed either the PCBFN or the NCBFN but only descriptive discussions.

In the present study, we still used the better spatial resolution imaging technique of functional MRI (fMRI) to test whether the small-world configuration of brain intrinsic organization is modulated during a post-task resting state? To further address the problem, (1) we still recorded BOLD signals from the two rests (pre- and post-task resting states) before and after subjects performed a simple semantic-matching task [28, 29]; (2) we constructed individual-level brain functional networks by a wide range of positive correlation thresholds during the two resting states; (3) finally, nine small-world properties were calculated, and compared between the two resting states under a statistic significant level.

2 Data Acquisition and Preprocessing

2.1 Subjects

Fifteen healthy subjects (7 males, 8 females; 23.8 $\pm$ 0.7 years old) from Beijing University of Technology participated in the study. All the subjects were right-handed and reported with no history of neurological or psychiatric disorders. Written informed consent was obtained from each subject. All the subjects were scanned during a semantic-matching task [29] and the two resting states before and after the task. During the rest scans, subjects were instructed to relax with their eyes closed and move as little as possible.

2.2 Data Acquisition

All subjects were scanned on 3.0 Tesla Siemens MRI scanner with the parameters: repetition time/echo time = 2000/31 ms, thickness/gap = 3.2/0 mm, matrix = 64 × 64, axial slices number = 32 and field of view = 200 × 200 mm^2. The functional images of the whole brain using an echo planar imaging (EPI) sequence were acquired over all sessions. The first and last sessions were at rest while the intermediate 3 sessions were on a semantic-matching task [29]. Each session lasted for 8 minutes and 14 seconds (244 volumes). In the present work, we still focused on the two resting states: the pre-task resting state (the first session) and the post-task resting state (the last session). To allow for magnetization equilibrium, subjects' adaptation to the circumstances and separation between two adjacent sessions, the first 4 volumes of EPI sequence of each session for each subject were discarded, with leaving 240 volumes for each session available for further processing.

2.3 Data Preprocessing

Image preprocessing was firstly carried out using the software package of statistical parametric mapping (SPM5, http://www.fil.ion.ucl.ac.uk/spm) by slice timing, realign and normalization (EPI template and resampled to 3 mm cubic voxels), without smoothing. Next, each brain image was parceled into 90 cortical and sub-cortical regions using the anatomically labeled template atlas (AAL atlas, 45 for each cerebral hemisphere [30]. Then, each regional time series were acquired by averaging the time series over all voxels within each region of interest (ROI), and then filtered into the frequency range of 0.01Hz∼0.08Hz to reduce the effects of low-frequency drift and high-frequency noise, followed by a multiple linear regression analysis to remove several sources of spurious variances from the estimated head-motion profiles (six parameters obtained from head-motion correction) and global brain signal [31]. The residual of the linear regression was considered the neuronal-induced signal of each corresponding region.

3 Construction of Brain Functional Networks

The 90 ROIs of the AAL atlas were defined as nodes of a large-scale brain functional network. Edges were determined by whether the strength of functional connectivity between any pair of ROIs exceeded a non-negative threshold to characterize their positive or synchronous couplings. To measure the functional connectivity between any two brain regions, we calculated Pearson correlation coefficients between any two residual time series (BOLD signals) extracted from the two ROIs, followed by a Fisher's r-to-z transformation [32] to improve the normality of the correlation coefficients. Then, a temporal correlation matrix

(90 × 90) was obtained for each subject corresponding to each resting state. Finally, all the correlation matrices were thresholded by a flexible threshold value $T(\geq 0)$, in which the elements were set to 1 if it exceeded T, otherwise to 0, then binary undirected graphs were resulted underlying the large-scale brain functional organization, in order to characterize the joint positive or synchronous couplings over the whole brain.

4 Small-World Properties

4.1 Basic Small-World Properties

Clustering coefficient (C_g) and characteristic path length (L_p) were originally used to describe small-world properties for a network by Watts and Strogatz [15]. The local clustering coefficient is a ratio of the number of actually existing connections among the nearest neighbors of a node to the number of all possible connections, which measures the local cliquishness of a typical neighborhood [15]. The global clustering coefficient of a network is the average of the local clustering coefficients over all nodes. Characteristic path length is the average of the shortest path distances between all pair of nodes. But in this study, the harmonic mean distance was used to evaluate the characteristic path length to deal with the bug when the graph is unconnected [33].

4.2 Information Efficiency

Network information efficiency was firstly used for estimating economical performance of small-world anatomical networks in a cat and a macaque cortex [34]. Then, Achard and Bullmore applied these metrics into the efficiency estimation of brain functional networks, and demonstrated that brain functional networks also had economical small-world performance in support of efficient parallel information transfer at relatively low cost [35]. Thus, global and local information efficiency (E_{global} and E_{local}) were defined to measure the ability of parallel information transfer at the global and local scopes in a network, respectively [18, 34, 35]. The followings are their formula definitions.

$$E_{global} = \frac{1}{n(n-1)} \sum_{i,j \in G \wedge i \neq j} d_{ij}^{-1}$$

$$E_{local} = \frac{1}{n} \sum_{i \in G} E_{global}(G_i)$$

where d_{ij} denotes the shortest path distance from node i to j, n is the number of nodes in the graph G, and G_i denotes the subgraph as composed of neighbors of node i in the graph G.

4.3 Scaling the Metrics with the Degree-Matched Random Networks

To evaluate the nine small-world characteristics, we generated 100 degree-matched random networks by a Markov-chain algorithm [22, 37, 38]. These metrics (C_g, L_p, E_{global} and E_{local}) of real networks were scaled by calculating the ratios with those averaged metrics of the corresponding random networks at each sparsity level. As reported by Watts and Strogatz (1998), small-world networks have short characteristic path distance (similar to random networks) and high clustering coefficient (similar to regular networks), that's to say, $\gamma = C_g^{real}/C_g^{random} > 1$ and $\lambda = L_p^{real}/L_p^{random} \approx 1$. Moreover, both E_{global} and E_{local} of real networks were also scaled with the averaged efficiency of the 100 degree-matched random networks to measure the relative efficiency of small-world brain functional network. Typically, the global efficiency in a small-world network is approximately equal to that in the corresponding random networks while the local efficiency is much higher ($E_{global}^{real}/E_{global}^{random} \approx 1$, $E_{local}^{real}/E_{local}^{random} > 1$). Finally, a scalar measurement was calculated for a summarized evaluation of "small-worldness" [19], $\sigma = \gamma/\lambda > 1$.

5 Statistical Analysis

5.1 Threshold Selection

In this study, we employed flexible correlation thresholds T (Fisher's r-to-z) to generate large-scale functional networks with the exactly same number of nodes and edges or connectivity, ensuring that any graph differences between two different behavioral states would be really because of specific connectivity variations in the intrinsic network, not the overall connectivity in network topology. In this study, the edges or connectivity were thresholded by a measurement of sparsity S ($0.05 \leq S \leq 0.46$, step by 0.01), which was defined by ratio of the number of existed edges to the number of all possible edges. With S decreased, lower-correlation edges were removed. The minimum S was empirically set to 0.05 [9, 15] while the maximum S of 0.46 was determined by the minimum value of the possibly maximum positive edges of the functional networks among all the subjects during the two resting states. As a result, a set (totally 42) of large-scale brain functional networks over such sequential sparsity levels ($0.05 \leq S \leq 0.46$) were produced for each subject during each behavioral state.

5.2 Statistical Comparisons

To determine whether there were significant differences in the small-world properties between the two resting states, two tailed paired t-tests were performed on all the individual entries over the 42 sequential sparsity levels across subjects, respectively. Thus, there was a multiple-comparison matrix: 9×42, in which the rows were tested items, and the columns were the 42 sequential sparsity levels. In this article, the overall statistical significance was corrected by a

Monte-Carlo correction method. The underlying principle is that the true difference for each tested item should tend to occur over a range of sequential sparsity levels (namely, sparsity segment length (SSL), or one-dimensional cluster size), whereas noise should have much less of a tendency to form a wide enough SSL. Therefore, a combination of thresholds of individual p and SSL could be used to enhance the overall multiple test power and achieve a desired overall significance level. This idea is very similar to that of the activation identification of voxel clusters in brains [36]. In the present study, we chose individual p thresholded by 0.05 to determine significant cells/elements in the multiple-comparison matrices, which would resulted in individually significant segments with a series of SSL. Next we set a threshold of SSL to 3, so that individually significant segments with SSL smaller than 3 were considered as noise and removed from the test resulting matrices of the multiple comparisons. Consequently, these processes can achieve a desired overall multiple significance level, $P < 0.05$.

6 Results

Figure 1 shows comparisons of the nine small-world properties (C_g, γ, L_p, λ, E_{global}, $E^{real}_{global}/E^{random}_{global}$, E_{local} and $E^{real}_{local}/E^{random}_{local}$) between the pre- and post-task resting states, and their original values during each resting state as functions of sparsity ($0.05 \leq S \leq 0.46$). The gray lines represent the 95% confidence intervals over the range of sparsity. For C_g in Fig. 1(a), the hollow pentagram indicates a point of individually significant ($p < 0.05$) difference but could be regarded as a noise in terms of the present Monte-Carlo correction. All the insets show the original values of the nine small-world properties during each resting state. In all the insets, the red lines represent the post-task resting state (PoTRS) while the blue lines represent the pre-task resting state (PrTRS)). The followings are the results of the small-world analysis with respect to the different resting states.

6.1 Robust Small-World Topology during Task-Free and Task-Dependent Resting States

The graph analysis revealed that, during the pre- and post-task resting states, the brain functional networks had all small-world topological properties ($\gamma = C^{real}_g/C^{random}_g > 1$ shown in the inset of Fig. 1(a), $\lambda = L^{real}_p/L^{random}_p \approx 1$ shown in the inset of Fig. 1(b), and $\sigma = \gamma/\lambda > 1$ shown in the inset of Fig. 1(e)) with economical local and global information efficiency ($E^{real}_{global}/E^{random}_{global} \approx 1$ shown in the inset of Fig. 1(c), $E^{real}_{local}/E^{random}_{local} > 1$ shown in the inset of Fig. 1(d)) over a wide range of sparsity ($0.05 \leq S \leq 0.46$). These small-world results of brain intrinsic organization during the two resting states were quantitatively consistent with previous brain functional network studies at rest based on AAL-atlas [6, 9, 35] and voxels [10] and during a task based on voxels [8]. On the whole, the economical small-world configuration in spontaneous intrinsic organization was robust during resting states regardless of preceding task influences.

6.2 Stable Small-World Topology across Task-Unrelated and Task-Dependent Resting States

Paired t-tests were performed on the nine small-world parameters between the pre- and post-task resting states (Fig. 1) over the 42 sequential sparsity levels. The Monte-Carlo simulation was used for the multiple comparison correction. There was almost no significant difference in the small-world topological properties of spontaneous intrinsic organization between the two resting states. Though there was an individually significant difference point of clustering coefficient (C_g) at the sparsity of 0.15 (Fig. 1(a)), it could be considered as a random noise in terms of the Monte-Carlo correction over the wide range of sparsity. On the whole, the human brain intrinsic organization exhibited stable small-world properties during the different resting states.

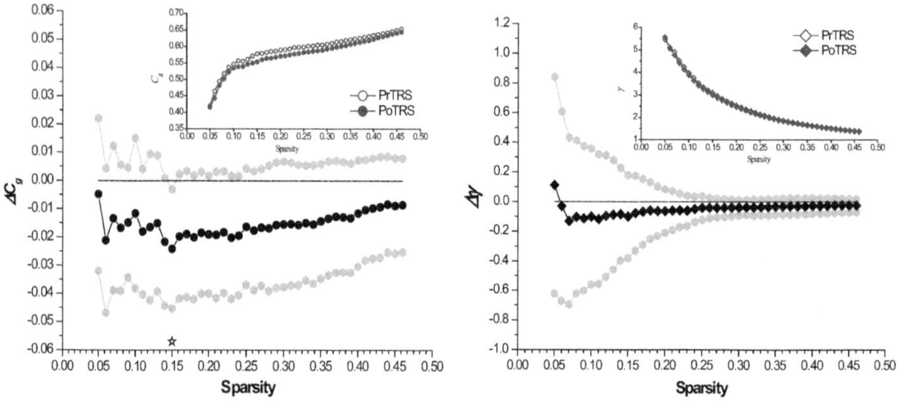

Fig. 1(a) Clustering coefficients (C_g) and ratios (γ)

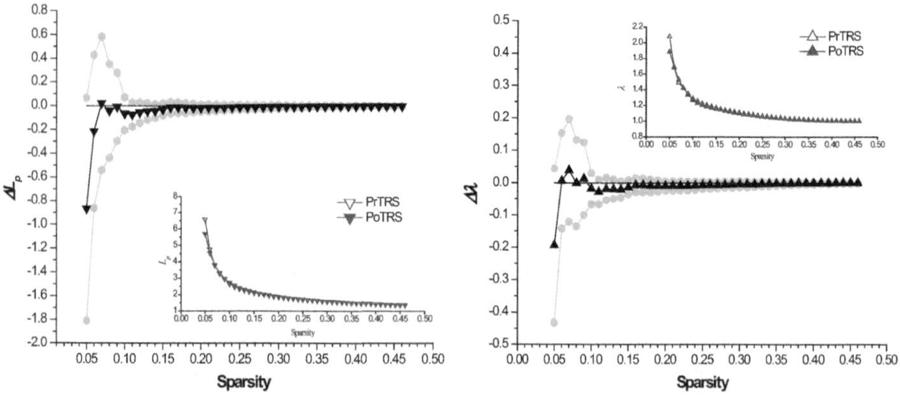

Fig. 1(b) Characteristic path distances (L_p) and ratios (λ)

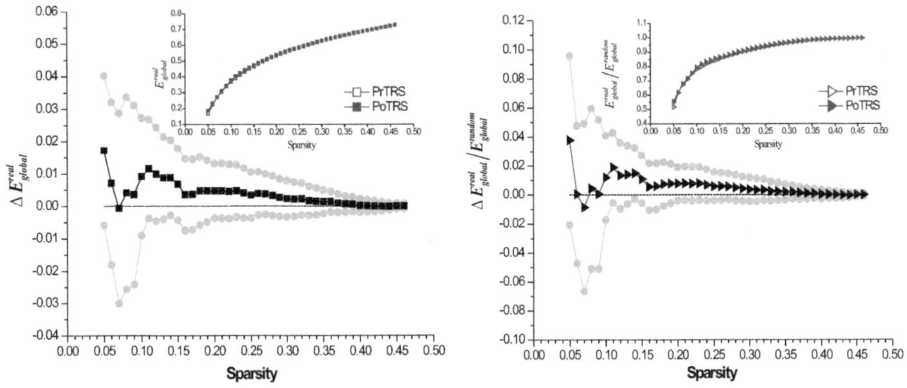

Fig. 1(c) Global information efficiencies (E_{global}) and ratios ($E_{global}^{real}/E_{global}^{random}$)

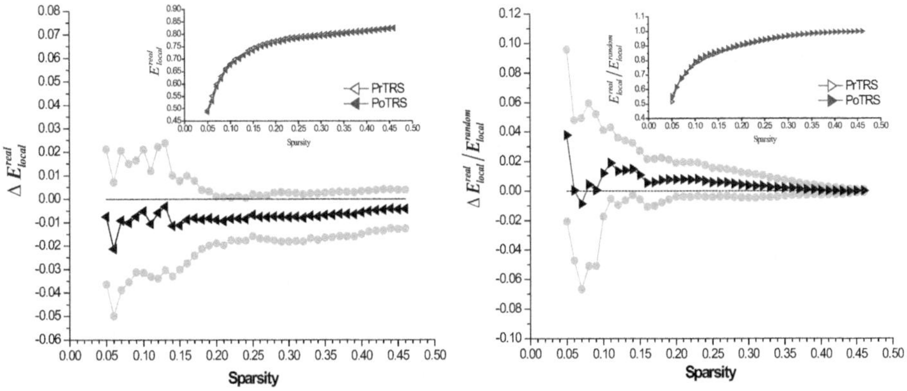

Fig. 1(d) Local information efficiencies (E_{local}) and ratios ($E_{local}^{real}/E_{local}^{random}$)

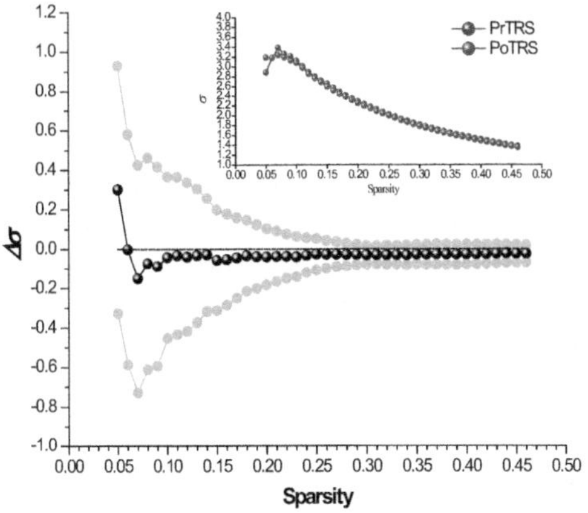

Fig. 1(e) Small-worldness (σ)

Fig. 1. Small-world analysis

7 Discussion

Functional connectivity serves a powerful approach to study the coupling mechanisms in brain intrinsic organization under different behavioral states. Previous resting-state brain functional network studies (AAL-based [6, 9, 35] and voxel-based [10]) demonstrated a small-world topology of the large-scale spontaneous intrinsic organization. Studies have revealed that the temporal coherence of spontaneous activity could be reshaped by learning effect during a post-task resting state within local spatial patterns, such as task-related and the default-mode networks [25–27]. However, to our best knowledge, it is still a lack of rigorous investigations that whether the small-world topology of spontaneous intrinsic organization remains robust and stable after influenced by a task. In the present study, we quantitatively investigated the preceding task influences on the small-world topology of brain intrinsic organization during the post-task resting state. We found that the small-world properties of brain intrinsic organization were robust and stable across the pre- and post-task resting states (Figure 1). That's to say, brain intrinsic organization maintains a robust and stable small-world configuration during resting states regardless of past-event influences.

Furthermore, functional segregation and integration are two fundamental organizational principles in brains [23, 24], which supports effective integration of multiple segregated sources of information over distributed cortical regions in real time [22] and a broad flexibility of cognitive processes (Sporns et al., 2004). As summarized by Rubinov and Sporns [39], clustering coefficient is a measure of functional segregation in the ability of specialized processing within densely interconnected groups of brain regions; while characteristic path distance is a measure of functional integration in the ability of rapidly combining specialized information from distributed brain regions. Hence, our results indicated that the post-task effect may not induce a modulation in the adaptive harmony balance between the local specialization and global integration of parallel information processing in brains.

However, does the topology of brain intrinsic organization during the pre-task resting state correspond to that during the post-task resting state? Future work should consider the issue, and we believe the answer is "no". Spontaneous intrinsic organization could have a slight reconfiguration of specific interregional connections related to past experiences underlying a tendency of a robust and stable global topology. The slight variability of intrinsic connectivity dependent on past experiences may be the critical driver for the evolution of brain organization.

Acknowledgments. The work is partially supported by the National Natural Science Foundation of China under Grant No.60875075 and Beijing Natural Science Foundation (No. 4102007).

References

1. Fox, M.D., Raichle, M.E.: Spontaneous fluctuations in brain activity observed with functional magnetic resonance imaging. Nat. Rev. Neurosci. 8, 700–711 (2007)
2. Raichle, M.E., Mintun, M.A.: Brain work and brain imaging. Annu. Rev. Neurosci. 29, 449–476 (2006)
3. Sporns, O., Chialvo, D.R., Kaiser, M., Hilgetag, C.C.: Organization, development and function of complex brain networks. Trends in Cognitive Sciences 8, 418–425 (2004)
4. Bassett, D.S., Bullmore, E.D.: Small-world brain networks. Neuroscientist 12, 512–523 (2006)
5. Bullmore, E.D., Sporns, O.: Complex brain networks: graph theoretical analysis of structural and functional systems. Nature Reviews Neuroscience 10, 186–198 (2009)
6. Salvador, R., Suckling, J., Coleman, M.R., Pickard, J.D., Menon, D., Bullmore, E.D.: Neurophysiological architecture of functional magnetic resonance images of human brain. Cereb. Cortex 15, 1332–1342 (2005a)
7. Salvador, R., Suckling, J., Schwarzbauser, C., Bullmore, E.D.: Undirected graphs of frequency-dependent functional connectivity in whole brain networks. Philos. Trans. R. Soc. Lond. B. Biol. Sci. 360, 937–946 (2005b)
8. Eguíluz, V.M., Chialvo, D.R., Cecchi, G.A., Baliki, M., Apkarian, A.V.: Scale-free brain functional networks. Phys. Rev. Lett. 94, 018102 (2005)
9. Achard, S., Salvador, R., Whitcher, B., Suckling, J., Bullmore, E.D.: A resilient, low-frequency, small-world human brain functional network with highly connected association cortical hubs. J. Neurosci. 26, 63–72 (2006)
10. Van den Heuvel, M.P., Stam, C.J., Boersma, M., Hulshoff Pol, H.E.: Small-world and scale-free organization of voxel-based resting-state functional connectivity in the human brain. Neuroimage 43, 528–539 (2008)
11. Stephan, K.E., Hilgetag, C.C., Burns, G.A.P.C., O'Neill, M.A., Young, M.P., Kö tter, R.: Computational analysis of functional connectivity between areas of primate cerebral cortex. Philos. Trans. R. Soc. Lond. B. Biol. Sci. 355, 111–126 (2000)
12. Micheloyannis, S., Pachou, E., Stam, C.J., Vourkas, M., Erimaki, S., Tsirka, V.: Using graph theoretical analysis of multi channel EEG to evaluate the neural efficiency hypothesis. Neuroscience Letters 402, 273–277 (2006)
13. Stam, C.J.: Functional connectivity patterns of human magnetoencephalographic recordings: a 'small-world' network? Neuroscience Letters 355, 25–28 (2004)
14. Bassett, D.S., Meyer-Lindenberg, A., Achard, S., Duke, T., Bullmore, E.: Adaptive reconfiguration of fractal small-world human brain functional networks. Proc. Natl. Acad. Sci. U.S.A. 103, 19518–19523 (2006)
15. Watts, D.J., Strogatz, S.H.: Collective dynamics of "small-world" networks. Nature 393, 440–442 (1998)
16. Sporns, O., Tononi, G., Edelman, G.M.: Theoretical neuroanatomy: relating anatomical and functional connectivity in graphs and cortical connection matrices. Cerebral Cortex 10, 127–141 (2000)
17. Hilgetag, C.C., Burns, G.A.P.C., O'Neill, M.A., Scannell, J.W.: Anatomical connectivity defines the organization of clusters of cortical areas in the macaque and the cat. Philos. Trans. R. Soc. Lond. B. Biol. Sci. 355, 91–110 (2000)
18. Latora, V., Marchiori, M.: Economic small-world behaviour in weighted networks. Euro. Phys. JB 32, 249–263 (2003)

19. Humphries, M.D., Gurney, K., Prescott, T.J.: The brainstem reticular formation is a small-world, not scale-free, network. Philos. Trans. R. Soc. Lond. B. Biol. Sci. 273, 503–511 (2006)

20. Hagmann, P., Kurant, M., Gigandet, X., Thiran, P., Wedeen, V.J., Meuli, R., Thiran, J.P.: Mapping the structural core of human cerebral cortex. PLoS ONE 2, e597 (2007)

21. Iturria-Medina, Y., Sotero, R.C., Canales-Rodriguez, E.J., Aleman-Gomez, Y., Melie-Garcia, L.: Studying the human brain ananatomical network via diffusion-weighted MRI and graph theory. NeuroImage 40, 1064–1076 (2008)

22. Sporns, O., Zwi, J.D.: The small world of the cerebral cortex. Neuroinformatics 2, 145–162 (2004)

23. Zeki, S., Shipp, S.: The functional logic of cortical connections. Nature 335, 311–317 (1988)

24. Tononi, G., Edelman, G.M., Sporns, O.: Complexity and coherency: integrating information in the brain. Trends in Cognitive Sciences 2, 474–484 (1998)

25. Waites, A.B., Stanislavsky, A., Abbott, D.F., Jackson, G.D.: Effect of prior cognitive state on resting state networks measured with functional connectivity. Human Brain Mapping 24, 59–68 (2005)

26. Albert, N.B., Robertson, E.M., Miall, R.C.: The resting human brain and motor learning. Curr. boil. 19, 1023–1027 (2009)

27. Lewis, G.M., Baldassarre, A., Committeri, G., Romania, G.L., Corbetta, M.: Learning sculpts the spontaneous activity of the resting human brain. Proc. Natl. Acad. Sci. U.S.A. 106, 17558–17563 (2009)

28. Wang, Z.J., Liu, J.M., Zhong, N., Qin, Y.L., Zhou, H.Y.: Two Perspectives to Investigate the Intrinsic Organization of the Dynamic and Ongoing Spontaneous Brain Activity in Humans. In: Proc. the 2010 International Joint Conference on Neural Networks (IJCNN 2010), pp. 1–4 (2010)

29. Zhou, H. Y., Liu, J. Y., Jing, W., Qin, Y.L., Lu, S.F., Yao, Y.Y., Zhong, N.: Basic level advantage and its switching during information retrieval: An fMRI study. In: Yao, Y., Sun, R., Poggio, T., Liu, J., Zhong, N., Huang, J. (eds.) BI 2010. LNCS, vol. 6334, pp. 427–436. Springer, Heidelberg (2010)

30. Tzourio-Mazoyer, N., Landeau, B., Papathanassiou, D., Crivello, F., Etard, O., Delcroix, N., Mazoyer, B., Joliot, M.: Automated anatomical labelling of activations in SPM using a macroscopic anatomical parcellation of the MNI MRI single-subject brain. Neuroimage 15, 273–289 (2002)

31. Fox, M.D., Snyder, A.Z., Vincent, J.L., Corbetta, M., Van Essen, D.C., Raichle, M.E.: The human brain is intrinsically organized into dynamic, anticorrelated functional networks. Proc. Natl. Acad. Sci. U.S.A. 102, 9673–9678 (2005)

32. Jenkins, G.M., Watts, D.G.: Spectral Analysis and Its Applications. Holden-Day, San Francisco (1968)

33. Newman, M.E.J.: The structure and function of complex networks. SIAM Rev. 45, 167–256 (2003)

34. Latora, V., Marchiori, M.: Efficient behaviour of small-world networks. Phys. Rev. Lett. 87, 198701 (2001)

35. Achard, S., Bullmore, E.: Efficiency and cost of economical brain functional networks. PLoS Comput. Biol. 3, e17(2007)
36. Ledberg, A., Akerman, S., Poland, P.F.: Estimation of the probabilities of 3D clusters in functional brain images. NeuroImage 8, 113–128 (1998)
37. Maslov, S., Sneppen, K.: Specificity and stability in topology of protein networks. Science 296, 910–913 (2002)
38. Milo, R., Shen-Orr, S., Itzkovitz, S., Kashtan, N., Chklovskii, D., Alon, U.: Network motifs: simple building blocks of complex networks. Science 298, 824–827 (2002)
39. Rubinov, M., Sporns, O.: Complex network measures of brain connectivity: Uses and interpretations. NeuroImage 52, 1059–1069 (2010)

Exploring Functional Connectivity Networks in fMRI Data Using Clustering Analysis

Dazhong Liu[1,2], Ning Zhong[1,3], and Yulin Qin[1]

[1] International WIC Institute,
Beijing University of Technology, Beijing China
[2] School of Mathematics and Computer Science,
Hebei University, Baoding China
[3] Dept. of Life Science and Informatics,
Maebashi Institute of Technology, Maebashi Japan
liudazhong@hbu.edu.cn, zhong@maebashi-it.ac.jp, yulinqin@gmail.com

Abstract. Some approaches have been proposed for exploring functional brain connectivity networks from functional magnetic resonance imaging (fMRI) data. Based on a popular algorithm K-means and an effective clustering algorithm called Affinity Propagation (AP), a combined clustering method to explore the functional brain connectivity networks is presented. In the proposed method, K-means is used for data reduction and AP is used for clustering. Without setting the seed of ROI in advance, the proposed method is especially appropriate for the analysis of fMRI data collected with a periodic experimental paradigm. The validity of the proposed method is illustrated by experiments on a simulated dataset and a human dataset. Receiver operating characteristic (ROC) analysis was performed on the simulated dataset. Results show that this method can efficiently and robustly detect the actual functional response with typical signal changes in the aspect of noise ratio, phase and amplitude. On the human dataset, the proposed method discovered brain networks which are compatible with the findings of previous studies.

1 Introduction

More recently, a new method is emerging in cognitive neuroscience that emphasizes the analysis of interactions within large-scale networks of brain areas. It focuses on exploring the structural and functional brain connectivity networks. The functional connectivity between two brain regions is defined as the temporal correlation between the brain region time courses, either in a resting state or when processing external stimuli [1, 2]. To find these networks from resting-state functional MRI (R-fMRI), many approaches such as ICA and PCA have been proposed [2, 3]. R-fMRI approaches are based on detecting temporally correlated patterns of low-frequency (< 0.1 Hz) fluctuations in the resting-state BOLD signal [4]. The technique has been proved to be a powerful tool for discovering connectivity network. The exploration of brain functional networks always begins with the choice of the seed region. However, inadequate seed region may lead

B. Hu et al. (Eds.): BI 2011, LNAI 6889, pp. 148–159, 2011.

to meaningless results. ICA need not choose some voxels as the seeds, and has been shown to be a promising data-driven method for the exploratory analysis of brain networks [3]. However, the method is limited to the linear mixture assumption [5]. In this study, we focus on another well-known data-driven method, unsupervised clustering methods. As a complement to the hypothesis-led statistical inferential methods, clustering methods have already been used in fMRI data analysis [6-13]. Few studies have investigated functional brain connectivity networks for subjects performing a given task using clustering methods. FMRI images are polluted by strong noises, such as subject movements, respiratory, heart artifacts and machine noise, hence BOLD signals in fMRI data has low signal-to-noise ratios (SNRs). Moreover, the whole brain datasets are usually very large with a very high dimensionality and a low sample size. This results in the detection and analysis of the BOLD effects being challenging.

To overcome these issues, we developed a completely data-driven approach combining two clustering methods for investigating the functional connectivity. Roughly speaking, it is a kind of two-stage clustering analysis (TSCA), and each clustering algorithm employs specific similarity measure. Every clustering method is appropriate for its corresponding situations. Being very easy and can deal with large data sets very quickly, K-means is used as the data reduction tool in the first stage. In the second stage, a new clustering approach named affinity propagation (AP) is selected as a refinement step. Because AP has several advantages of being able to avoid the a priori definition of the cluster number and the flexibility definition in similarity measure [14]. To test the TSCA method, Receiver operating characteristic (ROC) analysis was performed on the simulated dataset. Then, the method was applied to real data sets with a block-designed auditory task.

This paper is organized as follows. In Section 2, we introduce the dataset used in our experiment, define the similarity measure, and describe our method. K-means and AP are also reviewed. In Section 3, experimental results of the proposed approach are given. Finally, Section 4 gives discussion and concluding remarks.

2 Materials and Methods

2.1 Overview of K-Means and Affinity Propagation

K-means is regarded as one of the most popular clustering methods. K-means needs prescribed number of clusters at first, and then the algorithm will iteratively seek best partition of the data according to an optimal within-class inertia criterion [6, 15, 16]. The basic procedure of K-means is summarized as follows:

Given sample sets $D=\{x_1,..., x_n\}$, initialize K clusters $\{C_1,..,C_K\}$, $d(r_j, x)$ represents distance metric between the cluster center and the data vector.

Repeat
  % form clusters:
  for $k = 1, ..., K$

$C_k = \{x \in D \mid d(r_k, x) \leq d(r_j, x)$ for all $j = 1, ..., K, j \neq k\}$;
end;
% calculate the new center:
for k = 1, ..., K do
r_k = average vector of C_k
end;
Until C_k is stable.

K-means converges very fast and can deal with large-scale data sets easily.

AP has been applied to explore the problem of images of faces, detect genes in microarray data, airline travel etc [14, 17, 18]. AP has the power of using unusual measures of similarity which do not satisfy metric space conditions, and it can reach a small number of clusters automatically without a prior designated cluster number. This makes it suitable for exploratory data analysis. AP regards initially all the samples as potential exemplars, and then recursively refines this set by transmitting real-valued messages to minimize an energy function until a good set of exemplars and relative clusters emerge. The similarity matrix S and preferences parameters are taken as input. In general, for points x_i and x_k, $s(i,k) = -||x_i - x_k||^2$. The values $s(i,i)$ (that is, the diagonal entry) are set with a larger value to have a higher preference of being chosen as an exemplar. To produce a low number of clusters, one assign minimum similarities equal weights to all cluster centers. There are two kinds of message (i.e. responsibility$r(i,k)$ and availability $a(i,k)$) exchanged between data points. The responsibility $r(i,k)$, reflects the accumulated evidence for how point k suitably acts as the exemplar for point i. The availability $a(i,k)$ reflects the accumulated evidence for how fitting it would be for point i to choose point k as its exemplar.

Pseudo-code of the algorithm [14]:
Initially, the availabilities are set to be zero: $a(i,k) = 0$.
Repeat
Updating the responsibilities:

$$r(i,k) = s(i,k) - \max_{j:j \neq k}\{a(i,j) + s(i,j)\} \tag{1}$$

Updating the availabilities and the self-availability:

$$a(i,k) = \min\{0, r(k,k) + \sum_{j \notin \{i,k\}} \max\{0, r(j,k)\}\}; \tag{2}$$

$$a(k,k) = \sum_{j:j \neq k} \max\{0, r(j,k)\}. \tag{3}$$

Until the cluster centers stay constant for a fixed number of iterations.

The exemplars are identified by combined availabilities and responsibilities. For point i, the value of k that maximizes $a(i,k) + r(i,k)$ either identifies point i as an exemplar if $k = i$, or identifies the data point that is the exemplar for point i. After a fixed number of iterations or the messages fall below a threshold, the procedure may be terminated. It can be observed that a measure of similarity is a critical factor. We will give the similarity measure derived for fMRI datasets in the next subsection.

2.2 Proposed Analysis Methods

The purpose of this work is to discover functional brain connectivity networks in the block task design experimental paradigms, in which blocks of the task alternate with blocks of rest, or control in a periodic manner. In reaction to the experimental stimulus, some brain regions will change in the same periodic manner more or less. To explore this BOLD effect signals, a kind of two-stage clustering analysis (TSCA) was applied. It consists of two clustering algorithms K-means and AP, and each clustering algorithm employs specific similarity measure. Every clustering method is appropriate for its corresponding situations. For real dataset, preprocessing step was undertaken to enhance signals while suppressing noise. The low frequency components and polynomial drifts were removed for each voxel. The entire program was implemented using Matlab and SPM5 toolbox (http://www.fil.ion.ucl.ac.uk/spm/ext/). In this work, we used SPM5 to preprocess (realignment, normalization/registration and smoothing) the fMRI sequences. After that, a new 4-D dataset is obtained by calculating the autocovariance value series (AVS) of each voxel. Autocovariance value of voxel k is defined as follows:

$$R_l\left(k\right) = E\{\left(x_{n+l}\left(k\right) - \mu\left(k\right)\right)\left(x_n\left(k\right) - \mu\left(k\right)\right)\} \tag{4}$$

where $\{x_n(k)\}$ represents fMRI time series in the dataset, n is the time point,$\mu(k)$ denotes the mean values of time series for voxel k, and l is a lag time point [19].

The AVS of random noise has the feature that it decays rapidly as the lag increases, while the AVS of stimulus response signal decays slowly and will be periodic if the signal is periodic. K-means just uses the Euclidean-based distance of AVS of each voxel to partition the dataset into some groups. The AVS of random noise is quite different from that of periodic signal and can be distinguished easily. Other than the opposite situation, there are some vague series in the data set because of smoothing step or other reasons. Hence, initial cluster of K-means is set to be three. K-means is used to pick up the periodic response regions. For the next stage, AP is used to further partition the group with the fewest voxels, and explore the phases or amplitude of the signal in detail. Appropriate similarity measure plays a critical role in AP clustering. Given two fMRI voxels $i$and k, their similarity $s(i,k)$ is defined as follows:

$$d\left(i,k\right) = ||x_n(i) - x_n(k)||^2; s\left(i,k\right) = -exp(d\left(i,k\right)). \tag{5}$$

The procedure of the two stage clustering analysis method TSCA summarized in Fig.1.

Why should we use the two clustering algorithm? On the one hand, the whole brain 4-D dataset is quite large, and if AP is used solely, the similarity matrix will consume all the computer memory, while the K-means is not memory demanding. On the other hand, if we only use K-means, we can not determine

Preprocessing step using SPM5:
  Including: realignment, normalization/registration and smoothing;
Calculating AVS of the whole brain time series using (4);
Clustering AVS using K-means with the Euclidean-based distance measure;
Selecting the smallest group G, discovered by K-means;
Clustering the group G using AP with the similarity defined in (5);
Mapping the groups on the structure brain map.

Fig. 1. Proposed two-stage clustering method

the proper clustering number and the similarity measure is constrained by K-means. Therefore, we first use K-means to perform data reduction for reducing the sensitivity to noise, and then AP is used to explore the details of the brain activity.

2.3 Datasets

Simulated fMRI Data. To evaluate the properties of this method, fully artificially fMRI phantom was constructed similar to the one described by Yang J. et al [20]. The simulated dataset was constructed with three small activation foci of 21 voxels each. Three kinds of box-car like pattern signals with different period and amplitude were generated and added on each location. To simulate the actual situation, all the three kind of signals convolved with the hemodynamic response function (HRF) of SPM sampled at TP = 2 s, baseline Gaussian noise of zero mean value was added to the background, in which the noise deviation within the range of the SNR of real fMRI data varies from 0.2 to 3.5 corresponding to SNR from 0.93 to 0.22 [21]. All the length of the time series is 200.

Real fMRI Data. We illustrated our approach on a typical dataset: an auditory dataset from the Wellcome Department of Imaging Neuroscience of the University College London (http://www.fil.ion.ucl.ac.uk/spm/data/). Data were acquired on a on a modified 2T Siemens MAGNETOM Vision system. Functional images were collected using a gradient EPI pulse sequence with the following parameters: TR = 7 s; matrix size = 64x64x64 (3mm x 3mm x 3mm voxels). A T1-weighted high-resolution (1mm x 1mm x 1mm) scan was also required for anatomical reference and segmentation purpose. This data set was the first ever collected and analyzed in the Functional Imaging Laboratory. Each acquisition consisted of 64 contiguous slices. Acquisition took 6.05s, providing whole-brain coverage. A single subject participated in this study. The experiment consists of 96 acquisitions in blocks of 6 (42 seconds), giving 16 42s blocks.

The paradigm consisted of eight repeated cycles of rest and auditory stimulation, starting with rest. During stimulating states, the participant was presented with auditory stimuli with bi-syllabic words presented binaurally at a rate of 60 per minute. The functional data starts at acquisition 4. To avoid T1 effects in the initial scans of an fMRI time series, just as the Statistical Parametric Mapping SPM manual (http://www.fil.ion.ucl.ac.uk/spm/data/) suggested, the first complete cycle (12 scans) was discarded, leaving 84 scans to analyze.

3 Results

3.1 Results with Synthetic Data Set

We tested our analysis method on the synthetic fMRI data with different SNRs. Gaussian noise with standard deviation varying from 0.2 to 3.5 was added to the signal, which results in the SNR of the simulated data changing from 0.93 to 0.22. The data was smoothed spatially as commonly done for fMRI (FWHM = 4.5 mm = 1.5 voxel) at the preprocessing step, and then a cluster number was set for the K-means clustering stage. To evaluate the properties of our method, the most widely used receiver operating characteristic (ROC) analysis was performed on the dataset. ROC curve can be used to assess performance of method and determine the criterion for different conditions according to true-positive ratio versus false-positive ratio (i.e. sensitivity versus 1-specificity) at each point of the curve. Sensitivity is proportion of correctly detected from all added signals, and specificity is proportion of correctly recognized regions other than added signal regions. ROC curve are plotted under different thresholds by taking sensitivity as its y axis and 1-specificity as its x axis. Because we knew the locations and the sizes of the voxels of added signals, we were able to determine the true positive rate, and the false-positive rate at each threshold. An ideal algorithm would detect signals with 100% sensitivity and 100% specificity, and therefore its

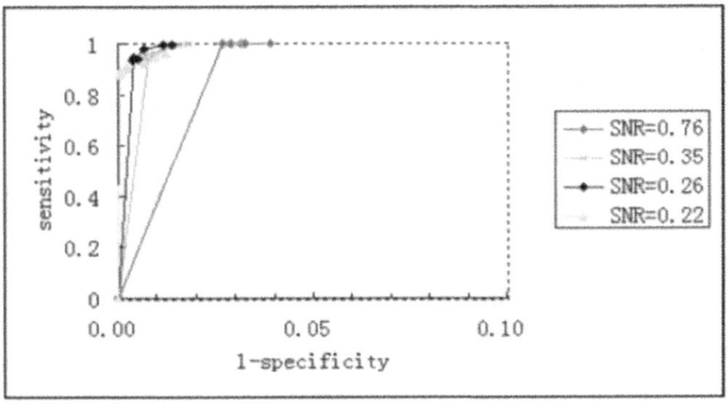

Fig. 2. ROC curves under SNR=0.76, 0.24 and 0.22 with K-means cluster numbers changing from 3 to 8

ROC curve would be closest to upper left corner of the plot. In the same way as [7], we chosen the K-means cluster number varied from 3 to 8 as the threshold. We perform the test at four noise levels, and the SNR are 0.76, 0.35, 0.26 and 0.22, respectively. The level SNR = 0.22 is the noisiest. The results are shown in Fig. 2. From the results, it can be seen that the ROC curve all pass near the upper left corner of the plot. In the condition of SNR = 0.76, the true-positive ratio is 1 with lower false-positive ratio, whose mean and standard deviation was 0.031±0.004. The performance of others have the true-positive ratio near 1 and quit lower false-positive ratio similar to SNR = 0.76. Each of the area under ROC curve (AUC) is greater than 0.979. An area of 1 means a perfect test. The plot also shows that the performance of the proposed method is not sensitive to the K-means cluster numbers. Therefore, we can choose the small number, say, three as the K-means cluster number.

3.2 Results with Human Data Set

For the real auditory fMRI data, we tested it on the whole brain time series (4-D) to illustrate the results. Initially, the real data sets were preprocessed just as presented in Section 2.2. In the analysis, SPM5 was used as a preprocessing tool. After the pre-processing steps, the two stage clustering analysis was carried out. The clustering groups are shown in Fig. 3. and Fig. 4 by using xjView (http://www.alivelearn.net/xjview/). In the first stage, K-means produced three groups, with 50626, 2426 and 12708 voxels in each group. The least group was further analyzed by AP and another three groups were acquired with 192, 1989 and 245 voxels in each group. To analyze further the three groups, the time series of each group is shown in Fig. 5. The orange group with 1989 voxels mainly

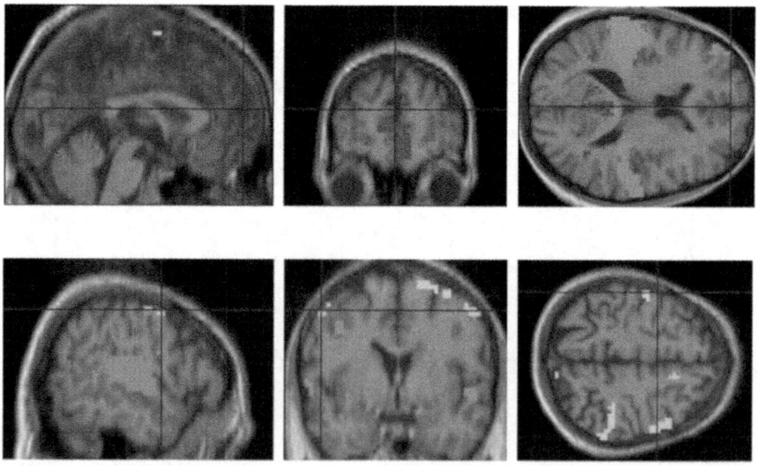

Fig. 3. The brain sagittal, coronal, and axial overlay maps of clustering results with z = 15 in top row and z = 51 in the bottom row

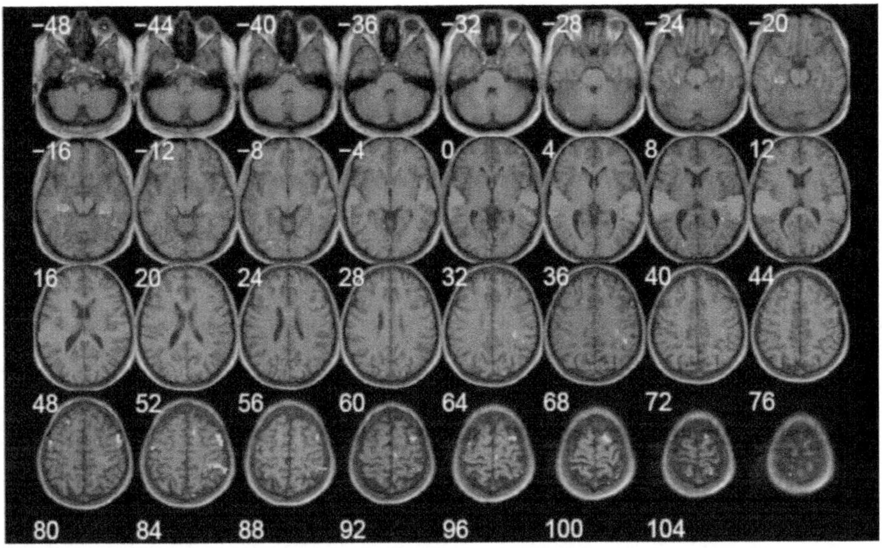

Fig. 4. The transaxial view of the three groups overlaid on the structural images

includes primary and association auditory cortices, the superior temporal gyrus and posterior insular. The blue group with 192 voxels mainly includes medial prefrontal cortex (MPFC), posterior cingulate cortex (PCC). The green group with 245 voxels mainly includes the frontal eye field (FEF), inferior parietal cortex. From Fig. 5, the time series of orange group is coherent with the box-car paradigm, the blue group time series and the box-car paradigm have opposite phase and the green group time series is coherent with the box-car paradigm in the first five blocks. From the two aspects, the blue group is the default mode network [22-24]; the green group belongs to the dorsal attention network [25-27]. The orange group is auditory network [28]. The TSCA discovered three networks at the same time.

4 Discussions and Conclusions

In this paper, a completely data-driven combined method was applied in exploratory functional connectivity analysis. Of course the combining strategy can be usually found in the area of data mining and machine learning. To our best knowledge, K-means and AP unified method has not been employed. In the proposed method, the initial cluster number for K-means was decided by domain knowledge, and we need not denote a cluster number for AP. The similarities used in AP do not necessarily satisfy the triangle inequality, however the similarity matrix will consume the memory for the 4-D fMRI dataset. Hence, data reduction should be adopted. K-means can be used solely in cascaded manner with two distance measures and two initial cluster number considered. Using the method, the default mode network (DMN) was discovered under task-induced

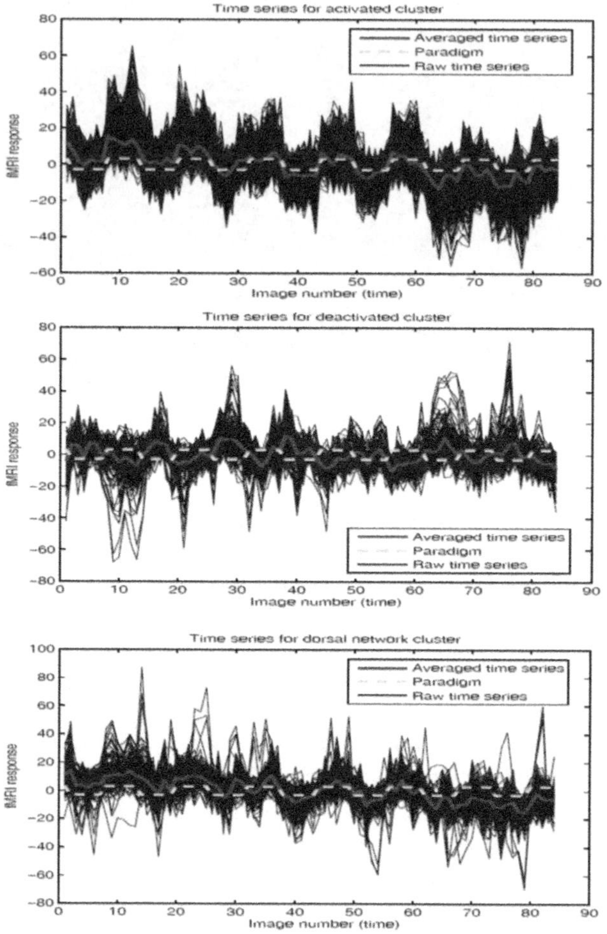

(a)

(b)

(c)

Fig. 5. The raw time series of members of one group were drawn in blue lines. The average time series of the raw time series of one group were drawn in thick red line. The yellow dashed line denotes box-car stimulus waveform. (a) The orange group; (b) The blue group; (c) The green group.

condition. DMN has been recently studied in the resting-state functional MRI (R-fMRI) [29]. In TSCA, the seed selection is not needed. On the other hand, the method needs not to choose HRF used in the model based method. The model free methods are always considered as a necessary complement to the hypothesis-led statistical inferential methods. Recently, supervised method (brain reading) has been applied in fMRI dataset. It emphasizes on cognitive state classification according to brain dataset [30-34]. Different from the supervised method, clustering method is considered as the unsupervised method trying to seek brain activity property under some cognitive states.

There are several works to do, including seeking the new data reduction strategy, confirming the method using many more real datasets, and functional connectivity presentation in future.

Acknowledgments. The work is supported by the National Natural Science Foundation of China under Grant No. 60875075, 60905027, and the Beijing Natural Science Foundation under Grant No. 4102007.

References

1. Friston, K.J., Frith, C.D., Liddle, P.F., Frackowiak, R.S.J.: Functional connectivity. The Principal Component Analysis of Large (PET) Data sets. J. Cereb. Blood Flow Metab. 13, 5–14 (1993)
2. Bressler, S.L., Menon, V.: Large-scale Brain Networks in Cognition. Emerging Methods and Principles. Trends in Cognitive Sciences 14(6), 277–290 (2010)
3. Zuo, X.-n., Kelly, C., Adelstein, J.S., Klein, D.F., Castellanos, F.X., Milham, M.P.: Reliable Intrinsic Connectivity Networks: Test – Retest Evaluation Using ICA and Dual Regression Approach. NeuroImage 49(3), 2163–2177 (2010)
4. Ogawa, S., Lee, T.M., Kay, A.R., Tank, D.W.: Brain Magnetic Resonance Imaging with Contrast Dependent on Blood Oxygenation. Proceedings of the National Academy of Sciences 87, 9868–9872 (1990)
5. Meyer-baese, A., Wismueller, A., Lange, O.: Comparison of Two Exploratory Data Analysis Methods for fMRI: Unsupervised Clustering versus Independent Component Analysis. IEEE Transactions on Information Technology in Biomedicine 8(3), 387–398 (2004)
6. Goutte, C., Toft, P., Rostrup, E., Nielsen, F.A., Hansen, L.K.: On Clustering fMRI Time Series. NeuroImage 9, 298–310 (1999)
7. Chuang, K., Chiu, M., Lin, C.C., Chen, J.: Model-free Functional MRI Analysis Using Kohonen Clustering Neural Network and Fuzzy C-means. IEEE Transactions on Medical Imaging 18, 1117–1128 (1999)
8. Baumgartner, R., Ryner, L., Richter, W., Summers, R., Jarmasz, M., Somorjai, R.: Comparison of Two Exploratory Data Analysis Methods for fMRI.: Fuzzy Clustering vs. Principal Component Analysis. Magnetic Resonance in Medicine 18, 89–94 (2000)
9. McKeown, M.J., Makeig, S., Brown, G.G., Jung, T.P., Kindermann, S.S., Bell, A.J., Spjnowski, T.J.: Analysis of fMRI Data by Blind Separation into Independent Spatial Components. Human Brain Mapping 6, 160–188 (1998)
10. Dimitriadou, E., Barth, M., Windischberger, C., Hornik, K., Moser, E.: A Quantitative Comparison of Functional MRI Cluster Analysis. Artificial Intelligence in Medicine 31, 57–71 (2004)

11. Fadili, M.J., Ruan, S., Bloyet, D., Mazoyer, B.: A Multistep Unsupervised Fuzzy Clustering Analysis of fMRI Time Series. Human Brain Mapping 10, 160–178 (2000)
12. Bandettini, P.A., Jesmanowicz, A., Wong, E.C., Hyde, J.S.: Processing Strategies for Time-course Data Sets in Functional MRI of the Human Brain. Magnetic Resonance in Medicine 30(2), 161–173 (1993)
13. Ye, J., Lazar, N.A., Li, Y.: Geostatistical Analysis in Clustering fMRI Time Series. Statistics in Medicine 28(19), 2490–2508 (2009)
14. Frey, B.J., Dueck, D.: Clustering by Passing Messages between Data Points. Science 315(5814), 972–976 (2007)
15. Duda, R.O., Hart, P.E.: Pattern Classification and Scene Analysis, pp. 189–225. John Wiley & Sons, New York (1973)
16. Wu, X., Kumar, V., Quinlan, J.R., Ghosh, J., Yang, Q., Motoda, H., et al.: Top 10 Algorithms in Data Mining. Knowledge and Information Systems, 1–37 (2008)
17. Sun, C., Wang, Y., Zhao, H.: Web Page Clustering via Partition Adaptive Affinity Propagation. In: Yu, W., He, H., Zhang, N. (eds.) ISNN 2009. LNCS, vol. 5552, pp. 727–736. Springer, Heidelberg (2009)
18. Li, C., Dou, L., Yu, S., Liu, D., Lin, Y.: Magnetic Resonance Image Segmentation Based on Affinity Propagation. In: Global Congress on Intelligent Systems, pp. 456–460 (2009)
19. Maas, L.C., Frederick, B.D., Yurgelun-Todd, D.A., Renshaw, P.F.: Autocovariance Based Analysis of Functional MRI Data. Biological Psychiatry 39, 640–641 (1996)
20. Yang, J., Zhong, N., Liang, P.P., Wang, J., Yao, Y.Y., Lu, S.F.: Brain Activation Detection by Neighborhood One-class SVM. In: Proceedings of the 2007 IEEE/WIC/ACM International Conferences on Web Intelligence and Intelligent Agent Technology – Workshops, pp. 47–51 (2007)
21. Friston, K.J.: Statistical Parametric Mapping.: The Analysis of Functional Brain Images. Academic Press, London (2006)
22. Buckner, R.L., Andrews-Hanna, J.R., Schacter, D.L.: The Brain's Default Network Anatomy, Function, and Relevance to Disease. New York Academy of Sciences 38, 1–38 (2008)
23. Fransson, P.: Spontaneous Low-frequency BOLD Signal Fluctuations: an FMRI Investigation of the Resting-state Default Mode of Brain Function Hypothesis. Hum. Brain Mapp. 26(1), 15–29 (2005)
24. Raichle, M., MacLeod, A., Snyder, A.: A default Mode of Brain Function. PNAS 98(2) (2001)
25. Mantini, D., Corbetta, M., Gianni, M., Luca, G., Del, C.: Large-scale Brain Networks Account for Sustained and Transient Activity During Target Detection. NeuroImage 44(1), 265–274 (2009)
26. Griffiths, T.D., Rees, G., Rees, A., Green, G.G.R., Witton, C., Rowe, D., et al.: Right Parietal Cortex is Involved in the Perception of Sound Movement in Humans. Nature Neuroscience 1(1) (1998)
27. Griffiths, T.D., Green, G.G.R., Rees, A., Rees, G.: Human Brain Areas Involved in the Analysis of Auditory Movement. Human Brain Mapping 9, 72–80 (2000)
28. Wise, R.J.S., Greene, J., Büchel, C., Scott, S.K.: Early Report Brain Regions Involved in Articulation. The Lancet 353, 1057–1061 (1999)

29. Biswal, B.B., Mennes, M., Zuo, X.-n., Gohel, S., Kelly, C., Smith, S.M., et al.: Toward Discovery Science of Human Brain Function. Proceedings of the National Academy of Sciences 107(10) (2009)
30. Haynes, J.-D., Rees, G.: Decoding Mental States from Brain Activity in Humans. Neuroscience 7, 523–534 (2006)
31. Mitchell, T.M., Shinkareva, S.V., Carlson, A., Chang, K.-m., Malave, V.L., et al.: Predicting Human Brain Activity Associated with the Meanings of Nouns. Science 320, 1191–1195 (2008)
32. Mitchell, T.O.M., Hutchinson, R., Niculescu, R.S., Pereira, F., Wang, X.: Learning to Decode Cognitive States from Brain Images. Machine Learning 57, 145–175 (2004)
33. Golland, Y., Golland, P., Bentin, S., Malach, R.: Data-driven Clustering Reveals a Fundamental Subdivision of the Human Cortex into Two Global Systems. Neuropsychologia 46, 540–553 (2008)
34. Chai, B., Walther, D., Beck, D.: Exploring Functional Connectivity of the Human Brain Using Multivariate Information Analysis. In: Neural Information, NIPS, pp. 1–9 (2009)

An Efficient Method for Odor Retrieval

Tsuyoshi Takayama[1], Shigeru Kikuchi[2], Yoshitoshi Murata[1], Nobuyoshi Sato[1], and Tetsuo Ikeda[3]

[1] Graduate School of Software and Information Science, Iwate Prefectural University
152-52, Sugo, Takizawa-Mura, Iwate020-0193, Japan
{takayama,y-murata,nobu-s}@iwate-pu.ac.jp
[2] F & B Solution Business Division, Ad-Sol Nissin Corp.
4-1-8, Kounan, Minato-Ku, Tokyo108-0075, Japan
Kikuchi.Shigeru@adniss.jp
[3] Administration and Informatics, University of Shizuoka
52-1, Yada, Suruga, Shizuoka, Shizuoka422-8526, Japan
t-ikeda@u-shizuoka-ken.ac.jp

Abstract. Recently, researchers have been increasingly interested in odor database retrieval using the sense of smell. However, it has two difficulties; different from sight- or hearing-sense database retrieval. One is that odor scientists have not yet been able to find a base component of odor, such as RGB or frequency. Therefore, smell-sense database retrieval cannot be conducted using a physical quantity. The other is that relevance tests of each retrieval result require a larger load. Conventional approaches have represented an odor by either a noun or impression word. It is more feasible if a user can efficiently obtain the relevant retrieval results by employing both nouns and impression words such as 'odor like slightly sweet coffee'. In this paper, we propose such an efficient method.

Keywords: Multimedia database, odor retrieval, impression-based retrieval.

1 Introduction

1.1 Characteristics of Odors and Smell Sense

Based on the studies [1]-[3], there exist a few hundred thousand types of odors in our world, of which an average human can sense about forty thousand. Odors and smell sense have several characteristics, compared to the sense of sight or hearing.

Characteristic 1: When an odor is present comprising a mixture of multiple elements, a human's sense of smell has a limited ability to distinguish them.

Generally, a single image contains some elements such as a human, an object, or a background. Moreover, in the case of sound, an orchestral piece contains the sounds of many kinds of instruments. It is not very difficult for a human to distinguish individual components in images or sounds. This is not the case for odors. Therefore, to simplify matters in the present study, we assumed that an odor originates from a single source. Under this assumption we have the following characteristics:

B. Hu et al. (Eds.): BI 2011, LNAI 6889, pp. 160–172, 2011.

Characteristic 2: Representing an actual sample is easier utilizing a single noun than in the case of an image or sound.

On the other hand,:

Characteristic 3: An odor can often be represented by an adjective.

When the phrase 'sweet odor' is used, it can pertain to a variety of situations, such as an odor like a 'rose', 'banana', or 'mother's perfume'. The methodology to classify them, however, has not yet been established. The paper [1][4] have empirically demonstrated the first instance of olfactory illusions created by words alone. More specifically,

Characteristic 4: Although odor scientists have tried to find a base element of odors fitting to theory and reality, it has remained elusive.

The next characteristic is a feature of odor.

Characteristic 5: Odor has the ability to improve the taste of food.

The following three characteristics (6–8) are negative aspects of odor.

Characteristic 6: The monetary cost of work related to odor is often high.

Characteristic 7: The sense of smell is easily fatigued.

Characteristic 8: When we continuously smell multiple odors, it is not always easy to eliminate the influence of the previously smelled odor.

1.2 Related Work

Many related studies have attempted to automatically recognize various odors and minimize human sensory testing[5]. The target areas of these studies include cosmetics, perfumes, beverage industries, environmental monitoring, food quality assessment, and medical diagnosis. Kwon *et al.* improve discrimination precision by employing neural networks[6]. Loutfi *et al.* propose an integration of an odor sensor with that of other visual or sound sensors. Their main target is a mobile robot, and they are able to detect a peripheral situation using a multi-sensor[5]. Yamada *et al.* propose and evaluate an olfactory display. If the user determines his/her position and an odor source, the corresponding odor is presented[7].

Conventional research has not been sufficient in the discussion of an odor database retrieval method. As one of the directions, several researchers have attempted to define an adequate impression word group. The study by Bannai *et al.*[8] is a typical example of this attempt and uses a membership value, from 0.0 to 1.0, for sixteen impression words. This method provides a retrieval condition using a single impression word without any value, and determines the most relevant odor and the second relevant one, based on the membership value. The common problem with this type of approach is that efficiency is insufficient, because no method exists that can select a noun or impression value as a specification method of the retrieval condition.

1.3 Study Purpose

The purpose of the present study is to propose an efficient method which allows a user to specify a retrieval condition using both a noun and impression value. Hereafter, based on the work by Katayose *et al.*[9], we treat 'retrieval by adjective' as 'retrieval by impression word'. We, hereafter, also refer to an odor sample simply as 'sample'. In the present study, for simplicity, we do not discuss odor composition[7], and set the output of a retrieval operation to an sample ID.

The rest of this paper is organized as follows. First, in Section 2, we generate noun and impression word groups for odor database retrieval, and determine a noun and impression value representing each sample. In Section 3, the main part of this paper, we propose a retrieval method able to specify a retrieval condition by both the noun and impression value. We introduce our preliminary system, and carry out an evaluation experiment in Section 4. Finally, in Section 5, we conclude our paper.

2 Generation of Noun and Impression Word Groups

In this section, we generate noun and impression word groups for specifying a retrieval condition. We also determine a noun and impression value representing each sample. Both of these are accomplished based on experiments using subjects and 101 different samples, including aromatics, teas, coffees, and spices.

2.1 1st Experiment: Generation of Noun and Impression Word Groups

Experiment Method. Thirty-one subjects (twenty-three men, and eight women; age range: 18–51 years) participated in the study. Each subject was instructed to smell each sample and write at least one noun and one adjective representing its odor. The number of subjects per sample was three, the reasoning for which is described in the following section. We process the obtained noun group as follows. If a certain noun occurs only once throughout the entire experiment, we exclude it from the noun group; it is considered to not be a noun commonly used to represent odor. We process the obtained adjective group as follows:

Step 1: If a certain adjective occurs only once throughout the entire experiment, we also exclude it, because it is not commonly used to describe odor.

Step 2: We reduce the remaining adjective group based on the study by Kumamoto *et al.*[10]. More specifically, we first use dictionaries to make an adjective set that contains words with similar meanings. Next, if there are two adjectives that have opposite meanings, we adopt them as a bipolar rating scale. In order to make the bipolar rating scale, we attempt to find a counterpart for an adjective from a dictionary. If an adjective has multiple counterparts that have different meanings or no counterpart, we adopt it as a monopole rating scale.

Experiment Result. A part of the noun table determined for each sample is shown in Table 1. For example, for sample ID = 2, 'soda' and 'lime' are adopted as a result of the reduction phase. We obtained a total of 66 types of nouns. For each sample, a mean number (2.89) of nouns were determined. Increasing the number of subjects to five per sample, we have obtained 67 types of nouns. Since 66 is 98.5% of 67, we concluded that sufficient types of nouns were obtained from three subjects per sample.

Table 1. A part of a noun table determined for each sample

ID	name	Noun					
1	maisyarudan kaorinokanzume lime	apple	lime	orange	lemon	lemon	orange
2	oheyano syousyuuriki ajianhabu 400ml	soda	lime	soda	(null)	(null)	(null)
3	bikkara apple	fragrant olive	peach	mint	lemon	(null)	(null)
...	...	...	...	...	...	...	...

The ten impression-rating scales adopted for the present study are shown in Table 2, and include six monopole and four bipolar scales. Increasing the number of subjects to five per sample gave similar results. Thus, we concluded that sufficient impression-rating scales were obtained from three subjects per sample.

Table 2. Ten impression-rating scales adopted for the present study

Monopole	Bipolar
sweet	grassy -- fragrant
sour	warm -- cool
bitter	hard -- soft
salty	refreshing -- discomfort
pungent	
astringent	

2.2 2nd Experiment: Determination of Impression Values

Experiment Method. The subjects were identical to those the participated in the first experiment. We set an impression value in a bipolar rating scale to seven levels in the same manner as that by Ikezoe *et al.*[11]. In this scale, the center '0' indicates 'neutral', and '+3' and '−3' each indicate the most extreme situations. For a monopole axis, we only use the positive side of the bipolar rating scale. Three subjects per sample provide impression values.

From the results of a preliminary experiment, providing impression values to odor samples differs from that for music[11]. More specifically, there are many cases when impression values of odor samples are not adequately represented by an impression axis. As a solution, we introduce 'N.A. (not adequate)' in addition to the seven impression values. Subjects were instructed to provide one impression value from the seven levels per sample on at least two axes from the possible ten.

We determine each impression value of a sample in the following manner. If half or more of the subjects assign 'N.A.' on an axis to a sample, we determine that its impression value is 'null'. Otherwise, we calculate the median of all data on each axis for a sample, round the median off to the nearest integer, and exclude outlying values.

Experiment Result. A part of the impression value table is shown in Table 3. The mean number (4.56) of impression values was determined. Increasing the number of subjects to five per sample changed the width of the impression value to within one from that obtained using three subjects at a ratio of 85.4%. Although we cannot conclude that three subjects per sample is perfect, it is not insufficient.

Table 3. A part of impression value table determined for each sample

ID	Name	Sweet	…	Grassy--fragrant	…	Refreshing--discomfort
1	maisyarudan kaorinokanzume lime	1	…	--3	…	0
2	oheyano syousyuuriki ajianhabu 400 ml	2	…	--1	…	--2
3	bikkara apple	1	…	--1	…	--2
…	…	…	…	…	…	…

3 Proposed Efficient Method

In this section, we first introduce four methods for relative comparison. Subsequently, based on the four methods, we describe our proposed method.

3.1 Methods for Relative Comparison

Method 1: Retrieval Method Using Only Noun (1) – 'NM(Noun Median) Method'. This method shows a page including selectable nouns on the screen(Fig. 1). If a user selects one of them, this method generates a retrieval result based on a distance from the point which corresponds to the selected noun in a multi-dimensional impression space(Fig. 2). If the noun corresponds to multiple samples, this method calculates its median from each impression value on an axis, and positions it at the basic point for distance calculation(Fig. 3-(a)). Hereafter, we call this method 1, the 'NM (Noun Median) method'.

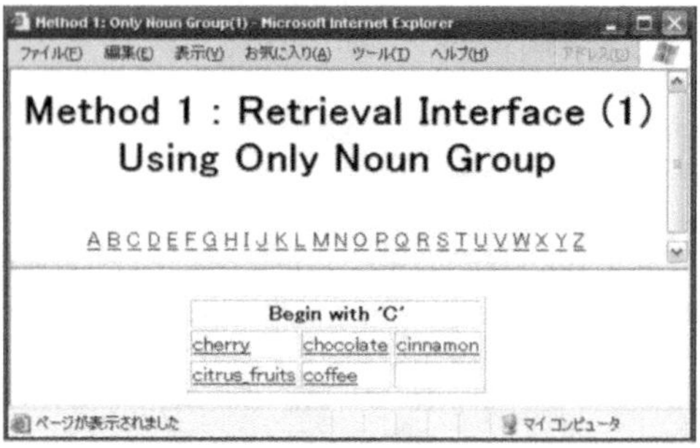

Fig. 1. Retrieval method using only noun (NM method)

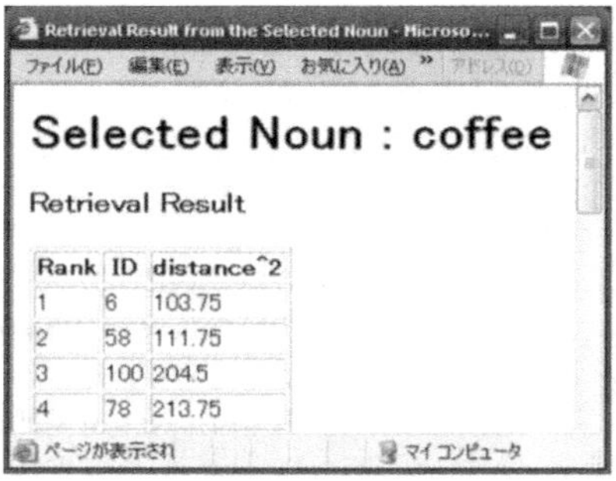

Fig. 2. Results page after retrieval shown in Fig. 1

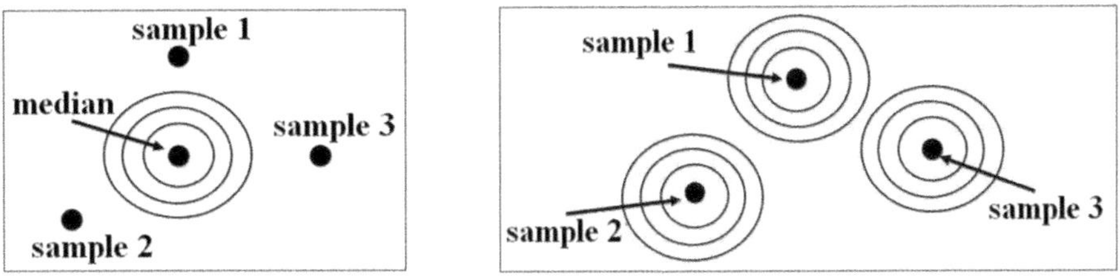

(a) The NM method (b) The NS Method

Fig. 3. Cases where a noun corresponds to multiple samples

Now, we define two common parameters d_* and d_0 for distance calculation in all methods. If one point p_1 on an axis has a concrete value and the other p_2 is 'null', we define their distance p_1p_2 on the axis as d_*. When both of the points are 'null', we define their distance p_1p_2 as d_0.

Method 2: Retrieval Method Using Only Noun (2) – 'NS(Noun Short) Method'. This method differs from the NM Method in only the following manner. If the selected noun corresponds to multiple samples, this method adopts the shortest distance from the multiple samples(Fig. 3-(b)). Hereafter, we call this method 2, the 'NS (Noun Short) method'.

Method 3: Retrieval Method Using Only Impression Word (1) – 'ID(Impression Distance) Method'. In this method, the user's input is an impression value which corresponds to a retrieval condition on each axis(Fig. 4). This method calculates a distance from the specified point, and displays the retrieval results(Fig. 5). Hereafter, we call this method 3, the 'ID (Impression Distance) method'.

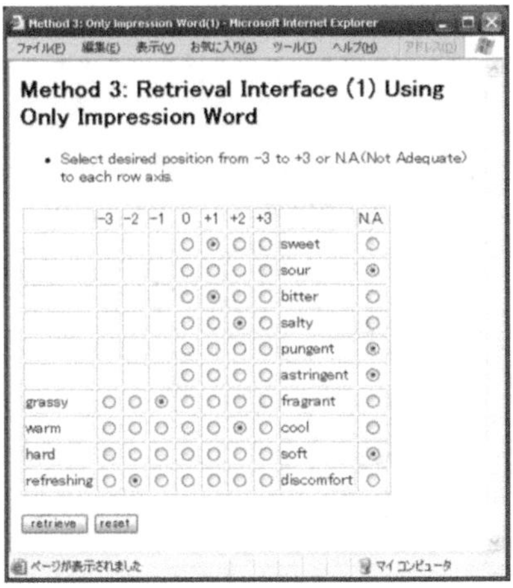

Fig. 4. Retrieval method using only an impression word (1) (ID method)

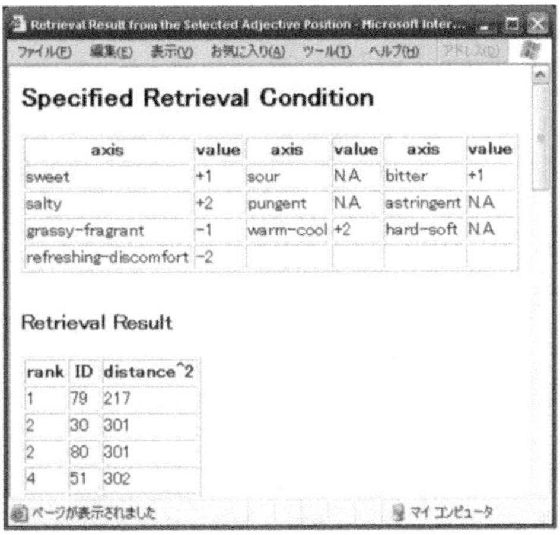

Fig. 5. Result page after retrieval shown in Fig. 5

Method 4: Retrieval Method Using Only Impression Word (2) – 'IC(Impression Cell) Method'. This method is a modification of the '2D-Oriented Retrieval Method with Basic Point' (2D-RIB) method[12] that is for music retrieval using impression. The features of 2D-RIB make it possible to look for a sample relevant to a user's retrieval intention while tracking the relationship with a known sample.

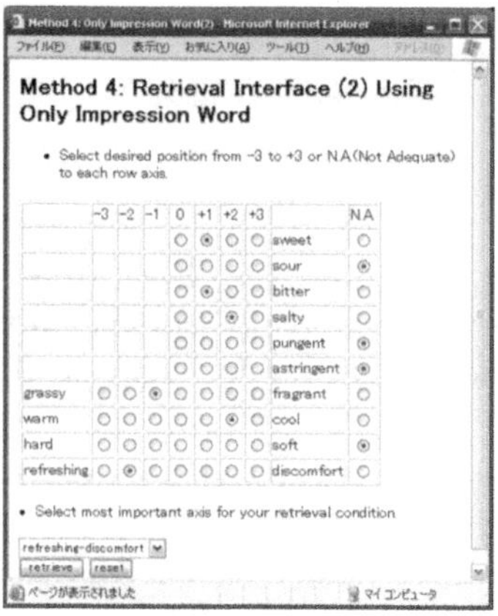

Fig. 6. Retrieval method using only an impression word (2) (IC method)

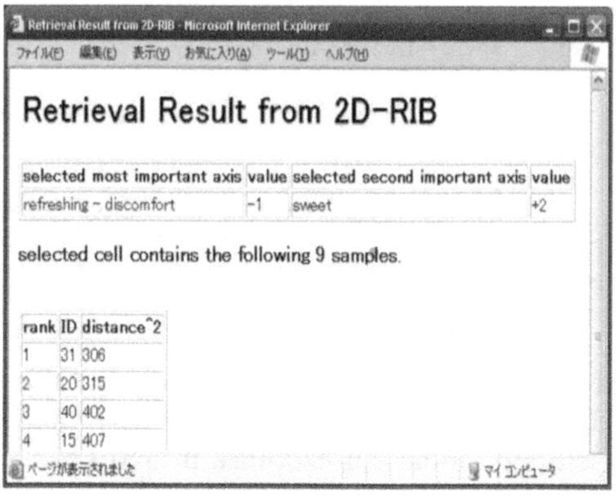

Fig. 8. Result page after retrieval shown in Fig. 7

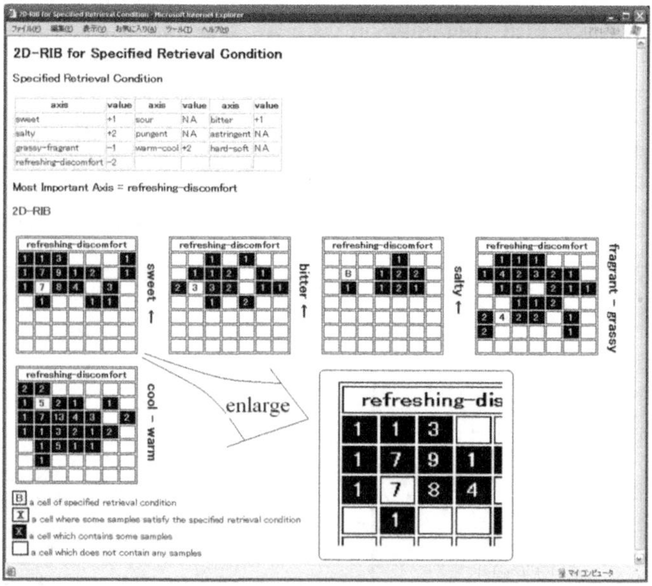

Fig. 7. 2D-RIB after page shown in Fig. 6

The user inputs an impression value which corresponds to a retrieval condition as in the case of the ID method. Moreover, the user inputs the most important impression axis (MIIA)(Fig. 6). This method displays a page including two-dimensional grids(Fig. 7). All horizontal axes are MIIA. Each vertical axis is one of the remaining axes except for MIIA. The number in each cell shows how many samples exist in the respective position. Black cells indicate the position where at least one sample exists. 'B' or the number on a white background shows the position of the impression value specified as a base. As an example, in the upper-left grid in Fig. 7, the upper-right cell of the basic point, with a number of nine, contains more little discomfort and sweeter sample than the basic position. The user selects the second important impression axis (SIIA) next to MIIA. The user then clicks a single cell on the two-dimensional grid whose horizontal axis is SIIA, and retrieve an odor which fits the user's intention. As shown in Fig. 8, this method displays the retrieval results in an order in which the distance from the basic position is from shortest to longest. We call this method 4, the 'IC (Impression Cell) method'.

3.2 Proposition of Efficient Retrieval Method

Using the four methods in the previous subsection, we explain our proposed retrieval method.

Method 5: Retrieval Method Using Noun and Impression Word (1) – 'NMI(Noun Median Impression) Method'. This method first shows the page as in the case of the NM method(Fig. 1). If the user selects a single noun, this method displays the page as in the case of the IC method on the lower half of the page(Fig. 9). The difference from the IC method is the meaning of the basic position. In each two-dimensional grid, the basic position means a cell which contains the noun specified as a retrieval condition. It is possible that multiple basic positions in a two-dimensional grid could arise. A sample table in the selected cell is generated from the distance calculation as in the NM method(Fig. 10). For example, if the user first selects 'coffee' in the noun selection, and clicks a cell whose 'sweet' axis equals '+1', he/she can retrieve 'odor like slightly sweet coffee'. Hereafter, we call this method 5, the 'NMI (Noun Median Impression) method'.

Method 6: Retrieval Method Using Noun and Impression Word (2) – 'NSI(Noun Short Impression) Method'. This method differs from the NMI method in only the following manner. The distance calculation after selection of a noun and clicking a cell in 2D-RIB is carried out identically to that in the NS method.

4 Preliminary System and Evaluation Experiment

4.1 Preliminary System

The development environment of our preliminary system is shown in Table 4. We set the parameter d_* and d_0 defined in subsection 3.1, to $d_*=10$ and $d_0=0$.

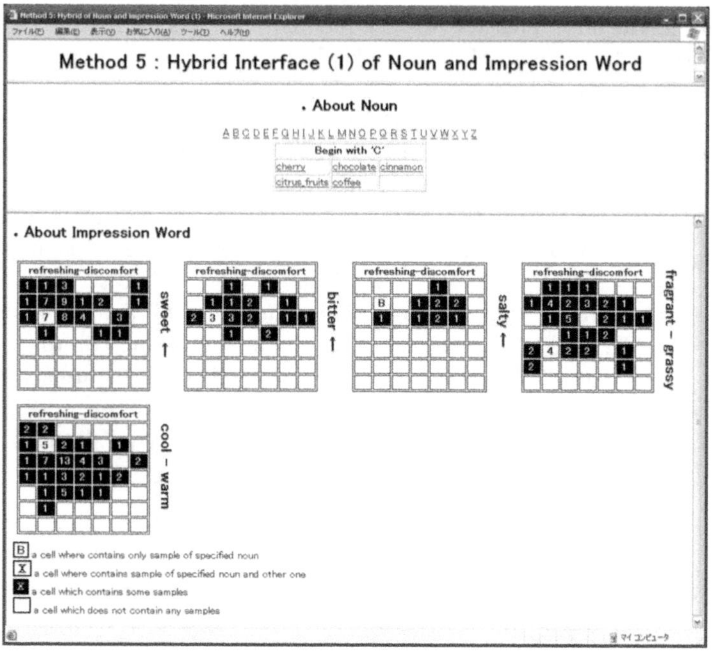

Fig. 9. Retrieval method using both noun and impression word (NMI method)

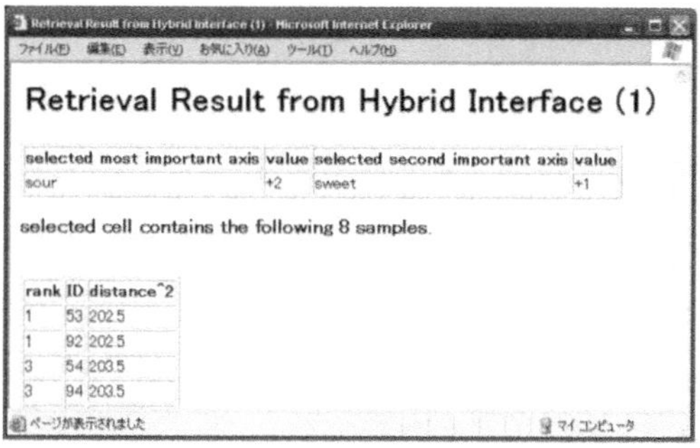

Fig. 10. Retrieval results after page shown in Fig. 9

Table 4. Development environment

OS	MS Windows 2003 Server SP2
DBMS	Oracle 9i
Servlet container	Tomcat 5.0.28
Web server	Apache 2.0.55
Web browser	MS Internet Explorer 6.0 SP2

4.2 3rd Experiment: Evaluation of Proposed Method

Experiment Method. The subjects were identical to those the participated in the first experiment. We use the evaluation method of Nakajima *et al.*[13]. We first provide the following to each subject: (i) odor of a goal sample, (ii) odor of a start sample, and (iii) retrieved page of the start sample. We then evaluate how many samples are smelled by the subject until arriving at the goal.

In the present study, in order to analyze the characteristics of each method in detail, we investigate two types of goal samples, 'easy sample' and 'difficult sample'. If at least one of the nouns assigned to a sample g_l in the experiment in Subsection 2.1 is included in g_l's goods name, we classify g_l as an 'easy sample'. Conversely, if we do not see such a noun, we classify g_l as a 'difficult sample'. We also investigate two types of start samples, 'cross sample' and 'uncross sample'. If there is at least one impression axis which has values along both a goal sample g and start sample s_l, we call s_l a 'cross sample' to the goal sample g. Conversely, if there is no such impression axis, we call s_l an 'uncross sample'. We evaluate the six methods described in Section 3 using the four retrieval types presented in Table 5.

Table 5. The combinations of start and goal samples

Start \ Goal	Easy	Difficult
Cross	Cross-Easy (CE)	Cross-Difficult (CD)
Uncross	Uncross-Easy (UE)	Uncross-Difficult (UD)

The actual sample provided to a subject is selected at random by an experiment supervisor. The subject looks for a goal sample from the above-mentioned '(iii) retrieved page of the start sample'. We use a start sample from the following two reasons. One is that we provide a subject with a sense where a method places a sample. The other is that we consider the following two situations to look for a sample: (a) from beginning without any sample and (b) after we have tried the other sample. We always try to set the latter situation. We avoid an advantage based on the former.

If "the subject feels that he/she had obtained a sample sufficiently close to the goal" or "the subject has already smelled nine samples including the start one", we finish the experiment using the combination of this goal sample and method. The parameters M_1 and M_2 for the subjective evaluation are described as follows:

- M_1: How much the subject feels to have been able to approach his/her goal until he/she had smelled two samples after the start sample. There are seven levels of this subjective evaluation, from '1: very close' to '7: very far'. '4' indicates 'neutral'.
- M_2: Sum of the number of samples smelled until the subject feels he/she has approached a sample sufficiently close to a goal.

The smaller the value of M_1 or M_2 becomes, the better the evaluation of its method becomes.

In addition, we record the following two types of data:

- retrieval condition which the subject provides at each try, and
- sample ID, the relevancy of which is tested against the goal sample in each retrieval result.

We objectively analyze the transition of the distance from the goal sample after the start sample. We also analyze the consistency between subjective and objective evaluations.

Experiment Result. First, we often observed that retrieval by noun contributes to a determination of rough position and retrieval by impression word contributes to detailed adjustment afterward.

The results of M_1 and M_2 are shown in Fig. 11 and 12. From the 'Total' shown in Fig. 11, we can determine the entire tendency based on M_1: the NMI and NSI methods obtain the best evaluation and the ID method is ranked third. We next analyze the results per each retrieval type. In Type UE, the NSI method is the best and the NMI method is ranked second. The NMI and NSI methods are ranked third or better than third in Types CE, CD and UD, too.

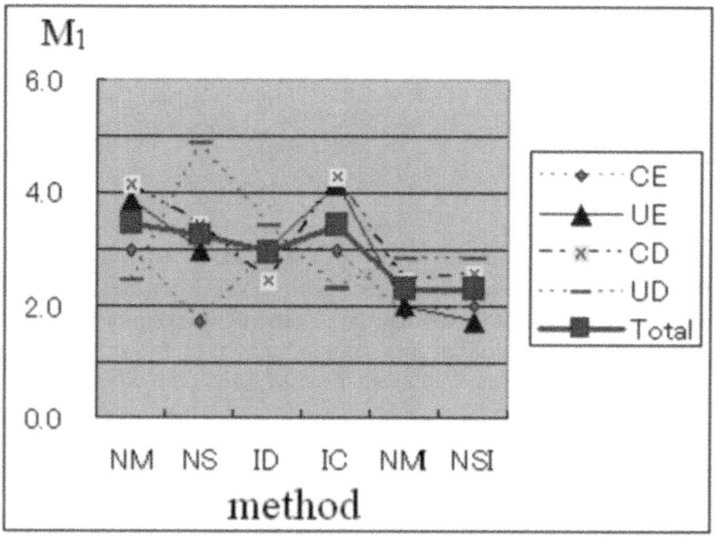

Fig. 11. Results of M_1

From the 'Total' in Fig. 12, we can determine the entire tendency based on M_2: the NMI and NSI methods also obtain the best evaluation and the NS method is ranked third. We next analyze the results per each retrieval type. In Types UE and UD, the NSI method is the best and the NMI method is ranked second. The NSI method is also the best and the NMI method is ranked third in Type CE. We can infer that the NS method is ranked second from the following. Since the goal sample is easy, it is easy to determine the rough position.

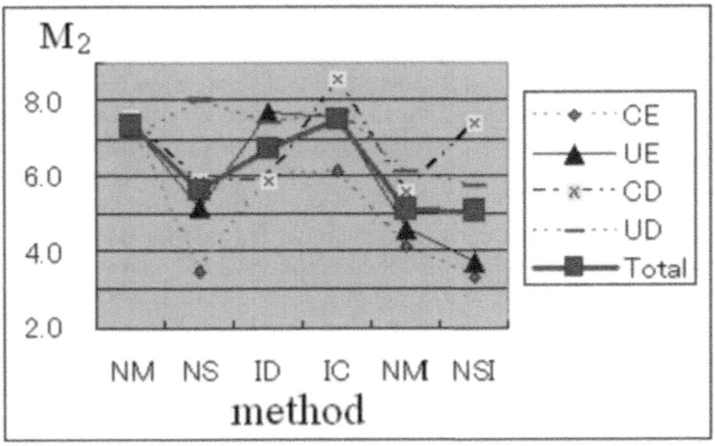

Fig. 12. Results of M_2

These results show that the proposed NMI and NSI methods are more feasible than the other four methods for odor retrieval relevant to the user's needs. Moreover, concerning the distance calculation from a noun, adopting the shortest distance obtains a better evaluation than the median. We can infer that, when we use the median, if there are other types of samples around the median, there is a danger in retrieving samples close to it.

Now we proceed to the results of the objective evaluation. From the graph in Fig. 13, we can determine the entire tendency. Concretely, the NMI and NSI methods relatively reduce the distance from each goal as the retrieval times increase, compared to the other methods. It does not contradict the one of subjective evaluation.

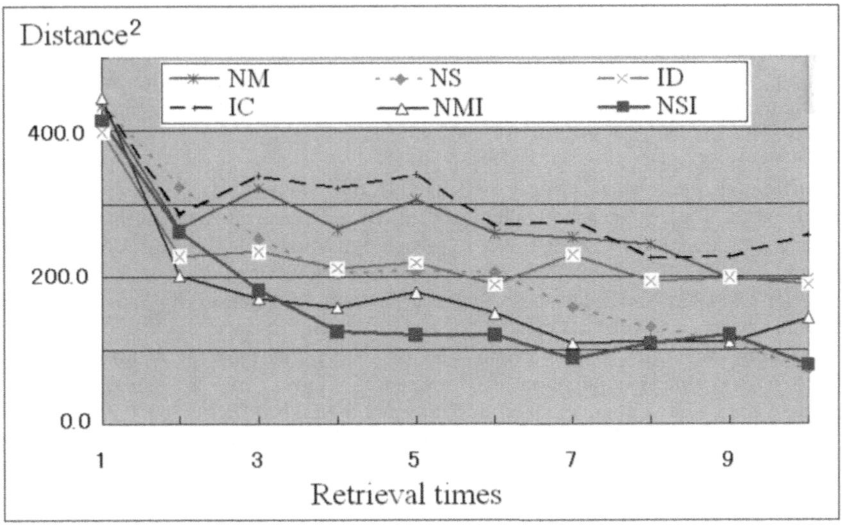

Fig. 13. Retrieval times vs. distance^2 from each goal

5 Concluding Remarks

In the present study, we have generated noun and impression word groups adequate for odor database retrieval. Based on these, we have proposed a database retrieval method which enables a user to specify a retrieval condition using both a noun and impression word. Our proposed method enables a user to carry out an efficient retrieval such as 'odor like slightly sweet coffee'. Results from evaluation experiments have shown that our method is more feasible for odor database retrieval relevant to a user's needs than the method employing only a noun or an impression word.

We are planning the following three future studies: (i) increasing the number of subjects in the experiments, (ii) personalizing the retrieval results, and (iii) investigating the sense of taste, that is closely related to the sense of smell.

References

1. Herz, R.S.: The Unique Interaction between Language and Olfactory Perception and Cognition. Tends in Experimental Psychology Research, 91–109 (2005)
2. Burr, C.: Emperor of Scent: A Story of Perfume, Obsession and the Last Mystery of the Senses. Arrow Books Ltd. (2004)
3. Plumacher, M., Holz, P.: Speaking of Colors and Odors (Converging Evidence in Language and Communication Research). John Benjamins Pub. Co., Amsterdam (2007)
4. Herz, R.S.: The Effect of Verbal Context in Olfactory Perception. J. Experimental Psychology: General 132, 595–606 (2003)
5. Loutfi, A., Coradeschi, S.: Odor Recognition for Intelligent Systems. J. IEEE Intelligent Systems 23(1), 41–48 (2008)
6. Kwon, K., Kim, N., Byun, H., Persaud, K.: On Training Neural Network Algorithm for Odor Identification for Future Multimedia Communication Systems. In: 2006 IEEE International Conference on Multimedia and Expo. (ICME), pp. 1309–1312 (2006)
7. Yamada, T.: Yokoyama, et al.: Wearable Olfactory Display: Using in Outdoor Environment. In: IEEE Virtual Reality Conference (VR 2006), pp. 199–206 (2006)
8. Bannai, Y., Ishizawa, M., Shigeno, H., Okada, K.: A Communication Model of Scents Mediated by Sense-descriptive Adjectives. In: Pan, Z., Cheok, D.A.D., Haller, M., Lau, R., Saito, H., Liang, R. (eds.) ICAT 2006. LNCS, vol. 4282, pp. 1322–1332. Springer, Heidelberg (2006)
9. Katayose, H., et al.: Kansei Music System. J. Comp. Music 13(4), 72–77 (1990)
10. Kumamoto, T.: Design and Evaluation of a Music Retrieval Scheme that Adapts to the User's Impressions. In: Ardissono, L., Brna, P., Mitrović, A. (eds.) UM 2005. LNCS (LNAI), vol. 3538, pp. 287–296. Springer, Heidelberg (2005)
11. Ikezoe, T., et al.: Music Database Retrieval System with Sensitivity Words Using Music Sensitivity space. J. IPSJ 42(12), 3201–3212 (2001) (in Japanese)
12. Takayama, T., Ikeda, et al.: Proposition of Direct Interface for Multimedia Database Retrieval by the Combination of Impression Values. In: 2003 IEEE Pacific Rim Conference on Communications, Computers and Signal Processing, pp. 609–612 (2003)
13. Nakajima, S., Kinoshita, S., et al.: Amplifying the Differences between Your Positive Samples and Neighbors. In: IEEE International Conference on Multimedia & Expo. (2003)

Multiplying the Mileage of Your Dataset with Subwindowing

Adham Atyabi, Sean P. Fitzgibbon, and David M.W. Powers

School of Computer Science, Engineering and Mathematics (CSEM)
Flinders University, Australia
{Adham.Atyabi,Sean.Fitzgibbon,David.Powers}@flinders.edu.au

Abstract. This study is focused on improving the classification performance of EEG data through the use of some data restructuring methods. In this study, the impact of having more training instances/samples vs. using shorter window sizes is investigated. The BCI2003 IVa dataset is used to examine the results. The results not surprisingly indicate that, up to a certain point, having higher numbers of training instances significantly improves the classification performance while the use of shorter window sizes tends to worsen performance in a way that usually cannot fully be compensated for by the additional instances, but tends to provide useful gain in overall performance for small divisors into two or three subepochs. We have moreover determined that use of an incomplete set of overlapping windows can have little effect, and is inapplicable for the smallest divisors, but that use of overlapping subepochs from three specific non-overlapping areas (start, middle and end) of a superepoch tends to contribute significant additional information. Examination of a division into five equal non-overlapping areas indicates that for some subjects the first or last fifth contributes significantly less information than the middle three fifths.

Keywords: Electroencephalogram, Window size, Overlapping window.

1 Introduction

Electroencephalography is one of the brain imaging and recording techniques that can be used to investigate human brain's activity, whilst Electroencephalogram (EEG) is the human brain's pattern that can be used to study the state of the brain, investigate medical conditions, monitor patients or research psychological phenomena. Recently Electroencephalogram (EEG) based Brain Computer Interface (BCI) has been an area of significant research activity with a variety of techniques being used to recognise and interpret brain events as a form of interface to a computer or other device, rather than for medical diagnosis or neuroscience research. Most commonly BCI is considered in terms of mental commands to control another device, and these may involve seeking to influence a particular brain rhythm, imagining a particular event or action, or even potentially a result of some direct intention or thought. BCI may also relate to

B. Hu et al. (Eds.): BI 2011, LNAI 6889, pp. 173–184, 2011.

unintended or automatic responses to events, or to recognition of particular cognitive states or levels of cognitive activity. This paper is presented in the context of BCI using single-trial EEG techniques, but the technique presented should be more generally applicable than the particular BCI-competition dataset and paradigm we have investigated.

Traditionally, a substantial period of time (a couple of seconds) is used as a single training or test instance, with an arbitrarily determined start and stop point. For a BCI trial in which the subject is seeking to maintain a desired brain state for a period of time, why should we treat this period of time, sometimes several seconds, as one trial or epoch? Indeed, at best, following the instruction to the subject there will be a latency of variable duration before they enter the state, a period of steady state maintaining the required mental process, and a point where the subject feels he has maintained the state for the requested time and ceases. In practice, subjects may take a while to satisfactorily reach the required brain state, may falter in their maintenance of the state, and may start and stop the state inside or outside of the arbitrarily selected constant time window used in the study. It is thus potentially useful to explore the information provided by different parts of this epoch, and the use of multiple smaller windows (subepochs) into the trial (superepoch).

For the purposes of training a neural network or other machine learning system, there is a general rule of the more data the better - at least to the point where we have fully generalised across all possible instances that might be expected. There is even evidence, a standard trick, that adding noise can improve the robustness and generalizability of the learned classifier, and in particular its resilience to noise. On the other hand, when collecting data, we tend to want to inconvenience (and pay) subjects as little as possible, so the less data the better, and this paper is about additional tricks that can be potentially used to multiply the effectiveness and increase the resilience of our classifiers. Our technique involves treating a single trial as a superepoch in which multiple subepochs are selected to multiply the number of examples in our dataset, whilst reducing the size and complexity of an individual training instance. We not only explore the use of covering nonoverlapping sets of subepochs, but consider the possibility of multiplying our data further by allowing overlap between subepochs, or of reducing training time and complexity by using noncovering sets of subepochs.

For this study, we consider only 10CV analysis of individual windowing patterns, but part of the unexplored potential of this work is the opportunity to train and fuse multiple classifiers.

2 Dataset

We used BCI competition dataset IVa [3]. The dataset contains EEG data that was collected from 5 healthy participants (with no indication of age or gender). During the data acquisition phase, subjects were seated in chairs with armrests and they were instructed to perform 280 task trails over four sessions. Random durations of 1.75 to 2.25 seconds have been used as intertrial interval. In each one of these 280 task trials, a visual cue has been presented to participants for 3.5 seconds during which they were instructed to perform either the right hand or left foot movement imagination based on the direction of the cue. To provide consistency with certain other studies done on the same dataset, the dataset is restructured to a common framework containing:

- The data acquired during the time that subject was performing a cognitive task (denoted as task in datasets).
- The data acquired outside of the time specified for performing the specified tasks during the instructions, blank screen, inter-trial and so on (denoted as non-task in datasets).
- The data acquired during the transition times when the subject is switching his/her state from non-task to task or vice versa (denoted as transition in datasets). This period nominally contained the first 0.5 seconds after the time that cue was presented to the subject and the 0.5 seconds before the end of the task.

The task period is labeled appropriately in a way to represent the performed motor imagery tasks. In this study, only task periods have been used for the purpose of feature extraction and classification. As a result, the dataset contains EEG data gathered from 5 subjects (aa,al,av,aw,ay), each containing 280 epochs with nominal 2.5s windows. each 2.5s window contains 2500 samples gathered from 118 electrodes. The sample rate is 1000Hz.

Table 1 provides details about the abbreviations used to describe the set of pre-processing methods applied to a dataset and its current status. In this study, a dataset is described using the following format : [type of referencing][demeaned or raw EEG data][sample rate]Hz[window size]s[percentage of the overlapping windows][number of sub-epochs][number of super-epochs].

Table 1. Table of Abbreviations

Definition	Description
CAR	Common Average Reference
D	Demeaned EEG data
R	Raw EEG data
s	Second
Hz	Hertz
OVLP	Overlapping windows
ROVLP	Reduced Overlapping windows
Red	Referenced to a particular sub-epoch by number

As an example, CARD1000Hz0.5s5*280 shows that common average reference is used and the data is demeaned. The sample rate is 1000Hz, with half a second window size (sub-epoch size), which results in having 5 time more epochs than the original 2.5 second windows (this is reflected in 5*280). No overlapping windows are used in this case.

CARD1000Hz0.3sOVLP25*280 shows that the demeaned and common average reference demeaned data is used. The sample rate is 1000Hz and 0.3 second window (sub-epoch size) is used but the windows/sub-epochs have 25% overlap (that is windows/sub-epochs are the same size (in terms of the time duration) starting from different offsets, with 75% delay and 25% overlap).

3 Results

Since any referencing of the dataset during the data acquisition is unknown, all the examples presented use EEG data that has been demeaned per electrode over the epoch, after common average referencing (CAR) across electrodes. In all figures, frequency features (FFT over the subwindow/subepoch) are used for classification, and LinearSVM is used as the classifier, as this is usually a good choice (in fact many other features and classifiers have been trialed, and certain other combinations work well, but this combination provides the most consistent performance in our tests). Furthermore, all results indicate the average value of Bookmaker informedness through 10-fold cross validation. Bookmaker is a chance-corrected measure that takes into account both sensitivity and specificity, and is a more informative method than accuracy, recall or precision for evaluating the performance, being computed from the true and false positive or negative rates [2]. The data used in this paper is dichotomous, that is we are seeking to distinguish only two conditions (when Bookmaker simplifies to Specificity + Sensititivity - 1 = tpr - fpr). However, Bookmaker informedness is also appropriate for discriminating multiple conditions whereas accuracy is not comparable across different experimental set ups, including changes in the number or prevalence of conditions.

In all experiments 10-fold cross-validation is used at the level of trials so that it is guaranteed that there is no repetition in terms of training and testing epochs - that is no trial used wholly or in part for learning will be used wholly or in part for evaluation. In all figures, averaged results are shown with errorbars spaced at one standard error from the mean, and non-overlap of the errorbars thus suggests significance of the difference of means. In many figures the errorbars are scarcely visible which means that any noticeable difference is potentially significant at the 0.05 level. However no explicit significance tests are performed and in particular no correction is made for the massive multiple testing we have performed. At 0.05 significance, chances are that 1 in 20 tests will show apparent significance due to chance (e.g. one method just happens to suit the specific dataset better). This risk is not fully mitigated by the use of 10CV.

3.1 Pre-processing: The Impact of Shorter vs. Longer Windows

This section describes a series of experiments to explore the effect of shorter time windows in combination with and in contrast with the number and choice of subepochs.

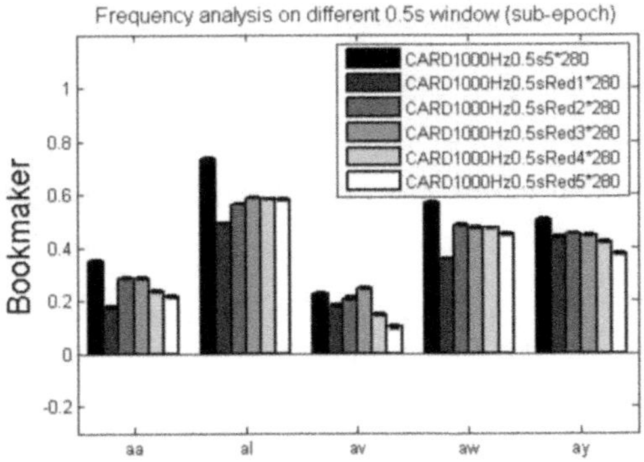

Fig. 1. The performance of 2.5s superepoch vs 0.5s subepochs at different offsets across different subjects (experiment 1a)

Experiment 1a - superepoch vs specific subepoch: Although our aim is to explore increasing the number of training instances through using shorter window sizes that may or may not overlap with each other, to see if we can improve the classification performance and/or reduce the training time required, it is useful to explore the variation in accuracy across epochs of different sizes and offsets within the trial. This will provide a baseline for understanding the results when we vary both the number of training epochs and the size of the epochs, and implicitly their offsets.

We illustrate that there is generally some loss of accuracy in reducing epoch size, and that there is some slight variability with change of offset, but that this can vary considerably across subjects. We present results for one specific case where reduction is achieved by dividing 2.5s windows into 5 0.5s windows and these are treated individually in separate 10CV runs. Each new epoch is called a subepoch while the 2.5s windows is considered as the superepoch. Viz. for this experiment, 5 new datasets are generated such that each contains only first, second, ..., or fifth sub epoch from each super epoch and a 10-fold cross validation is performed to create training and testing sets from each one of these five new datasets. The results are illustrated in Fig.1. In the figure, these new reduced sets are indicated as 'Red' and the following digit indicate the index number of the subepoch used. The results indicate that there is mostly little difference between a subject's performance in different 0.5s time-windows within the original 2.5s trial. However, the use of the entire 2.5s window benefits the classifier in all cases, but the central subepoch was marginally better for the weakest subject. This is evidently due to a preference for a more general picture of a subject's intention on the entire 2.5s window in compare with only 0.5s, however performance may be reduced because of the curse of dimensionality - the more attributes or features we have the harder it is to optimise the learner. The exception is likely due to the specific subject not reaching the desired state as quickly or maintaining it as long, and conforms to a general pattern that central subepochs tend to be give more consistent performance. Despite the observed performance improvement over a single 0.5s window, a 2.5s window is usually considered a long time period in human brain study and slightly shorter window sizes may be expected to provide better representation of the underlying pattern.

Experiment 1b - Covering non-overlapping Subepochs: As was mentioned earlier, the intention of this study is to investigate the impact of using multiple windows of shorter window sizes on the classifier's overall performance. To do so, a variety of windows sizes (0.1s, 0.2s, 0.3s, 0.4s, 0.5s, 0.6s, 0.8s, 1.25s, 2.5s) are applied to the demeaned signal so that essentially the entire 2.5s is used. Fig. 2 illustrates the frequency analysis results using this full set of time windows.

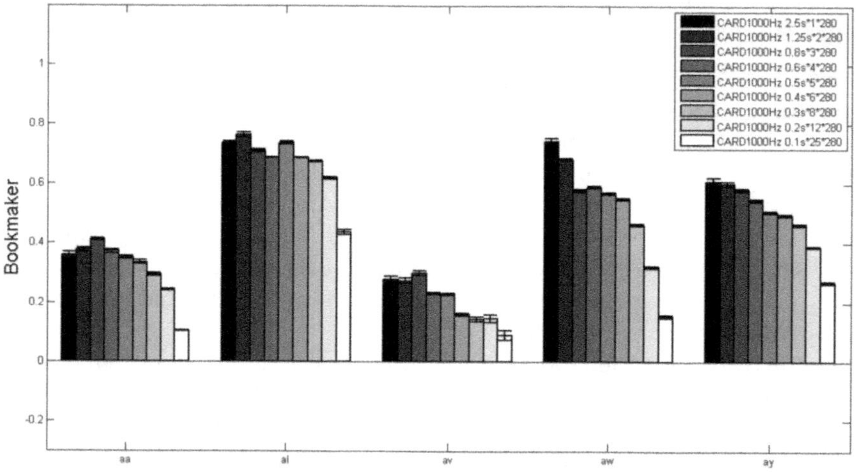

Fig. 2. The performance of full coverage subepoching across subjects (experiment 1b)

The results indicate that the classifier's performance is influenced by the window size. In addition, it suggests that even though shorter window sizes can benefit the classifier by providing higher number of training instances, very short window sizes (as in 0.2s and 0.1s) might be incapable of properly reflecting the subject's intention. On the other hand, the peak performance is always one of the long sizes (0.8s, 1.25s or 2.5s), but seldom the longest (2.5s). That is we normally do get a performance improvement (and/or reduction in variance) by using multiple subepochs where the subepoch length is around 1 second.

Experiment 1c - Random Partially Covering Subepochs: Even though the results achieved from the previous experiment indicate the impact of longer time windows on classifier performance, there remains the question of how much this is influenced by the multiplication of the effective number of epochs. It is thus useful to investigate the possibility of achieving a reasonable classification by using fewer training instances. This issue is investigated by reducing the number of sub-epochs by means of random selection for each of the investigated subwindow durations, rather than selecting specific intervals and durations as in experiment 1a. For each subepoch size, the process is to randomly select a total of 280 sub-epochs from each superepoch (2.5s windows), and in addition for the 0.1s size, with its rather high number of subwindows available (25), a selection of submultiples of 24 are tested in order to be comparable to their use with the corresponding fractions of the superepoch used in experiment 1b. Considering the fact that the shortest window size (0.1s) always generates higher number of instances, this time window is further investigated by applying different subepoch reduction rates (divisor k).

Note that for time domain analysis of a sequence of 0.1s windows we are essentially providing a bias of particular sensitivity to frequencies and harmonics of 10Hz, which will reinforce each other, where as other frequencies will have varying phase and tend to cancel out. In our time domain studies (not shown or discussed in this paper due to their generally reduced performance relative to the frequency domain) this is apparent with a dramatic spike up for 0.1s. Given we are mainly interested in frequencies up to 30Hz, and we see a strong reduction in informedness gain for smaller subepochs, it would seem advisable to restrict attention to subwindows of at least 0.3s.

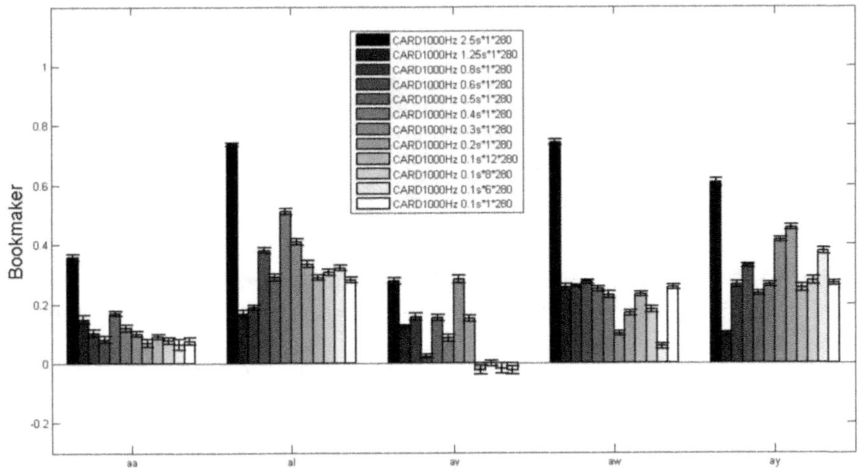

Fig. 3. The averaged results of sub-window reduction through random selection across different window sizes (experiment 1c)

The comparison of the achieved results between Fig.2 and Fig 3 indicates learning is far less stable and generally less effective when less than the full number of available subepochs is used, particularly for the randomly selected short intervals and the weakest subject (who is likely not maintaining the desired state stable throughout the 2.5 seconds). Clearly it is beneficial to make use of all the data, and even though the gain is not great, or guaranteed, in using k subepochs of 1/k window size, there is an expected gain of o(k) in the training and testing time, given we are using a learning algorithm that is linear in the number of training instances but quadratic in the number of attributes or samples.

In summary, for experiment 1 we have seen that for small divisors k (1 or 2) we can get an improvement in performance due to the increased number of training instances available, but we have not seen a strong reduction below 0.3s subwindows, and we have seen a slight reduction in between that might potentially be improved by additional training instances. We thus turn to look at the addition of overlapped training intervals for the central range of 0.8s down to 0.3s. Note that overlapping for k=1, or 50% overlapping for k=2, will not allow increasing the number of training epochs and so is not performed in the following series of experiments.

3.2 Preprocessing: The Impact of Overlapping

Although the above comparisons indicate that using shorter time window to increase the number of subepochs and reduce the number of training features does not consistently improve the classifier performance consistently across subjects for any particular multiplication/reduction factor k, there is still the further potential of using overlapping to increase the chance of positive classification by generating higher number of training instances while maintaining the same superepoch and subepoch size. Except for the specific case of a common frequency occurring across subepochs, we would expect non-overlapping subwindows to be uncorrelated. But for frequency domain analysis one would expect frequencies of interest to be represented across overlapped windows, in combination with other signal or 'noise' that is not of interest, and can help improve diversification and generalisation.

Experiment 2a - Investigation of Covering Overlapping Subwindows: Rather than just using shorter window sizes to provide a higher number of training samples, we investigate creating more training instances by overlapping the subepochs from 0.8s down to 0.3s. Considering the fact that EEG data contains a high level of contamination not only due to underlying noise in the signal but also due to receiving multiple instances of the same signal sent by various sources/cells on the brain and also their delayed versions, it is difficult to predict the underlying pattern of the brain wave. However, the idea of applying overlapping windows which cause multiple repetitions of some instances in the signal can help to capture this pattern more properly.
The following are considered as potential advantages of window overlapping:

- correcting sampling bias
- accommodating better for instability of intentional state
- accommodating better for impedance variation/drift
- improving the quality of EEG spectral analysis within Nyquist limits
- reproducing the fluidity of temporal data in the frequency domain.

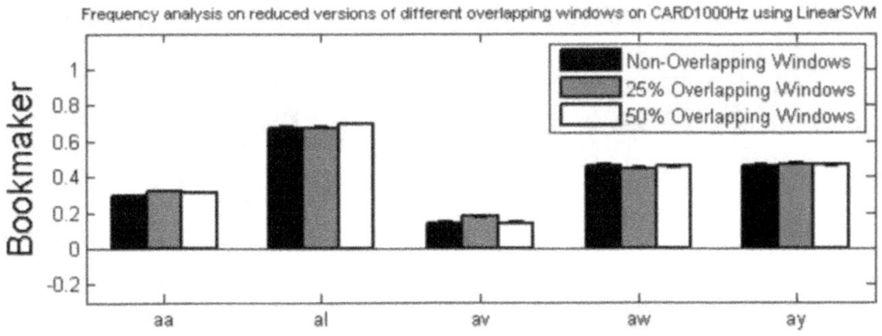

Fig. 4. The averaged results of various overlapping ratios across different time windows (experiment 2a)

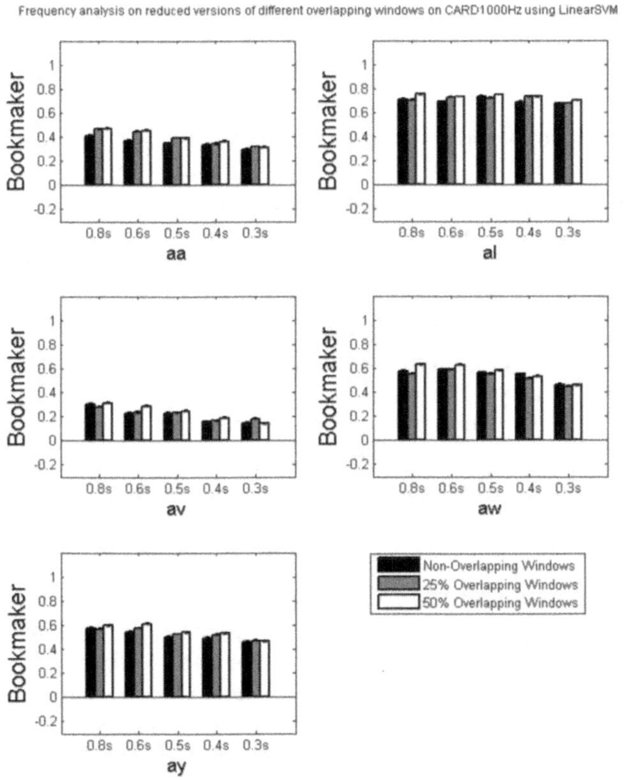

Fig. 5. The impact of various overlapping ratios across different time windows (experiment 2a)

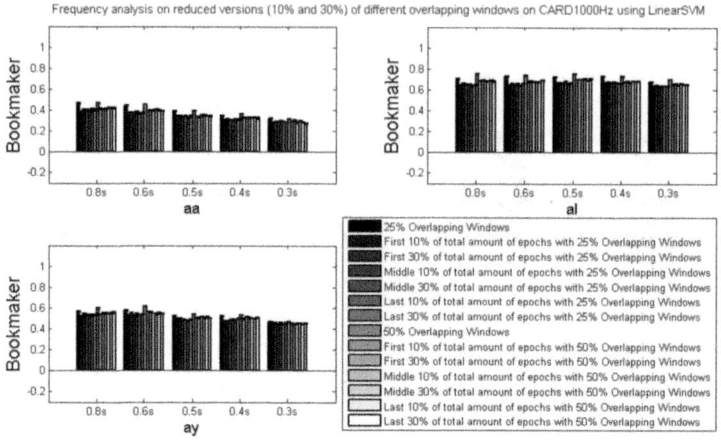

Fig. 6. The average classification results of the first, middle, and last 10% or 30% of the overlapped dataset versus all (overlapped by 0, 25% or 50%). The results are averaged across different time windows (experiment 2b).

In this section, the overlapping process is investigated with various window sizes. This is to further investigate the possibility of improving the overall classification performance through using shorter window sizes and having more training instances. To do so, frequency analysis is applied using LinearSVM on 25% and 50% overlapping windows using variety of window sizes. Note that using 50% overlap increases the number of subepochs by up to a factor of up to 2/1 (100%), whilst usage 25% overlap increases by a factor of up to 4/3 (33%). In general 1/c overlap increases the number of subepochs by a factor of up to c/(c-1) (and additive increase of 1/(c-1)).

The results in Figs 4 and 5 show that significant increases are achieved in general by increased amounts of overlap, and the corresponding increased number of effective epochs, often leading to the best result for a subject. For most subjects there is still a clear downward trend as we progress into the smallest intervals, but the optimum interval can be anything from 0.5s up.

Experiment 2b - Subsampled Overlapping Epochs: To further investigate the impact of having higher number of subepochs, the previous experiment is replicated by selecting only 10% or 30% of the dataset from its first, middle or last instances of overlapping windows from each 2.5s super epoch.[1] The procedure is similar to the experiment 1a. First, based on the required overlapping percentage (e.g., 25% or 50%), a new dataset of overlapped sub-epochs are created. Next, three new sets are generated in a way that each represents only the first, middle or last X% of the total amount of overlapping windows. X can ei-

[1] Another experiment with only 5 instances from either the first, middle or last segments of overlapping windows was also carried out. The results depicted poor (near chance level) classification performance which was due to having a small number of training instances that barely represent the underlying intention of the subjects.

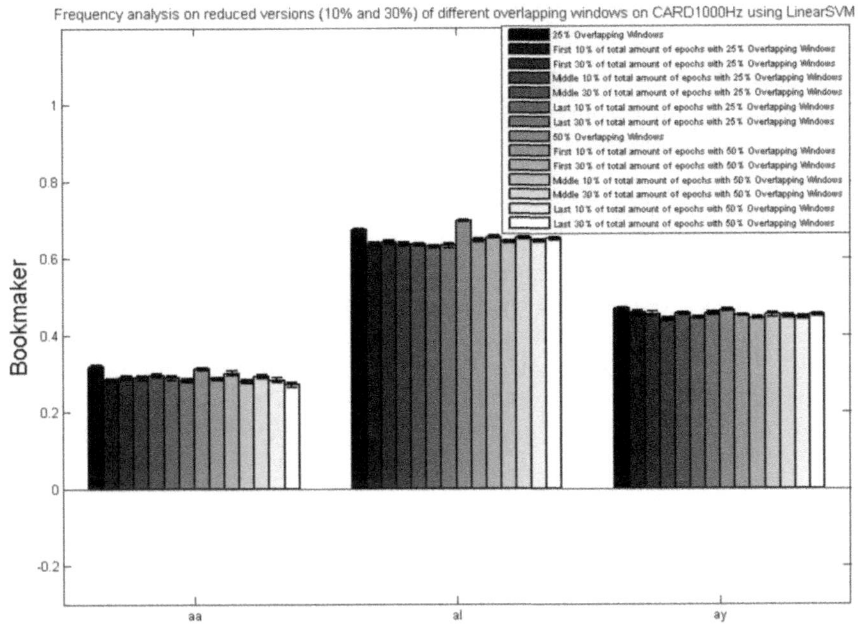

Fig. 7. The experimental results of reduced overlapping windows through choosing the first, middle, and last 10 and 30% overlapping windows (vs all) derived from each super-epoch (experiment 2b) across different window sizes and subjects

ther have 10 or 30 which results in only 10% or 30% of the maximum amount of overlapping windows. Consequently, in the new set that contains the first 10% of the overlapping windows, the other 90% are eliminated from the set and it mostly represents the start of the performed task. The results are demonstrated in Figs 6 and 7. Due to computational and space constraints, only 3 subjects are considered here (aa, al, and ay).

The results illustrate the possibility of improving the classification by providing higher numbers of training instances through the overlapping of shorter time windows. In addition, it represents the possibility of achieving a reasonable performance only using 10% or 30% of the data from the overlapped dataset, but emphasises the importance of representing the start, middle and end segments of the trial. There is no significant difference for inclusion level (10% or 30%) or for which single segment is sampled (first, middle or last), but there is a clear advantage when all possible overlap subintervals are included, and all three segments are covered, with our interpretation of the results indicating that coverage of these three segments (start, middle, end) is important.

4 Conclusion

This study is focused on investigating the idea of using shorter window sizes allowing a higher number of training instances. The data in non-overlapping windows is independent in one sense, but to the extent that consistent brain frequencies are present throughout a trial, but are not replicated across trials, the windows will correlate well in frequency space, with variation due to 'noise' that is not consistent throughout a trial. Results indicate that dividing the trial into two or three subepochs can produce a significant increase in performance when the full data is used, or apparently also when the start, middle and end of the trial are represented. However, it is clear that using shorter window sizes without increasing the number of epochs (training instances) tends to reduce the classification performance. Less clear is the role of overlap, which does appear to have some benefit in increasing the number of informative instances, but quickly saturates. For this dataset if a subject achieves 0.7 probability of an informed decision or above, the additional instances due to subwindowing or overlap are relatively unlikely to have an impact, but for subjects who achieve only 0.5 there is a good chance of improving considerably on this by using these techniques.

5 Future Work

This study is preliminary and further work is under way to automate feature selection and implement classifier fusion based on different sampling options as well as alternate classifier and preprocessing options. It is also worth teasing out and confirming the precise way in which the number of sampled overlapped and unoverlapped trials influences overall performance when constrained to sample across the start, middle and end thirds of the trial. These thirds evidently contain slightly different kinds of information, about the initiation, maintenance and termination of the target state, and thus classifiers trained separately on them should be fusable for better performance than simple concatenation (either as single superepochs, or sets of subepoch instances).

References

1. Fitzgibbon, S.: A Machine Learning Approach to Brain-Computer Interfacing. School of Psychology. Faculty of Social Sciences. Flinders University (2007)
2. Powers, D.M.W.: Recall and Precision versus the Bookmaker. In: International Conference on Cognitive Science (ICSC-2003), Sydney, Australia, pp. 529–534 (2003)
3. Blankertz, B., Muller, K.-R., Krusienski, D.J., Schalk, G., Wolpaw, J.R., Schlogl, A., Pfurtscheller, G., del Millan, J.R., Schroder, M., Birbaumer, N.: The BCI competition III:Validating alternative approaches to actual BCI problems. IEEE Trans. on Neural Syst. Rehabil. Eng. 14(2), 153–159 (2006)

Formal Specification of a Neuroscience-Inspired Cognitive Architecture

Luis-Felipe Rodríguez and Félix Ramos

Department of Computer Science, Cinvestav Guadalajara, México
{lrodrigue,framos}@gdl.cinvestav.mx

Abstract. Cognitive architectures allow the emergence of behaviors in autonomous agents. Their design is commonly based on multidisciplinary theories and models that explain the mechanisms underlying human behaviors, as well as on standards and principles used in the development of software systems. The formal and rigorous description of such architectures, however, is a software engineering practice that has been barely implemented. In this paper, we present the formal specification of a neuroscience-inspired cognitive architecture. Which ensures its proper development and subsequent operation, as well as the communication of its operational and architectural assumptions unambiguously. Particularly, we use the Real-Time Process Algebra to formally describe its architectural components and emerging behaviors.

Keywords: Cognitive Architecture, Neuroscience, Formal Description.

1 Introduction

Cognitive architectures (CAs) serve as the structural basis of autonomous agents (AAs.) They include a series of componentes that interoperate in order to produce certain types of behaviors [5, 7]. The design of such CAs usually adheres to a unifying approach, trying to embody a number of computational models of cognitive and affective functions in order to create artificial systems that achieve all kind of cognitive behaviors [6].

Through the development of CAs we are able to provide AAs with appropriate means for a favorable interaction with users and other agents. In particular, for developing AAs whose behaviors should resemble those observed in humans, the major challenge is to develop CAs that allow the emergence of realistic, believable, sociable, affective, cultural, anticipative, and intelligent behaviors. Because of the natural essence of these behaviors, CAs usually base their design on psychological and biological models which try to explain the mechanisms underlying human behaviors [4, 1]. Moreover, given their computational nature, CAs also take into account appropriate software tools and computational techniques and methodologies to carry out their development. However, a current drawback of most CAs is that their development is not supported with software engineering formalisms that ensure their correct design and subsequent implementation [5,1].

B. Hu et al. (Eds.): BI 2011, LNAI 6889, pp. 185–196, 2011.

In this paper, we present the formal specification of a neuroscience-inspired cognitive architecture previously proposed and described by Rodríguez et al. [7]. This CA allows the simulation of *human brain functions* by implementing a series of components that replicate the functioning and architecture of *brain structures*. In this manner, it is intended to provide human-like behaviors to AAs. However, in order to achieve working models of these brain functions, the internal operations and architecture of the components of the CA have been subject of further refinements. Therefore, in order to unambiguously understand the fundamental assumptions and design of the CA, a formal description of its architectural components and behaviors is required. Furthermore, such formal descriptions allows developing architectural modules separately and their subsequent integration seamlessly.

The structure of the paper is as follows. The next section highlights the importance of formally describing cognitive architectures. The formal method used to specify the CA's is then explained in section 3. The architecture and behaviors of the CA are formally described in section 4 and 5 respectively. Finally, section 6 provides some concluding remarks.

2 Formalizing Cognitive Architectures

Although a software system can initially be specified using high level languages, such as the natural language, more precise means are required to obtain a reliable final specification. In this sense, formal methods are used for the modeling and specification of software systems in a rigorous, precise, and correct way [2].

In particular, CAs can widely benefit from this practice. They are integrated systems with a number of components embodying complex architectures and behaviors. However, CAs have barely been developed using formal methods and languages. For example, ACT-R [1], an integrative cognitive theory that explains coherent cognition through the implementation of a CA, has not presented any formalization of their architecture or functionality. Similarly, Soar [4], a symbolic CA based on knowledge, has evolved without a formal and rigorous basis. This has probably impacted on the fact that although many contributions have been proposed to Soar, getting a unified working system with all these new components running at the same time has become a difficult task [4].

The CA we focus here has been previously proposed by Rodríguez et al. [7]. Its desing is based on three fundamental assumptions: (1) it is appropriate for implementing AAs that show human-like behaviors, (2) its implementation can be totally based on theories and models formulated in disciplines concerned with understanding the human brain operations and architecture, and (3) by following an integrative perspective, it imitates the nature of the operation and architecture of the brain.

The formal description of this type of CAs is necessary for several reasons. First, it contributes to an easy translation of theoretical cognitive and affective models to a computational one. Then, since a CA follows a unified approach, its design and implementation becomes very complex, thus, its formalization allows controlling and facilitating its constantly evolution. Similarly, an unambiguous description of its components and behaviors permits developers to understand the same way its general functioning, allowing them to make their own contributions in a transparent manner and adhering, at the same time, to the design and main assumptions of this architecture.

3 Real-Time Process Algebra

For the specification of the CA we use the Real-Time Process Algebra (RTPA) [8]. This is a proper mathematical structure useful for the formal specification of software systems in terms of their *architecture* and *static* and *dynamic behaviors* [9]. RTPA allows to algebraically denote and manipulate systems and human behavioral processes. For the modeling of the system architecture it provides 17 primitive types: Natural number, Integer, Real, String, Boolean, Byte, Hexadecimal, Pointer, Time, Date, Date/Time, Run-time determinable type, System architectural type, Event, Timing, Interrupt, and Status (fig. 1, part 1), as well as a set of Abstract Data Types such as Stack, Record, Array, List, and Queue [8]. For the modeling of elemental system behaviors the following meta-processes are given: Assignment, Evaluation, Addressing, Memory allocation, Memory release, Read, Write, Input, Output, Timing, Duration, Increase, Decrease, Exception detection, Skip, Stop, and System (fig. 1, part 2.) Complex behaviors can be modeled using 17 relational process operations: Sequence, Jump, Branch, Switch, While-loop, Repeat-loop, For-loop, Recursion, Function call, Parallel, Concurrence, Interleave, Pipeline, Interrupt, Time-driven dispatch, Event-driven dispatch, and Interrupt-driven dispatch (fig. 1, part 3.)

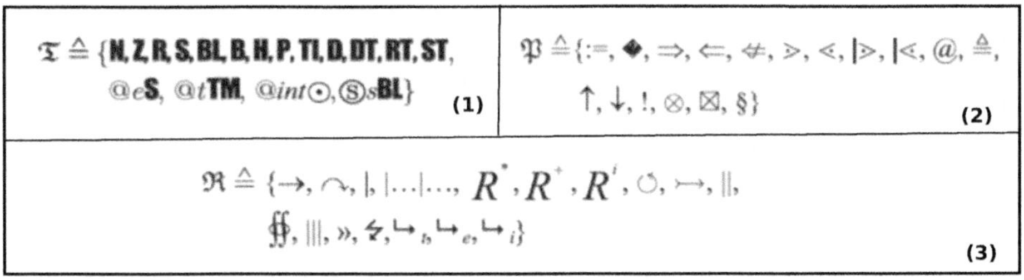

Fig. 1. RTPA notations

The RTPA methodology is based on the conception that a software system is specified via a number of systematic refinements in a top-down approach. This methodology uses a three-level process for the modeling, specification, and refinement of software architectures and behaviors [8, 9]. According to this, a system can be specified by its architectural components, static and dynamic behaviors, as well as their interactions. The refinement steps for architectural specifications are system architecture, data schemas, and data objects. For static behaviors are system static behaviors, process schemas, and process implementations. Finally, for the specification of dynamic behaviors are process priority allocation, process deployment, and process dispatching models [8].

Architectural components are specified using *Unified Data Models* (UDMs), which are abstract schemas composed of records that include the fields used in a specific architectural component, their types, and constraints (as shown in section 4). Static behaviors are specified using *Unified Process Models* (UPMs), which are a composition of a finite set of n processes representing the structure of a program (as shown in section 5) [9].

Details of RTPA notations, methodology, and models for specification are given elsewhere [8, 9]. In order to follow them, we carry out the formal description of the cognitive architecture (CogArch) by considering it as a software system composed of two subsystems: *architectural components* and *operational behaviors*. Thus, the top level framework of the system is specified as follows:

$$\begin{aligned}\S(\mathbf{CogArch}) \triangleq\ & \text{CogArch}\S.\text{Architecture}\mathbf{ST} \\ & \parallel \text{CogArch}\S.\text{Behaviors}\mathbf{PC}\end{aligned}$$

The following two sections deal with the refinement process of both subsystems. Section 4 presents the UDMs for to the CogArch§.Architecture**ST**, and section 5 introduces the UPMs corresponding to the CogArch§.Behaviors**PC**.

4 Specifications of the Architecture of the CA

The structural design of the CA was carried out so that the implementation of behaviors with the characteristics mentioned in the introduction were possible. Because these behaviors are mainly observed in humans, the simulation of *brain processes* as a result of the joint operation of *architectural components* was proposed [7,3]. The brain functions to be simulated are: Perception, Learning, Memory, Attention, Emotions, Planning, Decision-Making, and Motor-Action [7]. Thus, the architectural design of the CA consists of those components that enable the simulation of these cognitive and affective processes.

A direct translation of these brain functions into architectural components is unsuitable. Actually, this is not the way the brain works; the brain is not composed of a perception or learning component, but of a set of *brain structures* that work and interact in order to generate these functions [3]. Thus, considering these brain functions as requirements, the components included in the CA were designed so that they resemble the functioning and anatomy of brain structures. These structures are: Sensory System, Olfactory Bulb, Thalamus, Sensory Cortex, Association Cortex, Hippocampus, Amygdala, Prefrontal Cortex, Basal Ganglia, and Motor Cortex [7].

Due to the modular nature of the CA design, each brain function can be separately modeled and implemented. However, in order to achieve a working system, all architectural components may be refined and new data structures proposed. As a consequence, the formal schemes (i.e., UDMs and UPMs) introduced in this paper are developed so that they provide a general and functional description of the CA.

(1)

CogArch§.Architecture**ST** ≜
<SensorySystem : **ST** | [1]>
‖ <OlfactoryBulb : **ST** | [1]>
‖ <Thalamus : **ST** | [1]>
‖ <SensoryCortex : **ST** | [1]>
‖ <AssociationCortex : **ST** | [1]>
‖ <Hippocampus : **ST** | [1]>
‖ <Amygdala : **ST** | [1]>
‖ <Prefrontal : **ST** | [1]>
‖ <BasalGanglia : **ST** | [1]>
‖ <MotorCortex : **ST** | [1]>

(2)

Architecture**ST**.Thalamus**ST** ≜
<LateralGeniculateNucleus : **ST** | [1]>
‖ <MedialGeniculateNucleus : **ST** | [1]>
‖ <Ventrobasal : **ST** | [1]>
‖ <VentralPosteriorMedialNucleus : **ST** | [1]>

Architecture**ST**.SensoryCortex**ST** ≜
<VisualCortex : **ST** | [1]>
‖ <GustatoryCortex : **ST** | [1]>
‖ <SomatosensoryCortex : **ST** | [1]>
‖ <AuditoryCortex : **ST** | [1]>
‖ <OlfactoryCortex : **ST** | [1]>

Architecture**ST**.PrefrontalCortex**ST** ≜
<OrbitoFrontalCortex : **ST** | [1]>
‖ <DorsolateralCortex : **ST** | [1]>
‖ <VentromedialCortex : **ST** | [1]>

Fig. 2. High level architectural framework of the CA

In this manner, the high-level architectural framework of the CA's design is depicted in figure 2 (part 1), where the Thalamus**ST**, SensoryCortex**ST**, and PrefrontalCortex**ST** receive further refinement (figure 2 part 2).

In addition to the components of the CA shown in figure 2, an external Environment**ST** module is considered. The rest of this section provides a description of all these components and their respective UDMs, which support the formal description of their internal structure.

Environment: this component generates a variety of stimuli that will reach the SensorySystem**ST** (i.e., visual, gustatory, somatosensory, auditory, and olfactory stimuli.) It includes one structure called DataSource**ST** that contains five fields used to communicate the stimuli being elicited. Next is its UDM:

Environment**ST** ≜ (
<DataSource**ST**(
<VisualDataID : **N** | $0 \leq$ VisualDataID ≤ 100000 >
<GustatoryDataID : **N** | $0 \leq$ GustatoryDataID ≤ 100000 >
<SomatoSDataID : **N** | $0 \leq$ SomatoSDataID ≤ 100000 >
<AuditoryDataID : **N** | $0 \leq$ AuditoryDataID ≤ 100000 >
<OlfactoryDataID : **N** | $0 \leq$ OlfactoryDataID ≤ 100000 >) >)

Sensory System: it captures and organizes the data caught from the environment, which will be processed by other modules. Fields for data flow control are at least required in this module, they are shown in its corresponding UDM:

SensorySystem**ST** ≜ (
<TypeStimuli : **N** | TypeStimuli**N** = {(0, Visual), (1, Gustatory),
(2, Somatosensory), (3, Auditory), (4, Olfactory)}>

<VisStim : **Queue**[SE_1**N**, SE_2**N**, SE_3**N**, ..., SE_n**N**] >
<GustStim : **Queue**[SE_1**N**, SE_2**N**, SE_3**N**, ..., SE_n**N**] >
<SomaStim : **Queue**[SE_1**N**, SE_2**N**, SE_3**N**, ..., SE_n**N**] >
<AudiStim : **Queue**[SE_1**N**, SE_2**N**, SE_3**N**, ..., SE_n**N**] >
<OlfaStim : **Queue**[SE_1**N**, SE_2**N**, SE_3**N**, ..., SE_n**N**] >)

(α) ***Olfactory Bulb:*** by filtering olfactory data received from the SensorySystem**ST**, this module helps with the discrimination of synthetic odors. It includes one field for representing and identifying the input data, one for sensing its operational conditions, and one for preparing the outputs:

OlfactoryBulb**ST** ≜ (
<RecOlfaDataID : **N** | 0 ≤ RecOlfaDataID**N** ≤ 100000>
<DataStatus : **BL** | DataStatus**BL** = {(0, Normal), (1, Faulty)}>
<OlfaDataToSC : **Array** | OlfaDataToSC**Array** = [x**N**]>)

Thalamus: the four subcomponents of this module detect and interpret the most salient features of the data captured by the SensorySystem**ST** (except the olfactory.) Each of them includes at least four fields: one for the control of received data, one for sensing its internal state, and two for preparing outputs. Next is the UDM of one subsystem, the others are similar:

LateralGeniculateNucleus**ST** ≜ (
<RecVisDataID : **N** | 0 ≤ RecVisDataID**N** ≤ 100000>
<DataStatus : **BL** | DataStatus**BL** = {(0, Normal), (1, Faulty)}>
<VisDataToSC : **Array** | VisDataToSC**Array** = [x**N**] >
<VisDataToAmy : **Array** | VisDataToAmy**Array** = [x**N**]>)

Sensory Cortex: the subsystems of this module provide full interpretation to the stimuli filtered by the Thalamus**ST** and the OlfactoryBulb**ST**. At least four fields are required in each subsystem: two for the received data, one for the state of the data being processed, and the last for the outputs. The following UDM corresponds to one subsystem, the others are similar:

AuditoryCortex**ST** ≜ (
<RecAudiStimID : **N** | 0 ≤ RecAudiStimID**N** ≤ 100000>
<DataFromHippoID : **N** | 0 ≤ DataFromHippoID**N** ≤ 100000>
<DataStatus : **BL** | DataStatus**BL** = {(0, Normal), (1, Faulty)}>
<AudiDataProc : **Array** | AudiDataProc**Array** = [x**N**]>)

(λ) ***Association Cortex:*** it provides a perceptual model of the world by combining and organizing the interpretations made by the SensoryCortex**ST**. This brain structure has a variety of fields for managing its inputs and outputs:

AssociationCortex**ST** ≜ (
<DataTypeReceived : **N** | DataTypeReceived**N** = {(0, Visual), (1, Gustatory), (2, Somatosensory), (3, Auditory), (4, Olfactory)}>
<RecHippoDataID : **N** | 0 ≤ RecHippoDataID**N** ≤ 100000 >
<RecAmyDataID : **N** | 0 ≤ RecAmyDataID**N** ≤ 100000 >

<RecDlpcDataID : **N** | 0 ≤ RecDlpcDataID**N** ≤ 100000 >
<AssociatedStimu : **Array** | AssociatedStimu**Array** = [x**N**]>)

(μ) ***Hippocampus:*** it manages the encoding, storage, and retrieval of memories, and creates a context with all stimuli processed and previously stored. Fields for controlling the data inputs and outputs must be at least considered:

Hippocampus**ST** ≜ (
<DataTypeRec : **N** | DataTypeRec**N** = {(0, Visual), (1, Gustatory), (2, Somatosensory), (3, Auditory), (4, Olfactory)}>
<SentMemSC : **Array** | SentMemSC**Array** = [x**N**] >
<RecAmyLevel : **N** | 0 ≤ RecAmyLevel**N** ≤ 9 >
<RecLearnDataID : **Array** | RecLearnDataID**Array** = [x**N**] >
<RecDlpcDataID : **N** | 0 ≤ RecDlpcDataID**N** ≤ 100000 >
<SentMemAmy : **Array** | SentMemAmy**Array** = [x**N**] >
<SentAcMemID : **Array** | SentAcMemID**Array** = [x**N**] >
<GoalDlpcID : **Array** | GoalDlpcID**Array** = [x**N**] >)

(ν) ***Amygdala:*** this component is responsible for interpreting all incoming stimuli from an affective perspective. Fields for controlling received data and affective processed data are required as shown in its UDM:

Amygdala**ST** ≜ (
<DataTypeRec : **N** | DataTypeRec**N** = {(0, Visual), (1, Gustatory), (2, Somatosensory), (3, Auditory), (4, Olfactory)}>
<FastEmoReact : **N** | 0 ≤ FastEmoReact**N** ≤ 100 >
<AdjustedEmoReact : **N** | 0 ≤ AdjustedEmoReact**N** ≤ 100 >
<GlobalEmoStatus : **N** | 0 ≤ GlobalEmoStatus**N** ≤ 9 >
<ActualRewardLevel : **N** | 0 ≤ ActualRewardLevel**N** ≤ 9 >
<RecHippoMem : **Array** | RecHippoMem**Array** = [x**N**] >)

(ξ) ***Orbitofrontal Cortex:*** this component processes affective information in order to allow cognitive functions such as planning and decision-making make use of proper affective stimuli. At least three fiels are required in this component:

OrbitoFrontalCortex**ST** ≜ (
<RecAmyDataID : **N** | 0 ≤ RecAmyDataID**N** ≤ 100000 >
<DataStatus : **BL** | DataStatus**BL** = {(0, Normal), (1, Faulty)}>
<EmoVmpcID : **N** | 0 ≤ EmoVmpcID**N** ≤ 100000 >)

(o) ***Dorsolateral Prefrontal Cortex:*** this is the room for the process that creates plans and is responsible for communicating the next action to perform. Its UDM shows some of the required data for its proper functioning:

DorsolateralCortex**ST** ≜ (
<RecHippoMem : **Array** | RecHippoMem**Array** = [x**N**] >
<SentVmpfDataID : **N** | 0 ≤ SentVmpfDataID**N** ≤ 100000 >
<RecVmpfDataID : **N** | 0 ≤ RecVmpfID**N** ≤ 100000 >
<NextActionID : **N** | 0 ≤ NextActionID**N** ≤ 100 >

<TempMem : **Array** | TempMem**Array** = [x**N**]>
<PlanState : **Array** | PlanState**Array** = [x**N**]>
<ExpectedRewardLevel : **N** | 0 ≤ ExpectedRewardLevel**N** ≤ 9 >
<RationalPlan : **BL** | RationalPlan**BL** = {(**T**, Ok), (**F**, Rejected)}>
<EmoPlan : **BL** | EmoPlan**BL** = {(**T**, Ok), (**F**, Rejected)}>)

(π) ***Ventromedial Prefrontal Cortex:*** its main function is to select the next action to perform. Its corresponding UMD is:
VentromedialCortex**ST** ≜ (
<RecHippoMemID : **Array** | RecHippoMemID**Array** = [x**N**] >
<EmoData : **Array** | EmoData**Array** = [x**N**]>
<RationalData : **Array** | RationalData**Array** = [x**N**]>
<GeneralViewWorld : **Array** | GeneralViewWorld**Array** = [x**N**]>
<SentDlfcID : **N** | 0 ≤ SentDlfcID**N** ≤ 100000 >)

(ρ) ***Basal Ganglia:*** selects movable components to carry out an action. It requires at least four fields for receiving, sending, storing, and managing data:
BasalGanglia**ST** ≜ (
<ReceivedAction : **N** | 0 ≤ ReceivedAction**N** ≤ 100 >
<DataStatus : **BL** | DataStatus**BL** = {(0, Normal), (1, Faulty)}>
<SelectedComp : **Array** | SelectedComp**Array** = [x**N**]>
<BasalMem : **Array** | BasalMem**Array** = [x**N**]>)

(σ) ***Motor Cortex:*** this module makes the needed calculations to control movable components selected by the BasalGanglia**ST** and complete an action:
MotorCortex**ST** ≜ (
<ReceivedBgID : **N** | 0 ≤ ReceivedBgID**N** ≤ 100000 >
<CurrentPositions : **Array** | CurrentPositions**Array** = [x**N**, y**N**, z**N**]>
<DataCalculation : **Array** | DataCalculation**Array** = [x**N**, y**N**, z**N**]>
<MotorMem : **Array** | MotorMem**Array** = [x**N**]>)

5 Specifications of the Behaviors of the CA

In this section we refine the CogArch§.Behaviors**PC** subsystem. We first provide a high-level description of the behaviors implemented in the CA and then detail their operations by developing their corresponding UPMs. As explained before, such behaviors synthesize the operations and architecture of the following brain functions: Perception, Learning, Memory, Attention, Emotions, Planning, Decision-Making, and Motor-Action [7], which are the result of the interoperation of the architectural components specified in section 4.

Perception: the stimuli captured by the SensorySystem**ST** are classified according to their modality and then sent to the Thalamus**ST** and OlfactoryBulb**ST**, which filter such stimuli in order to detect their salient features and then project to the SensoryCortex**ST**. This component uses memories retrieved from the Hippocampus**ST** and derives a high-level interpretation of each type of stimulus. Then, this information is sent to the AssociationCortex**ST** to create an internal representation of the world. Its UPM formally describes this process:

Perception**PC** ≜ { *// 1. Data source is classified*
↣ Classify(DataSource**ST**)
// 2. Data source is adapted to be processed by sensory system
↣ Adapt(DataSource**ST**.VisualDataID**N**) > VisStim**Queue**
↣ Adapt(DataSource**ST**.GustatoryDataID**N**) > GustStim**Queue**
↣ Adapt(DataSource**ST**.SomatoSDataID**N**) > SomaStim**Queue**
↣ Adapt(DataSource**ST**.AuditoryDataID**N**) > AudiStim**Queue**
↣ Adapt(DataSource**ST**.OlfactoryDataID**N**) > OlfaStim**Queue**
// 3. Thalamus and Olfactory bulb filter captured stimuli
↣ ThalFilter(VisStim**Queue**) > VisDataToSC**Array**[x**N**]
↣ ThalFilter(GustStim**Queue**) > GustDataToSC**Array**[x**N**]
↣ ThalFilter(SomaStim**Queue**) > SomaDataToSC**Array**[x**N**]
↣ ThalFilter(AudiStim**Queue**) > AudiDataToSC**Array**[x**N**]
↣ BulbFilter(OlfaStim**Queue**) > OlfaDataToSC**Array**[x**N**]
// 4. Interpretation is done by Sensory Cortex's subsystems
↣ VisCortex(VisDataToSC**Array**[x**N**]) > VisDataProc**Array**[x**N**]
↣ GustCortex(GustDataToSC**Array**[x**N**]) > GustDataProc**Array**[x**N**]
↣ SomaCortex(SomaDataToSC**Array**[x**N**]) > SomaDataProc**Array**[x**N**]
↣ AudiCortex(AudiDataToSC**Array**[x**N**]) > AudiDataProc**Array**[x**N**]
↣ OlfaCortex(OlfaDataToSC**Array**[x**N**]) > OlfaDataProc**Array**[x**N**]
// 5. Association Cortex organizes all information
↣ Association(VisDataProc**Array**[x**N**], GustDataProc**Array**[x**N**],
SomaDataProc**Array**[x**N**], AudiDataProc**Array**[x**N**],
OlfaDataProc**Array**[x**N**]) > AssociatedStimu**Array**[x**N**] }

Emotions: the Amygdala**ST** receives and uses little processed information from the Thalamus**ST** to produce fast emotional reactions. In order to generate an emotional state and regulate emotions, this component retrieves memories from the Hippocampus**ST** and receives highly processed stimuli from the SensoryCortex**ST** and the AssociationCortex**ST**. The following UPM formally describes such procedures:

Emotions**PC** ≜ { *// 1. Fast reactions are generated*
↣ FastReactions(VisDataToAmy**Array**[x**N**], GustDataToAmy**Array**[x**N**],
SomaDataToAmy**Array**[x**N**], AudiDataToAmy**Array**[x**N**],
OlfaDataToAmy**Array**[x**N**], SentMemAmy**Array**[x**N**]) > FastEmoReact**N**[x**N**]
// 2. Adjustments for reactions are generated
↣ ReactionAdjustments(VisDataProc**Array**[x**N**], GustDataProc**Array**[x**N**],
SomaDataProc**Array[xN]**, AudiDataProc**Array[xN]**, OlfaDataProc**Array**[x**N**],
AssociatedStimu**Array**[x**N**], SentMemAmy**Array**[x**N**]) > AdjustedEmoReact**N**[x**N**]
// 3. General emotional evaluation
↣ EmoEvaluation(VisDataProc**Array**[x**N**], GustDataProc**Array**[x**N**],
SomaDataProc**Array**[x**N**], AudiDataProc**Array**[x**N**], OlfaDataProc**Array**[x**N**],
AssociatedStimu**Array**[x**N**], SentMemAmy**Array**[x**N**]) > GlobalEmoStatus**N** }

Attention: once emotional information is derived in the Amygdala**ST**, such structure projects to the SensoryCortex**ST** and AssociationCortex**ST**, where interpretations of the external environment are being conducted. In this manner, emotional signals determine which stimuli must be attended. Its UPM is:

Attention**PC** ≜
{ *// 1. Influencing individual senses*
↣ VisAtt(VisDataProc**Array**[x**N**], FastEmoReact**N**, GlobalEmoStatus**N**)
↣ GustAtt(GustDataProc**Array**[x**N**], FastEmoReact**N**, GlobalEmoStatus**N**)
↣ SomaAtt(SomaDataProc**Array**[x**N**], FastEmoReact**N**, GlobalEmoStatus**N**)
↣ AudiAtt(AudiDataProc**Array**[x**N**], FastEmoReact**N**, GlobalEmoStatus**N**)
↣ OlfaAtt(OlfaDataProc**Array**[x**N**], FastEmoReact**N**, GlobalEmoStatus**N**)
// 2. Influencing the creation of world representation
↣ GlobalAtt(AssociatedStimu**Array**[x**N**], FastEmoReact**N**, GlobalEmoStatus**N**) }

Memory: in this process, the sensory memory temporarily stores information held in the SensoryCortex**ST** and AssociationCortex**ST**. The working memory at the DorsolateralCortex**ST** receives data from the Hippocampus**ST**, AssociationCortex**ST**, and VentromedialCortex**ST** to temporarily store limited data and make up an overall view of the agent's internal and external status. The episodic memory uses the Hippocampus**ST** to permanently store experiences. The semantic memory stores knowledge about facts without considerations of time and space. The procedural memory stores procedures useful for the achievement of common tasks using the BasalGanglia**ST** and the Hippocampus**ST**.

Memory**PC** ≜ { *// 1. Managing five types of memories*
↣ SensoryMem(VisDataProc**Array**[x**N**], GustDataProc**Array**[x**N**], SomaDataProc**Array**[x**N**], AudiDataProc**Array**[x**N**], OlfaDataProc**Array**[x**N**], AssociatedStimu**Array**[x**N**], GlobalEmoStatus**N**) ⋗ RecLearnDataID
↣ WorkingMem(TempMem**Array**[x**N**], GlobalEmoStatus**N**) ⋗ RecLearnDataID
↣ EpisodicMem(VisDataProc**Array**[x**N**], GustDataProc**Array**[x**N**], SomaDataProc**Array**[x**N**], AudiDataProc**Array**[x**N**], OlfaDataProc**Array**[x**N**], AssociatedStimu**Array**[x**N**], GlobalEmoStatus**N**) ⋗ RecLearnDataID
↣ SemanticMem(VisDataProc**Array**[x**N**], GustDataProc**Array**[x**N**], SomaDataProc**Array**[x**N**], AudiDataProc**Array**[x**N**], OlfaDataProc**Array**[x**N**], AssociatedStimu**Array**[x**N**], GlobalEmoStatus**N**) ⋗ RecLearnDataID
↣ ProceduralMem(BasalMem**Array**[x**N**], MotorMem**Array**[x**N**], GlobalEmoStatus**N**) ⋗ RecLearnDataID }

Learning: in order to determine what information will be learned, there must be a discrepancy between the expected rewards and the actual acquired rewards managed by the Amygdala**ST**, which arise from the interaction of the agent with its environment. For this process, the Hippocampus**ST** collects and stores current stimuli interpretations conducted by the SensoryCortex**ST** and AssociationCortex**ST**, as well as their corresponding emotional level. If no discrepancy occurs, the already stored memories are only strengthened:

Learning**PC** ≜ { *// Checking discrepancies and updating or creating memories*
→ (? ActualRewardLevel ≠ ExpectedRewardLevel
    ↣ StoreUpdateMem(AssociatedStimu**Array**[x**N**], GlobalEmoStatus**N**)
  | ? ∼
    ↣ StrengthenMem(AssociatedStimu**Array**[x**N**], GlobalEmoStatus**N**) }

Planning: plans are created at the DorsolateralCortex**ST**. It receives a rational representation of the world from the SensoryCortex**ST** and AssociationCortex**ST**. Once these information is classified according the current goal (provided by the Hippocampus**ST**), it is sent to the VentromedialCortex**ST** to be combined with emotional data received from the OrbitoFrontalCortex**ST**. These data is then returned to the DorsolateralCortex**ST**, which generates new states for the plan being constructed. These states are passed to the SensoryCortex**ST** and to the Amygdala**ST** to perform a rational and emotional evaluation. When such evaluated states reaches again the DorsolateralCortex**ST**, it is linked to the previous state, and the new planning sequence is used to start again the same cycle.

  Planning**PC** ≜ { *// 1.Getting rational and emotional states*
↣ RationInfo(AssociatedStimu**Array**[x**N**], GoalDlpcID**Array**[x**N**])
⋗ RationalData**Array**[x**N**]
↣ EmoInfo(EmoVmpcID**N**) ⋗ EmoData**Array**[x**N**]
  // 2. Combining rational and emotional view of the world
↣Comb(RationalData**Array**[x**N**],EmoData**Array**[x**N**])⋗GeneralViewWorld**Array**[x**N**]
  // 3. Creating new states and evaluating them
↣ NewPlanState(GeneralViewWorld**Array**[x**N**]) ⋗ PlanState**Array**[x**N**]
↣ RationalEvState(PlanState**Array**[x**N**]) ⋗ RationalPlan**BL**
↣ EmotionalEvState(PlanState**Array**[x**N**]) ⋗ EmoPlan**BL**
  // 4. The planning process is called again
↣ Planning**PC** }

Decision Making: to take a decision, the VentromedialCortex**ST** receives emotional data from the OrbitoFrontalCortex**ST** and rational data from the DorsolateralCortex**ST**. In addition, based on the current goal, the next action to perform is sent to the BasalGanglia**ST** through the DorsolateralCortex**ST**.

  DecisionMaking**PC** ≜ { *// Deciding what action to take*
↣ NextAction(RationalData**Array**[x**N**], EmoData**Array**[x**N**],
GoalDlpcID**Array**[x**N**]) ⋗ NextActionID**N** }

Motor Action: assisted by the AssociationCortex**ST**, the BasalGanglia**ST** senses the current physical status of the agent and selects the appropriate body movements. This information is then sent to the MotorCortex**ST**, which with continuous feedback from the SomatosensoryCortex**ST** carries out the action.

MotorAction**PC** ≜ { *// Deciding what action to take*
↣ CompMovSelect(ReceivedAction**N**, AssociatedStimu**Array**[x**N**])
> SelectedComp**Array**[x**N**]
↣ ExecAct(SelectedComp**Array**[x**N**], CurrentPositions**Array**[x**N**, y**N**, z**N**]) }

6 Conclusion

The formal specification of a neuroscience-inspired cognitive architecture was elaborated using a formal methodology called Real-Time Process Algebra. Its architectural components and behaviors were rigorously described, allowing thus a clear understanding of the high-level functioning of the cognitive architecture and enabling the unambiguous communication of its important characteristics and essential assumptions. Furthermore, this proposal represents an attempt to create biological-inspired models that rigurously conform to the principles and standards established for the development of software systems.

Acknowledgments. The authors would like to acknowledge the PhD scholarship (CONACYT grant No. 229386) sponsored by the Mexican Government for their partial support to this work. We would like to thank the anonymous reviewers for their valuable comments and suggestions.

References

1. Anderson, J.R., Lebiere, C.: The atomic components of thought. Lawrence Erlbaum Associates, Mahwah (1998)
2. Hinchey, M., Bowen, J.P., Rouff, C.A.: Introduction to formal methods. In: Rouff, C., Hinchey, M., Rash, J., Truszkowski, W., Gordon-Spears, D. (eds.) Agent Technology from a Formal Perspective. NASA Monographs in Systems and Software Engineering, pp. 25–64. Springer, Heidelberg (2006)
3. Kandel, E.R., Schwartz, J.H., Jessell, T.M.: Principles of Neural Science, 4th edn. McGraw-Hill, New York (2000)
4. Laird, J.E.: Extending the soar cognitive architecture. In: Proceeding of the 2008 Conference on Artificial General Intelligence, pp. 224–235. IOS Press, Amsterdam (2008)
5. Langley, P., Laird, J.E., Rogers, S.: Cognitive architectures: Research issues and challenges. Cognitive Systems Research 10(2), 141–160 (2009)
6. Newell, A.: Unified theories of cognition. Harvard University Press, Cambridge (1990)
7. Rodríguez, F., Galvan, F., Ramos, F., Castellanos, E., García, G., Covarrubias, P.: A cognitive architecture based on neuroscience for the control of virtual 3D human creatures. In: Yao, Y., Sun, R., Poggio, T., Liu, J., Zhong, N., Huang, J. (eds.) BI 2010. LNCS, vol. 6334, pp. 328–335. Springer, Heidelberg (2010)
8. Wang, Y.: The real-time process algebra (rtpa). Annals of Software Engineering 14(1-4), 235–274 (2002)
9. Wang, Y.: Software Engineering Foundations: A Software Science Perspective. Auerbach Publications (2008)

Computational Modeling of Brain Processes for Agent Architectures: Issues and Implications

Luis-Felipe Rodríguez[1], Félix Ramos[1], and Gregorio García[2]

[1] Department of Computer Science, Cinvestav Guadalajara
{lrodrigue,framos}@gdl.cinvestav.mx
[2] Department of Psychology, Benemérita Universidad Autónoma de Puebla
gregorio.garcia@correo.buap.mx

Abstract. Cognitive architectures are integrative frameworks that include a series of components that interoperate to generate a variety of behaviors in autonomous agents. Commonly, such components attempt to synthesize the operations and architecture of brain functions, such as perception and emotions. To carry out this, they embody computational models whose development is based on theories explaining cognitive and affective functions as well as on principles and standards established for the development of software systems. Unfortunately, such theories and software principles are not always available or entirely adequate. In this paper, we analyze and discuss fundamental issues associated to the development of these type of architectural components. We focus on the problems that arise throughout their development cycle and identify some improvements for the tools used in their construction.

Keywords: Computational Models, Brain processes, Cognitive Architectures.

1 Introduction

The brain is a complex system that allows humans to perceive, integrate, and process internal and external stimuli, allowing thus the generation of appropriate actions as responses to determined situations [9]. A multidisciplinary study of the brain has identified a number of brain functions that interact in order to produce such behaviors. Furthermore, specific brain structures have been identified as architectural components of these brain processes [19].

The operation and architecture of the human brain can be studied at different levels. As described above, it can be considered as a system constituted of several brain structures that communicate and implement specific tasks (e.g., the hippocampus, the thalamus, and the amygdala) [19]. Similarly, at a lower level, the brain can be addressed as a body of nerve cells (or neurons) that are organized in a way that allows the generation of behaviors [9]. However, regardless of how the human brain is studied, it seems a complex system that processes information efficiently, effectively, and with high performance and reliability [3, 9].

The study of brain functions has been addressed in various disciplines. For example, neuroscience and cognitive psychology have developed theoretical models

B. Hu et al. (Eds.): BI 2011, LNAI 6889, pp. 197–208, 2011.

that explain the mechanisms and structures underlying human brain processes [9, 19]. Artificial intelligence (AI) has also developed computational and formal models of cognitive and affective functions [15, 31]. While neuroscientists and psychologists use the computational modeling as a powerful tool for testing and complete their theories [28], computer scientists use theoretical models that explain human behaviors to create intelligent systems [6].

In particular, cognitive architectures (CAs) include computational models of brain processes (CMBs) to allow autonomous agents (AAs) implementing behaviors with specific characteristics, such as sociable, affective, and intelligent [10, 27]. These CMBs are implemented in CAs as behaviors that emerge from the operation of a set of architectural components that usually embody algorithms that simulate the functioning and anatomy of brain structures. Figure 1 illustrates such conception using a framework based on levels.

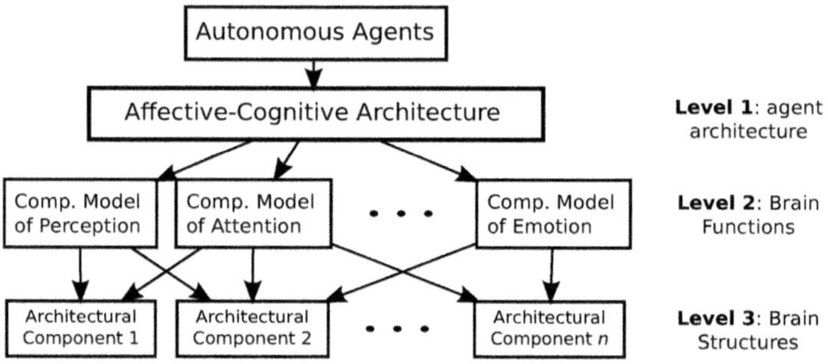

Fig. 1. Cognitive architecture as basis of autonomous agents

The development of these CMBs has a theoretical and a computational basis. Their theoretical basis validates their internal mechanisms and external behaviors by conforming to theories that explore human cognitive and affective processes [9, 19]. Similarly, their computational basis ensures the quality and adequacy of their development by following principles and standards established for the development of software systems [25]. However, many difficulties arise throughout the development of such CMBs. The main source of these problems comes from this dual nature. Although theoretical and computational approaches have provided adequate models to explain and simulate human behaviors, most have been developed without a full collaboration between the two areas [27]. Therefore, an integrated approach to create CMBs definitely gives rise to a number of new and diverse problems.

In this paper, we explore and discuss the issues that limit the proper development of CMBs. We explain the nature of these problems and provide some examples in section 2. Then, we analyze how these issues affect the particular phases of their development cycle in section 3. Additionally, we review some proposals for the construction of appropriate tools for this type of developments. Finally, section 4 provides some concluding remarks.

2 Fundamental Issues in the Development of CMBs

The translation of human brain functions into artificial processes has become one of the main objectives in several subareas of computer sciences [7, 20, 27]. As a result, many formal and computational models of cognitive and affective processes have been implemented [15, 17, 31]. As we explained above, these models are mainly intended to be included in agent architectures in order to improve the believability and autonomy of virtual and physical agents.

A variety of constraints, however, makes the synthesis of brain processes a complex task. We devote this section to briefly discuss the issues that hinder the development of CMBs, which are mainly derived from three aspects that are central to their construction:

1. *Computational basis*: we explore whether software engineering tools and methodologies have the potential to deal with these type of developments.
2. *Theoretical basis*: the design of CMBs inherits the problems in the theories in which they are based. We explain why and how it happens.
3. *Architectural basis*: we examine the benefits and disadvantages that involve the two main approaches followed to design CMBs.

2.1 Computational Basis

After all, the synthesis of human brain processes must be addressed, in general, as a software engineering project. As such, it must be subject to the rules, methods, techniques, and all those fundamental principles involved in the development of software systems [25].

When we refer to software engineering (SE), we talk, among many other aspects, about the quality of software, methodologies, software processes, architectural designs, and formal specifications [25, 32]. For the development of conventional software projects (e.g., those for industry), all those concepts are very familiar and useful, however, for projects related to building CMBs they can hardly be applied. Nevertheless, the application of SE principles and the adequate use of assistive software tools is essential to achieve a successful software project development [21].

There are many factors that prevent the proper use of SE tools and methodologies in the development of CMBs. These tools and methodologies have been designed under the assumption that all system requirements are established by users, however, for computational models of cognitive and affective processes additional types of requirements are considered. In this case, part of the requirements comes from user's observations of human behaviors, but others must be formulated from formal and well-founded evidence about the functioning of brain processes. In this manner, nonsensical specifications are prevented by considering theories and models developed in disciplines concerned with understanding the mechanisms and procedures that underlie human behaviors. Unfortunately, few tools recognize these needs and properly assist the development of CMBs [1, 4].

Appropriate tools and methodologies to assist this type of developments are yet to be constructed [1, 32]. However, this does not only depend on the developers' skills, many other factors are involved. For example, a detailed, precise, and complete specification of the process these SE tools are intended to automate is necessary. In the case of most brain functions, detailed explanations of their internal operations and architecture are not yet available or fully covered. As an instance, the computational modeling of human emotions can lead to inconsistencies, complications, or even contradictions due to the wide variety of theories that address the emotional process from different perspectives. Most of these theories and models disagree on the set of components that are considered part of this process. Furthermore, a universal definition of the term "emotions" has not been clearly established [16].

Accordingly, although many conventional software tools can be used in the development of CMBs, they rather represent an starting point toward the construction of new extraordinary tools. For example, most tools and methodologies developed in AI and SE to build autonomous agents have proven useful for implementing "intelligent" AAs, but they are little concerned in supporting the construction of emotional, social, and cultural agents [22, 25]. What's more, they are not committed with the development of intelligent systems based on theoretical models, in particular, those addressing the internal processing that underlie human behaviors [32]. Similarly, in the area of Agent Oriented Software Engineering (AOSE), the main interest is to develop tools and methodologies to create Multi-Agent Systems (MAS), minimizing the importance of constructing proper internal architectures for the autonomous agents that inhabit these environments [18]. Thus, although SE, AOSE, and AI have developed tools and methodologies to create intelligent systems, they are not yet ready to meet all demands posited by the dual nature of the development of CMBs.

2.2 Theoretical Basis

The inquiry on the brain operation and its internal architecture is complex by nature. However, several disciplines have devoted considerable work to this endeavor, such as philosophy, cognitive psychology, and neuroscience. This multidisciplinary study has resulted in a number of theories and models that explain diverse cognitive and affective phenomena such as the perception, attention, decision-making, and emotional process [3, 11, 19].

Because CMBs are intended to simulate human brain functions, they must adhere to the actual functioning of these processes by implementing theories and models that explain their internal mechanisms and architecture. Most CMBs have been based on psychological and neuroscientific theories [8, 14, 29, 30]. On the one hand, psychology provides theories and models that study human behaviors from a functional and high level perspective. These theories are not intended to reveal the internal mechanisms inside the brain, but on finding associations between stimuli and responses. On the other hand, neuroscience theories and models contribute with more detailed descriptions of internal mechanisms underlying human behaviors; they usually specify which operations and structures are involved in the brain process they are addressing [19].

However, there are usually several theories explaining the same phenomenon [16, 23]. They usually differ in (1) the levels of abstraction used to study brain processes, (2) the components they consider as part of the process they are exploring, and (3) the nature of such brain functions. Ron Sun [26] recognizes four different levels of analysis based on the level of abstraction that different disciplines use to study models, see table 1 and refer to [26] for further explanations.

Table 1. Four levels of analysis [26]

Object of analysis	Type of analysis	Model
Inter-agent/collective processes	Social/cultural	Collections of agent models
Agents	Psychological	Individual agent models
Intra-agent processes	Componential	Modular construction of agent models
Substrates	Physiological	Biological realization of modules

As a particular instance, in the computational modeling of human emotions a useful approach has been to classify emotions as primary and secondary (also known as basic and nonbasic emotions) [2, 30]. While primary emotions are supposed to be innate, instinctive, and with an evolutionary basis, secondary emotions are learned through experience [5, 12]. Although most theories agree in the nature of the two types of emotions, many of them disagree on how secondary emotions arise from the primary ones. Some theories assume that they are derived from primary emotions by a variety of combinatorial methods, however, other models consider that they follow the primary emotions, but their construction is independent of them [5, 12].

As a consequence, CMBs are likely to inherit such variability in their internal designs. That is, decisions of what elements, what levels of abstraction, and what interactions are necessary to achieve a working application are carried out by developers subjectively, which leads to the creation of CMBs whose internal mechanisms and external behaviors differ in several aspects, making it difficult to create assessment frameworks to evaluate and compare them.

As another example, although we are now able to handle more clearly some terms used in the specification of affective models such as mood and personality, a precise definition for them has not been determined. Most of the times, their definition depends on the affective model under study or on the influence of researchers. Since the design of CBEs makes extensive use of terms formulated in psychology and neuroscience, the inherent ambiguity of these terms seems to be inherited. This issue greatly contributes to the difficulty of understanding computational models without understand the theories in which they are based.

2.3 Architectural Basis

Computational models of cognitive and affective processes are commonly included in CAs by following two perspectives: as stand-alone models, and as integrated models. The former refer to components that are built separately and then included as extensions for existing cognitive frameworks or architectures, thus providing them with the necessary mechanisms for affective and cognitive processing [6, 24]. The second ones have to do with models that are designed and implemented as part of cognitive frameworks. They are implemented on several architectural components [8].

The benefits and disadvantages of each approach vary. On the one hand, to include stand-alone models in CAs brings many advantages. For example, they allow the use of previously tested components as well as a fast and easy integration of additional processes into CAs. Existing architectures use these components by sending them some raw data and receiving back processed information, which is then used to influence the normal behavior of some other functions [24]. As an instance, emotional components can be included in architectures of conversational agents in order to adjust the selection of appropriate emotional expressions as responses in social situations [6]. Nonetheless, this approach also presents many disadvantages. For example, when designing AAs whose behaviors should display those characteristics observed in humans, several types of processed data is required in order to influence a variety of processes. In this case, specialized components may not be able to process all the required data for the fulfillment of all the requirements.

On the other hand, for CMBs designed and implemented in integrated environments such as CAs, the problems and advantages are different. The development of this type of models follows a more natural design, therefore, they are not built as individual architectural extensions, but as processes that emerge from the joint operation of multiple mechanisms [7, 8, 27]. Its construction becomes more complicated, and as many other aspects inherent to the architecture in which they are included should be understood, their implementation is more prone to errors. In addition, they are the most likely to inherit the problems from their underlying theories (as explained above.) Many benefits can also be gained by using this approach. For example, because these models are built based on how cognitive and affective functions actually arise in the human brain, they can be more easily adapted to include other processes such as personality, mood, and perception, without having to make many changes in the already implemented mechanisms.

As a particular instance, the incorporation of computational models of emotions into CAs as individual components can be disadvantageous. This interpretation leads to think that emotional processing is handled by a single process, but since these models are grounded on theories that deal with the mechanisms that govern human emotions, this approach becomes contradictory. Multidisciplinary studies have demonstrated that emotions are a process that emerges from the interoperation of many brain structures [9]; they are not the result of a single component that receives raw inputs and delivers emotional outputs. Additionally, to talk about the interactions between emotions and cognition contributes to perceive emotions as separate from cognition. Although this independence has been used to achieve organized designs [6, 7], it is far from reality. Furthermore, although it seems (and is widely accepted) that some brain structures process more cognitive information than affective, and vice versa, the most accepted theory is that cognitive and affective processes emerge from the same brain structures operations [9, 13].

3 Implications for the Development Cycle of CMBs

In this section, we briefly discuss particular problems faced at each stage of the development cycle of CMBs, and analyze how a variety of available software instruments can be improved to become useful in their construction. Suggestions to improve the performance of these phases and the tools used are given based on two aspects: (1) how to *maximize the use of existing theoretical knowledge* about the operation and architecture of cognitive and affective processes, and (2) how to follow the development of CMBs to *create more integrative models*. Additionally, the last subsection presents some software tools and methodologies that have been developed to aid the construction of nature-inspired models.

In order to provide a coherent analysis, we examine these implications and tools according to the phases in the software development cycle: specification, design, and implementation.

3.1 Specification

This is one of the most critical phases of the software development cycle. It has to do with formal and informal specifications of the behaviors of a software system in terms of its expected functionality, desirable features, and operational constraints [21, 25]. Software tools and methodologies used in this phase focus on defining clearly and unambiguously the system requirements and restrictions, as well as on achieving complete and coherent system specifications. Under the assumption that the requirements of a system are mainly specified by users, these tools work seamlessly. However, when the software system to be specified has to do with the modeling of cognitive and affective processes, the system requirements have to be expanded to capture the essence of the operations and restrictions of the internal mechanisms of brain functions. Therefore, inaccurate and nonsensical requirements can be prevented when the software tools used are adequate to assist the collection of these two types of requirements.

However, as we explained in the previous sections, there are many factors that hinder the proper collection of detailed descriptions about the functioning of brain processes. In addition, current tools are not able to properly handle the various theories that explain a specific brain process, nor have the strategies needed to create complete and consistent specifications from incomplete theories.

In this sense, new software tools should enable us to correctly specify the interactions between the processes we are modeling, the influences they exert on each other, and the type of the data they communicate. These procedures, however, must conform to solid theories so that inconsistencies and contradictions regarding the nature of such processes will be prevented. For example, in order to specify the computational process of learning in a CA, a suitable software tool should allow us to correctly establish that, for example, the process of emotions can represent reinforcers, and that as a result, the retention of memories about high emotional events will be strongly consolidated. That is, such new tools should be aware of many theories that explain the processes we are intended to model, allowing us to create specifications that are totally valid and that encompass important processes and restrictions according to the functioning and architecture of the actual processes in the human brain.

3.2 Design

This phase delivers a more formal specification of the behaviors expected in a software system, as well as a detailed description of the components that constitute its underlying architecture. At this stage, it is necessary to establish the interfaces of each component as well as the data structures used to enable their communication [21, 25]. The tools used in the design process range from those that allow the creation of simple architectural diagrams to methodologies that facilitate the transition from the system specification to its architectural design [21].

When designing CMBs many questions should be addressed. For example, which are the essential elements that should be considered to construct these models, which of them are mandatory and which not, and how they should interact in order to meet the specifications. To answer these questions it is necessary to analyze the requirements given in the specification stage, however, unlike conventional software projects, evidence explaining the mechanisms underlying brain processes should be also considered.

Furthermore, a direct translation of the specification of a CMB to an architectural design is unsuitable. That is, even though a requirement establishes that decision making is influenced by emotions, usually, the resulting architectural design will not represent this with two components corresponding to emotions and decision-making. Instead, an architectural design based on the architecture of the brain should best be addressed. In this manner, the system would be constituted by components imitating brain structures and their interactions. A direct consequence of this approach, however, is that common strategies for grouping similar requirements in a single subsystem, or in the contrary, decomposing them to facilitate the design process cannot be deliberately applied [25]. For CMBs, these strategies can be addressed by strictly following composition (or decomposition) methods based on the nature of operation of the human brain.

Accordingly, by using the results of multidisciplinary theories, current tools can be greatly improved. For example, such tools may guide the creation of architectural designs by providing the necessary knowledge to establish which are the structures involved in the particular cognitive or affective process to be modeled, as well as their possible interactions with other brain structures. In this way, specifications can appropriately be grouped or separated conforming to theories that validate such procedures.

Similarly, the type and content of the data structures used to communicate architectural components have to be determined by two constraints. First, computational aspects establish what are the necessary data to manage the software constraints in the system. Second, natural aspects influence the composition of these structures by determining the cognitive-affective data that mechanisms should exchange in order to operate adequately.

3.3 Implementation

While the specification and design phases are vital to understand the expected functionality of a system, the implementation phase is concerned with transforming such specifications and architectural designs to an executable system [25].

Although the quality and style of the code lies in the skills of, and good practices implemented by, software developers, the success of the implementation phase also depends on the computational techniques, methodologies, and tools used. Many strategies are available to assist this stage, for example, software reuse and automatic code generation. Furthermore, for the implementation of CMBs a number of computational techniques have proven useful, such as fuzzy sets and logic, classifiers, evolutionary algorithms, neural networks, and symbolic systems [7, 20].

Since some sub-processes operate similarly in many conventional software projects, they can be adapted for reuse. This approach brings a variety of benefits, for example, the cost of the software development decreases, the system maintenance becomes easier, well tested products are used, and in general the development cycle is faster. Unfortunately, this technique is hardly used when implementing CMBs. There exists several reasons to support such argument, some of them are derived from the inherent complexity of the brain processes (already discussed above), as well as due to the ambiguity of the terms used to describe them. These issues make it difficult to create specialized and well defined reusable components. Furthermore, it makes impossible to create programming environments that offer pre-made pieces of code embodying models of brain processes. Therefore, standards should be proposed to enable the development of reusable components that implement theories and models of human processes.

Nonetheless, some current approaches can help to create reusable components for CMBs. For example, in [14] has been abstracted the execution cycle of computational models of emotions as a process of three stages: appraisal derivation, affect derivation, and affect consequences; the implementation of components corresponding each of these phases under standards that restrict the meaning of the terms, concepts, and mechanisms used can surely allow their reuse. Similarly, reusable components can be achieved by including meta-information about the terms, concepts, and theories considered. In this manner, before using them, we can realize if they manage the terminology and functions according the model we attempt to build. As a consequence of a reuse of nature-inspired software components, suitable programming environments could be developed.

3.4 Contemporary Software Tools

Research done on understanding and facilitating the computational modeling of cognitive and affective processes has led to the creation of new tools and methodologies. Cognitive Objects within a Graphical EnviroNmenT (COGENT) [4] is a software tool with a visual environment for the computational design and modeling of high-level cognitive processes. COGENT allows the creation and testing of cognitive models using box-arrow diagrams constituted of functional components with their respective interactions. Conceptually, these components represent cognitive processes such as memory systems, knowledge networks, and decision procedures, which are embodied in computational structures such as memory buffers, knowledge bases, and connectionist networks. This tool provides an appropriate environment for executing and testing the developed models.

The Emotion Markup Language (EmotionML) is a general purpose annotation language for representing affective aspects in human-machine interactive systems [1]. It is proposed by the W3C Multimodal Interaction Working Group as an attempt to standardize the description of emotions in three main contexts: (1) manual annotation of texts, videos and anything that involves emotional data, (2) accurate representations of emotional aspects captured from user's expressions, postures, speech, etc., and (3) for comprehensible generation of emotional responses from user interfaces. Although a specification of the syntax of EmotionML is still in progress, several elements may already be used.

For the rigorous and formal description of cognitive-affective processes and nature-inspired systems, a set of denotational mathematics has been proposed [32]. These are expressive mathematical means that emerge in the framework of cognitive informatics, a discipline concerned with the internal information processing mechanisms of natural intelligence. Two particular instances of denotational mathematics are *concept algebra* and *real-time process algebra*. The former is appropriate to rigorously manipulate abstract concepts in a formal and coherent framework, which leads to the construction and treatment of more complex knowledge representations. The latter has been developed as a coherent notation system and formal methodology to algebraically denote and model the behaviors and architectures of systems and human cognitive and affective processes [31, 32].

4 Conclusion

In this paper we discussed the fundamental issues that hinder the computational modeling of cognitive and affective processes. We focus on computational models that are part of cognitive frameworks such as cognitive architectures for autonomous agents. Three main aspects that are essential to their construction were identified as the main sources of such issues; they are their computational basis, their theoretical basis, and their architectural design. We explored the effects of these problems in the particular phases of their development cycle, and examined the appropriateness of current tools to aid such phases. Finally, improvements were proposed for the creations of new tools and a better realization of their construction.

Acknowledgments. The authors would like to acknowledge the PhD scholarship (CONACYT grant No. 229386) sponsored by the Mexican Government for their partial support to this work. We would like to thank the anonymous reviewers for their valuable comments and suggestions.

References

1. Baggia, P., Burkhardt, F., Oltramari, A., Pelachaud, C., Peter, C., Zovato, E.: Emotion markup language (emotionml) 1.0 (July 2010), `http://www.w3.org/TR/emotionml/`
2. Becker-Asano, C.W., Wachsmuth, I.: Affective computing with primary and secondary emotions in a virtual human. In: Autonomous Agents and Multi-Agent Systems, vol. 20(1), pp. 32–49 (2010)
3. Carter, R.: Mapping the Mind. University of California Press, Berkeley (2000)
4. Cooper, R., Fox, J.: Cogent: A visual design environment for cognitive modeling. Behavior Research Methods 30(4), 553–564 (1998)
5. Damasio, A.R.: Descartes' error: Emotion, Reason, and the Human Brain, 1st edn. Putnam Grosset Books, New York (1994)
6. Gebhard, P.: Alma: a layered model of affect. In: AAMAS, pp. 29–36 (2005)
7. Gray, W.D. (ed.): Integrated Models of Cognitive Systems, 1st edn. Oxford University Press, Oxford (2007)
8. Hudlicka, E.: Beyond cognition: Modeling emotion in cognitive architectures. In: Proceedings of the International Conference on Cognitive Modeling (ICCM), CMU, Pittsburgh (2004)
9. Kandel, E.R., Schwartz, J.H., Jessell, T.M.: Principles of Neural Science, 4th edn. McGraw-Hill, New York (2000)
10. Langley, P., Laird, J.E., Rogers, S.: Cognitive architectures: Research issues and challenges. Cognitive Systems Research 10(2), 141–160 (2009)
11. LeDoux, J.E.: The Emotional brain: The Mysterious Underpinnings of Emotional Life. Simon and Schuster, New York (1993)
12. Lewis, M., Sullivan, M.W., Stanger, C., Weiss, M.: Self development and self-conscious emotions. Child Development 60(1), 146–156 (1989)
13. Marinier, R.P., Laird, J.E., Lewis, R.L.: A computational unification of cognitive behavior and emotion. Cognitive Systems Research 10(1), 48–69 (2009)
14. Marsella, S., Gratch, J., Petta, P.: Computational models of emotion. In: Scherer, K.R., Bänziger, T., Roesch, E.B. (eds.) Blueprint for Affective Computing: A Source Book, 1st edn. Oxford University Press, Oxford (2010)
15. Marsella, S.C., Gratch, J.: Ema: A process model of appraisal dynamics. Cognitive Systems Research 10(1), 70–90 (2009); Modeling the Cognitive Antecedents and Consequences of Emotion
16. Moors, A.: Theories of emotion causation: A review. Cognition and Emotion 23, 625–662 (2009)
17. Nuxoll, A., Laird, J.E.: A cognitive model of episodic memory integrated with a general cognitive architecture. In: ICCM, pp. 220–225 (2004)
18. Padgham, L., Winikoff, M.: Prometheus: A methodology for developing intelligent agents. In: Giunchiglia, F., Odell, J., Weiß, G. (eds.) AOSE 2002. LNCS, vol. 2585, pp. 174–185. Springer, Heidelberg (2003)
19. Phepls, E.A.: Emotion and cognition: Insights from studies of the human amygdala. Annual Review of Psychology 57, 27–53 (2006)

20. Plaut, D.C.: Methodologies for the computer modeling of human cognitive processes. In: Boller, F., Rizzotti, J.G. (eds.) Handbook of Neuropsychology, 2nd edn. Elsevier, Amsterdam (2000)
21. Pressman, R.S.: Software Engineering: A Practitioner's Approach, 6th edn. McGraw-Hill, New York (2005)
22. Russell, S.J., Norvig, P.: Artificial Intelligence: A Modern Approach. Pearson Education, London (2003)
23. Scherer, K.R.: Psychological models of emotion. In: Borod, J. (ed.) The Neuropsychology of Emotion, pp. 137–166. Oxford University Press, Oxford (2000)
24. Sollenberger, D., Singh, M.: Koko: an architecture for affect-aware games. In: Autonomous Agents and Multi-Agent Systems, pp. 1–32 (2010)
25. Sommerville, I.: Software Engineering, 8th edn. Addison Wesley, Reading (2006)
26. Sun, R.: Cognitive architectures and the challenge of cognitive social simulation. In: Zhong, N., Liu, J., Yao, Y., Wu, J., Lu, S., Li, K. (eds.) Web Intelligence Meets Brain Informatics. LNCS (LNAI), vol. 4845, pp. 190–204. Springer, Heidelberg (2007)
27. Sun, R.: The importance of cognitive architectures: an analysis based on clarion. J. Exp. Theor. Artif. Intell. 19, 159–193 (2007)
28. Sun, R. (ed.): The Cambridge Handbook of Computational Psychology. Cambridge University Press, Cambridge (2008)
29. Sun, R.: Cognition and Multi-Agent Interaction: From Cognitive Modeling to Social Simulation, 1st edn. Cambridge University Press, New York (2008)
30. Velásquez, J.D.: A computational framework for emotion-based control. In: Proceedings of SAB 1998 Workshop on Grounding Emotions in Adaptive Systems (1998)
31. Wang, Y.: On the cognitive processes of human perception with emotions, motivations, and attitudes. International Journal of Cognitive Informatics and Natural Intelligence 1(4), 1–13 (2007)
32. Wang, Y.: Software Engineering Foundations: A Software Science Perspective. Auerbach Publications (2008)

Analysis of Gray Matter in AD Patients and MCI Subjects Based Voxel-Based Morphometry

Zhijun Yao[1], Bin Hu[1,2,*], Lina Zhao[1] and Chuanjiang Liang[1]

[1] The School of Information Science and Engineering, Lanzhou University, Lanzhou, China
[2] School of Computing, Telecomminications and Networks, Birmingham City University, Birmingham, UK
bh@lzu.edu.cn, bin.hu@bcu.ac.uk
{yaozj,zhaoln10,liangchj07}@lzu.edu.cn

Abstract. In recent years, pathological researches of mild cognitive impairment (MCI) subjects and the Alzheimer's disease (AD) patients have gained a great deal of attention. In this study, we used the voxel-based morphometry (VBM) method to analyze the Magnatic Resonance Imaging (MRI) data of gray matter volumes in 98 normal controls (NCs), 91 AD patients and 113 MCI subjects. The measurements of gray matter volumes were calculated for each of the three groups respectively. We found that compared with MCI subjects, AD patients had further atrophy in the following brain regions: right insula, left hippocampus, right fusiform and bilateral middle temporal gyrus. Compared with NCs, AD patients and MCI subjects shared some abnormal brain regions such as bilateral parahippocampal gyrus, bilateral hippocampus, left amygdala and left fusiform. The results provided additional evidences to support the viewpoint that MCI is the transitional stage between normal aging and AD.

Keywords: Alzheimer's disease; mild cognitive impairment; voxel-based morphometry.

1 Introduction

As people aging, the morbidity of dementia shows faster growth. AD, the most common style of dementia, is associated with neurodegenerative disease characterized histologically by the presence of neurofibrillary tangles and neuritic amyloid plaques. It represents a serious health problem for the elderly, with about 15% of those over 65 years old demonstrating some degree of dementia [1]. MCI has been considered to be a transitional state between NCs and a diagnosis of clinically probable AD [2]. MCI subjects have a memory loss greater than expected for people matched with age and educational level and have intact daily living activities [3]. The study of differences between AD patients and MCI subjects can improve our understanding of the progression from MCI to AD. Recently, many research groups have studied AD and MCI from various perspectives, attempting to understand the pathogenesis with a goal

[*] Corresponding author.

B. Hu et al. (Eds.): BI 2011, LNAI 6889, pp. 209–217, 2011.

of discovering effective therapies, such as the abnormal cortical networks and the decreased cortical thickness [4, 5]. VBM method, proposed by Friston and Ashburner [6] is an automated image analysis technique that offers improvised, rapid and unbiased whole brain survey [7]. Using the VBM method, many studies have indicated that AD is associated with atrophy of gray matter volume mainly in parahippocampal gyrus, medial temporal lobe, insula and thalamus [8]. MCI subjects also have atrophy brain regions in frontal lobe, temporal lobe and parietal lobe [9]. However, many studies only focused on gray matter volume in AD patients and MCI subjects respectively [8, 9], the differences of gray matter volume between AD patients and MCI subjects are still largely unexplored. In the present study, we used VBM to analyze gray matter volume in AD patients, MCI subjects and NCs respectively. The primary goal of this study is to investigate the progression from MCI to AD, which can provide the key knowledge about the formation of AD related pathology as well as the insight into the nature of MCI itself.

2 Materials and Methods

2.1 Subjects

This study included 98 NCs, 113 MCI subjects, and 91 AD subjects. Alzheimer's disease Neuroimaging Initiative (ANDI) database (http://www.loni.ucla.edu/ADNI/) provided all the subjects used in this study. The detailed information about the participants was summarized in Table 1.

Table 1. Demographic features of the participants

Group	Number of subjects	Age range	Mean age	Standard deviation	Female: Male
NCs	98	70.02-90.74	77.27	4.66	49:49
MCI	113	56.28-55.73	75.12	7.60	34:79
AD	91	55.73-90.20	76.16	7.81	41:50

2.2 Data Acquisition

All of the data in our study included standard T1-weighted MR images acquired sagittally using volumetric 3D MPRAGE with 1.25×1.25mm in-plane spatial resolution and 1.2mm thick sagittal slices. All the high-resolution magnetic resonance images were obtained using 1.5 T scanners. Images using 3T scanners were excluded to remove the discrimination that might be introduced by using different magnetic field strengths. All scans were downloaded in the DICOM format and finally converted to the NIFTI format. Detailed information about the MR acquisition procedures is available at the ADNI website.

2.3 Data Analysis

Structural images were preprocessed using VBM implemented with Statistical Parametric Mapping software (SPM5) running under Matlab 7.0. VBM is a whole- brain, unbiased, semiautomatic, neuroimaging analysis technique that allows the investigation of between-group differences in brain volume [7]. In brief, the gray matter volume was obtained for each subject with the following steps. Firstly, the native MRI images were corrected for intensity non-uniformity which caused by gradient distortions and different positions of cranial structures within the MRI coil [10]. Secondly, the corrected images were registered into an asymmetric T1-weighted template in Montreal Neurological Institute (MNI) stereotactic space. Thirdly, the registered and corrected structural images were segmented into gray matter, white matter, cerebrospinal fluid and background with the help of an advanced neural-net classifier. Fourthly, the normalized, segmented images were smoothed using an 8-mm FWHM isotropic Gaussian kernel to allow for individual gyral variation and to increase the signal-to-noise ratio [11]. The preprocessed data were analyzed using statistical parametric mapping (SPM5). Specific differences in gray matter among the NCs, MCI subjects and AD patients were assessed statistically using the two-sample t-tests [12], namely testing for an decreased voxel containing gray matter. The level of significance for clusters was set at $p<0.001$.

3 Results

The reduction of gray matter volume was calculated to measure the cerebral atrophy for the MCI subjects and AD patients. The results of three groups were shown in Figure 1. Compared with the normal aging, AD patients showed significant atrophy of gray matter volume in following regions: bilateral parahippocampal gyrus, bilateral hippocampus, left amygdala, left fusiform, left orbital-frontal gyrus, bilateral olfactory and left temporal gyrus. The reduction of gray matter volume in right cerebrum and left cerebrum were symmetrical to some extent (Figure 1-A).The MCI subjects revealed significant atrophy in bilateral parahippocampal gyrus, bilateral hippocampus, left amygdala and left fusiform compared with the normal aging (Figure 1-B). These results were consistent with previous studies, which showed abnormal brain regions in AD and MCI [8, 13-16]. The AD group showed significant atrophy in the following regions: right insula, left hippocampus, right fusiform and bilateral middle temporal gyrus when compared with the MCI group (Figure 1-C). Furthermore, we also found the increased gray matter volume in MCI and AD.

Table 2. The first row showed shared abnormal brain regions in MCI and AD compared with NCs. The second row listed further atrophy brain regions when we made a comparison in AD patients and MCI subjects ($p<0.001$).

Shared abnormal brain regions by AD and MCI comparison with NCs		
Bilateral parahippocampal gyrus	Bilateral hippocampus	
Left amygdala	Left fusiform	
Further atrophy brain regions in comparison of AD and MCI		
Right insula	Left hippocampus	Right fusiform
Bilateral middle temporal gyrus		

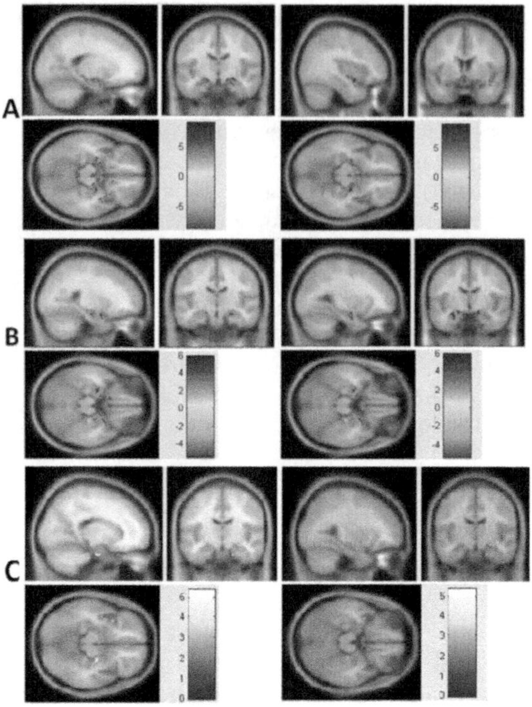

Fig. 1. The atrophied brain regions showed in the AD and MCI. The color bars mean T-values which indicate the significant level of the gray matter atrophy. A. Differences between AD patients and normal aging. B. Differences between MCI subjects and normal aging. C. Differences between AD patients and MCI subjects ($p<0.001$).

4 Discussion

In this large population-based cohort study, we used VBM method to identify the abnormal gray matter volume in MCI subjects and AD patients [17-19]. The present results showed that the gray matter volumes of the following brain regions were reduced in both MCI subjects and AD patients: bilateral parahippocampal gyrus, bilateral hippocampus, left amygdala and left fusiform. Moreover, we also measured the gray matter volume between MCI subjects and AD patients. We found the further atrophy which existed in the following structures of AD patients: right insula, left hippocampus, right fusiform and bilateral middle temporal gyrus.

4.1 Shared Abnormal Brain Regions by AD and MCI

The results we found in MCI and AD fitted nicely with the previous studies [9, 16, 20-22]. These different regions are known to be some of the first to be involved in the progression of AD pathology [23] and had been implicated in previous VBM studies in MCI subjects [17, 24, 25]. The pattern of loss was bilateral although slightly greater on the left. Many previous researches similarly showed left-sided patterns of cerebral atrophy in AD [11, 14]. These results might indicate the asymmetric atrophy in the progression from normal aging to AD.

The atrophy of parahippocampal gyrus has been observed in previous MCI and AD studies [16, 20, 22]. Our results showed the obvious volume atrophy of the parahippocampal gyrus in MCI subjects and AD patients. Previous studies have reported that the parahippocampal gyrus played an important role in transmitting information from other areas of the cortex into the hippocampus, the limbic circuit and the fusiform gyrus. Moreover, it was also related to the memory encoding and retrieval [26, 27].We suggested that the issue loss likely indicated the worsening cognitive functioning that showed obviously in the progression of AD.

The symmetrical atrophy of hippocampus has been reported in many previous related researches [3, 9, 16, 21, 22, 24, 25, 28]. Hippocampal atrophy has been consistently described as a feature in dementia [29]. Fox et al. found the progressive hippocampal atrophy over time and with disease severity in subjects with AD [21]. Previous VBM study has also shown a greater degree of hippocampal atrophy in subjects with AD and MCI [9]. Many studies have shown that hippocampus played important roles in the consolidation of information from short-term memory to long-term memory, cognitive function and spatial navigation [20, 30-32]. Moreover, hippocampal atrophy has been shown to discriminate AD from controls with a high sensitivity and high specificity [33]. This result fitted nicely with the faster decline in memory and other cognitive functions in the early stage of AD [16, 19, 20, 22].

In the present study, the atrophy of left amygdala was found both in MCI and AD. This region was known to be a part of the limbic system and was connected with generating and processing emotional reactions such as fear and desire [34-36]. In addition, previous study has reported that the left amygdale was one of the regions that first identified the gray matter losses in subjects 3 years before progression to AD [16]. Andrew et al. found the atrophic change of the left amygdala in the people who developed AD [37]. The reduced volume in the left amygdala in MCI and AD might be responsible for the clinical symptoms in MCI and AD, such as the lack of initiative, selfishness, aloneness, reduced interests in environment and people around and irascibility.

The fusiform gyrus which is also known as the occipitotemporal gyrus is a part of the temporal lobe. The atrophy of gray matter volume in this region has been reported in many previous researches of AD patients of mild to moderate severity [38, 39]. In this study we detected the atrophy in the left fusiform which was consistent with the results that Rombouts et al. found in 2000 [40]. Similarly, Hiroshi Matsuda et al. also found the significant reduction of gray matter volume in left fusiform gyrus in AD patients compared with healthy volunteers at the baseline study [41]. The results suggested that the left fusiform atrophy might lead to the decline of the face recognition and the semantic comprehension.

4.2 Further Atrophy Brain Regions in Comparison of AD and MCI

We found that the atrophy regions were asymmetric and most regions only existed in the comparison of AD and MCI, such as the right insula, the right fusiform and the bilateral middle temporal gyrus. So we hypothesized that these regions might play an important role in the conversion from MCI to AD.

Insula has been reported related to the emotion or the regulation of the body's homeostasis included perception, motor control, self-awareness, cognitive functioning, and interpersonal experience [42]. In the present study, we detected the significant atrophy of the right insula which was consistent with the results Karas et al. and Shiino et al. found in patients with AD. Previous studies have indicated the right insula was associated with AD. Chetelat et al. found the marked hypometabolism and atrophy of the gray matter in the right insula [43]. Similarly, Shannon et al. reported that MCI-Converters had significantly reduced gray matter relative to MCI-Stable in the medial temporal lobe region, with a global maximum in the right insula [44]. These results suggested that the right insula was the critical brain region in the conversion from MCI to AD.

Many previous studies have noted the particular effects of the left hippocampus in the progression from MCI to AD. Andrew et al. found something about left hippocampus when they explored the basal forebrain atrophy in AD. They reported that when the left hippocampus was also atrophic, the onset of dementia typically occurred earlier than in case in which the atrophy was confined to basal forebrain [37]. Similarly, some studies using hippocampal atrophy surface mapping showed that left hippocampus was the only significant predictor of conversion to AD [45, 46]. These results indicated that left hippocampal volume in particular discriminated between converting and stable MCI [47]. The reduction of the regional cerebral blood flow in the right fusiform was detected from the one year to two years follow-up studies of AD patients and this region was related to processing of color information, face and word recognition [41, 48, 49]. The result might indicate the asymmetric atrophy in the progression to AD and be related to the decline of the cognitive function in patients with AD.

Though previous study has reported that middle temporal gyrus subserved language and semantic memory processing, visual perception, recognition of known faces and multimodal sensory integration, the exact function of this area is not clear [50]. Leube et al. found that the atrophy in the middle temporal gyrus correlated closely with episodic memory performance when they used the VBM method to explore the brain atrophy in patients with MCI and AD [51]. Whitwell et al. indicated that middle temporal gyrus was involved in the atrophy of the temporal lobe by the time the subjects were one year before the diagnosis of AD. In contrast, it didn't significantly appear by the time 3 years before the diagnosis of AD [16]. In addition, a recent study by Karas et al. investigated the structural differences on MRI and the development of clinical AD in patients with amnestic MCI at 3-year follow-up [52]. They noted that converters had more atrophy in middle temporal gyrus than stable patients with MCI. Similarly, Chetelat et al. also reported that middle temporal was in the significant regions of gray matter loss in converters relative to non-converters [24]. These results all suggested that the atrophy of middle temporal gyrus might herald the presence of future AD among non-demented individuals.

Finally, we noted that there was increased gray matter volume in the comparison of MCI and AD (Figure 1-A, Figure 1-B). These increased gray matter volume might indicate the progression to AD is a long and complicated process.

The strength of this study is that we have a relatively large number of clinically well-characterized subjects which can allow us to investigate the progression of gray matter atrophy from NCs to AD. Likewise, by generating three between-group comparisons we found the regions of atrophy both in MCI and AD and the further atrophy in AD.

However, several possible limitations of our study need to be addressed. First, the gender of these groups didn't match very well. Second, we will use the MR images acquired from a higher magnetic intensity in the future study.

In summary, the present study suggested that VBM can be used to map the progression of gray matter loss in subjects with MCI and AD. These results might offer an additional insight into the conversion to AD and contribute to understanding the pathogenesis of MCI and AD.

Acknowledgements. This work was supported by National Natural Science Foundation of China (grant no.60973138, 61003240), the EU's Seventh Framework Programme OPTIMI (grant no. 248544), and Gansu Provincial Science & Technology Department (grant no. 1007RJYA010), and The Study of Brain Network of The Group of Mild Cognitive Impairment (grant no. Lzujbky-2011-61), and National Basic Research Program of China (973 Program) (No.2011CB711001).

References

1. Neuman, M.A., Cohn, R.: Prevalence and malignancy of Alzheimer disease. Arch. Neurol. 33(10), 730 (1976)
2. Gauthier, S., et al.: Mild Cognitive Impairment Represents. Lancet 367, 1262–1270 (2006)
3. John, C., Morris, M., et al.: Mild Cognitive Impairment Represents Early-Stage Alzheimer Disease. Arch. Neurol. 58, 397–405 (2001)
4. Yao, Z., et al.: Abnormal Cortical Networks in Mild Cognitive Impairment and Alzheimer's Disease. PLoS Computational Biology 6(11), 1–11 (2010)
5. Julkunen, V., et al.: Cortical Thickness Analysis to Detect Progressive Mild Cognitive Impairment: A Reference to Alzheimer's Disease. Dement. Geriatr. Cogn. Disord. 28, 404–412 (2009)
6. Ashburner, J.: Voxel-Based Morphometry—The Methods. Neuroimage 11(6), 805–821 (2000)
7. Good, C.D., et al.: A voxel-based morphometric study of ageing in 465 normal adult human brains. Neuroimage 14(1), 21–36 (2001)
8. Chetelat, G., et al.: Mapping gray matter loss with voxel-based morphometry in mild cognitive impairment. Neuroreport 13(15), 1939–1943 (2002)
9. Karas, G.B., et al.: Global and local gray matter loss in mild cognitive impairment and Alzheimer's disease. Neuroimage 23(2), 708–716 (2004)
10. Mechelli, A.: Structural Covariance in the Human Cortex. Journal of Neuroscience 25(36), 8303–8310 (2005)
11. Karas, G.B., et al.: A comprehensive study of gray matter loss in patients with Alzheimer's disease using optimized voxel-based morphometry. Neuroimage 18, 895–907 (2003)
12. Salmond, C.H., et al.: Distributional Assumptions in Voxel-Based Morphometry. Neuroimage 17(2), 1027–1030 (2002)

13. Convita, A., de Asis, J., de Leon, M.J.: Atrophy of the medial occipitotemporal, inferior, and middle temporal gyri in non- demented elderly predict decline to Alzheimer's disease. Neurobiology of Aging 21, 19–26 (2000)
14. Baron, J., Chetelat, C., Desgranges, B.: In Vivo Mapping of Gray Matter Loss with Voxel-Based Morphometry in Mild Alzheimer's Disease. Neuroimage 14(2), 298–309 (2001)
15. den Heijer, T., et al.: A 10-year follow-up of hippocampal volume on magnetic resonance imaging in early dementia and cognitive decline. Brain 133, 1163–1172 (2010)
16. Whitwell, J.L., et al.: 3D maps from multiple MRI illustrate changing atrophy patterns as subjects progress from mild cognitive impairment to Alzheimer's disease. Brain 130(7), 1777–1786 (2007)
17. Narr, K.L.: Mapping Cortical Thickness and Gray Matter Concentration in First Episode Schizophrenia. Cerebral Cortex 15(6), 708–719 (2004)
18. Robbins, S.M.: Anatomical standardization of the human brain in euclidean 3-space and on the cortical 2-manifold: School of Computer Science. McGill University, Montreal (2004)
19. Singh, V., et al.: Spatial patterns of cortical thinning in mild cognitive impairment and Alzheimer's disease. Brain 129(11), 2885–2893 (2006)
20. Dickerson, B.C., et al.: MRI-derived entorhinal and hippocampal atrophy in incipient and very mild Alzheimer's disease. Neurobiology of Aging 22, 747–754 (2001)
21. Fox, N.C., et al.: Presymptomatic hippocampal atrophy in Alzheimer's disease. A longitudinal MRI study. Brain 119, 2001–2007 (1996)
22. Teipel, S.J., et al.: Multivariate deformation-based analysis of brain atrophy to predict Alzheimer's disease in mild cognitive impairment. NeuroImage 38, 13–24 (2007)
23. Braak, H., Braak, E.: Evolution of the neuropathology of Alzheimer's disease. Acta Neuro. Scand. Suppl. 165, 3–12 (1996)
24. Chetelat, G., et al.: Using voxel-based morphometry to map the structural changes associated with rapid conversion in MCI: a longitudinal MRI study. Neuroimage 27, 934–946 (2005)
25. Bozzoli, M., et al.: The contribution of voxel-based morphometry in staging patients with mild cognitive impairment. Neurology 67, 453–460 (2006)
26. Ferriera, N.F., et al.: Analysis of parahippocampal gyrus in 115 patients with hippocampal sclerosis. Arq. Neuropsiquiatr. 61, 707–711 (2003)
27. Mc Donald, B., Highley, J.R., Walker, M.A.: Anomalous asymmetry of fusiform and parahippocampal gyrus gray matter in schizophrenia: A postmortem study. Am. J. Psychiatry 157, 40–47 (2000)
28. Lyketsos, C.G., et al.: Prevalence of neuropsychiatric symptoms in dementia and mild cognitive impairment: results from the cardiovascular health study. JAMA 288(12), 1475–1483 (2002)
29. Summerfield, C., et al.: Structural Brain Changes in Parkinson Disease With Dementia: A Voxel-Based Morphometry Study. Arch. Neurol. 62, 281–285 (2005)
30. Broglio, C., et al.: Hallmarks of a common forebrain vertebrate plan: Specialized pallial areas for spatial, temporal and emotional memory in actinopterygian fish. Brain Res. Bull. 57, 397–399 (2002)
31. Broyer, P., et al.: Hippocampal abnormalities and memory deficits: new evidence of a strong pathophysiological link in schizophrenia. Brain Res. Rev. 54, 92–112 (2007)
32. Burke, S.N., Barnes, C.A.: Neural plasticity in the ageing brain. Nat. Rev. Neurosci. 7, 30–40 (2006)
33. Scheltens, P., et al.: Atrophy of medial temporal lobes on MRI in "probable"Alzheimer's disease and normal ageing: diagnostic value and neuropsychological correlates. J. Neurol. Neurosurg. Psychiatry 55, 967–972 (1992)

34. Amunts, K., et al.: Cytoarchitectonic mapping of the human amygdala, hippocampal region and entorhinal cortex: intersubject variability and probability maps. Anat. Embryol (Berl.) 210, 343–352 (2005)
35. Paton, Joseph: The primate amygdala represents the positive and negative value of visual stimuli during learning. Nature 439, 865–870 (2005)
36. Killcross, S., Robbins, T.W., Everitt, B.J.: Different types of fear-conditioned behaviour mediated by separate nuclei within amygdala. Nature 388, 377–380 (1997)
37. Hall, A.M., et al.: Basal forebrain atrophy is a presymptomatic marker for Alzheimer's disease. Alzheimer's & Dementia 4, 271–279 (2008)
38. Frisoni, G.B., et al.: Detection of grey matter loss in mild Alzheimer's disease with voxel based morphometry. J. Neurol. Neurosurg. Psychiatry 73, 657–664 (2002)
39. Whitwell, J.L., et al.: Temporoparietal atrophy: A marker of AD pathology independent of clinical diagnosis. Neurobiology of Aging (2009)
40. Rombouts, S.A.R.B., et al.: Unbiased whole-brain analysis of gray matter loss in Alzheimer's disease. Neurosci. Lett. 285, 231–233 (2000)
41. Hiroshi Matsuda, M., et al.: Longitudinal Evaluation of Both Morphologic and Functional Changes in the Same Individuals with Alzheimer's Disease. J. Nucl. Med. 43, 304–311 (2002)
42. Bamiou, D.E., Musiek, F.E., Luxon, L.M.: The insula (Island of Reil) and its role in auditory processing. Brain Res. Rev. 2, 143–154 (2003)
43. Chetelat, G., et al.: Direct voxel-based comparison between grey matter hypometabolism and atrophy in Alzheimer's disease. Brain 131, 60–71 (2008)
44. Risacher, S.L., et al.: Baseline MRI Predictors of Conversion from MCI to Probable AD in the ADNI Cohort. Current Alzheimer Research 6, 347–361 (2009)
45. Csernansky, J.G., et al.: Preclinical detection of Alzheimer's disease: Hippocampal shape and volume predict dementia onset in the elderly. Neuroimage 25(3), 783–792 (2005)
46. Thompson, P.M., et al.: Mapping hippocampal and ventricular change in Alzheimer disease. Neuroimage 22(4), 1754–1766 (2004)
47. Eckerström, C., et al.: Small baseline volume of left hippocampus is associated with subsequent conversion of MCI into dementia: The Göteborg MCI study. Neurological Sciences 272, 48–59 (2008)
48. McCarthy, G.: Face-specific processing in the fuman fusform gyrus. J. Cognitive Neuroscicence 9, 605–610 (1997)
49. Radua, J., et al.: Neural response to specific components of fearful faces in healthy and schizophrenic adults. Neuroimage 49, 939–946 (2010)
50. Toshiaki Onitsuka, M.D., et al.: Middle and Inferior Temporal Gyrus Gray Matter Volume Abnormalities in Chronic Schizophrenia: An MRI Study. Am. J. Psychiatry 161, 1603–1611 (2004)
51. Leube, D.T., et al.: Neural correlates of verbal episodic memory in patients with MCI and Alzheimer's disease–a VBM study. Int. J. Geriatr. Psychiatry 23, 1114–1118 (2008)
52. Karas, G., et al.: Amnestic Mild Cognitive Impairment: Structural MR Imaging Findings Predictive of Conversion to Alzheimer Disease. AJNR Am. J. Neuroradiol. 29, 944–949 (2008)

Fundamental Study for Human Brain Activity Based on the Spatial Cognitive Task

Shunji Shimizu[1], Noboru Takahashi[2], Hiroyuki Nara[3], Hiroaki Inoue[2] and Yukihiro Hirata[1]

[1] Tokyo University of Science, Suwa
shun@rs.suwa.tus.ac.jp
[2] Graduate School, Tokyo University of Science, Suwa
jgh10614@ed.suwa.tus.ac.jp
[3]Hokkaidou University

Abstract. Recently, there is a pressing need to develop a new system which assists and acts for car driving and wheelchair for the elderly as the population grows older. In terms of developing a new system, examining human spatial recognition is important implications. We pay attention to determine direction as well as spatial, especially left and right, perceptions. The final goal of our measuring brain activity research is to contribute to developing new interfaces with functions that are responsive like human. So, we have performed experiments for investigating human spatial perception by measuring brain blood flow when subjects perform driving tasks. In virtual experiment using driving movies, we measured brain activity when T-junctions in driving movies were shown to subjects. In this time, we performed experiment in which brain activities were measured during actual car driving. We will report on these analysis and comparison results between virtual one and actual one.

1 Introduction

Human movements change relative to his environment. Nevertheless, he/she recognizes a new location and decides what behavior to take. It is important to analyze the human spatial perception for developing autonomous robots or automatic driving.

The relation of the theta brain waves to the human spatial perception was discussed in [1, 2]. When humans perceive space, for example, try to decide the next action in a maze, the theta brain waves saliently appear. This means we have a searching behavior to find a goal at an unknown maze. From the side of human navigation E.A. Maguire et.at.al measures the brain activations using complex virtual reality town [3]. But every task is notional and the particulars about the mechanism that enables humans to perceive space and direction are yet unknown. From researches we performed, there were significant differences at dorsolateral prefrontal cortex in left hemisphere when subjects turned a steering wheel at T-junction [4, 5, 6].

Brain activities concerned with cognitive tasks during car driving have been examined. For example, there was a report about brain activity when disturbances were given to subjects who manipulated driving simulator. And power spectrums increased in beta and theta bands. However, there is little report on the relationship among right

B. Hu et al. (Eds.): BI 2011, LNAI 6889, pp. 218–225, 2011.

and left perception and driving task. It is well known that higher order processing is done such as of memory, judgment, reasoning, etc in the frontal lobe. We tried to grasp the mechanism of information processing of the brain by analyzing data about human brain activity during car driving. The goal of this study is to find a way to apply this result to new assist system. To achieve the goal, the brain activity of frontal lobe, which is related to behavioral decision-making, was discussed from the viewpoint of human spatial perception. Therefore, we measured the brain activity of frontal lobe when subjects performed action of car driving. Furthermore, we examined the mechanism of information processing of the brain and human spatial perception by analyzing experimental data concerning human brain activity during car driving using NIRS.

2 Experimental Method

2.1 Brain Activity on Virtual Driving

The subjects for this experiment were eight males aged 22 to 24. The average age was 22.7 and the age of standard deviation was 0.74. All of the subjects were right handed. They were asked to read and sign an informed consent regarding the experiment.

NIRS (Hitachi Medical Corp ETG-100) with 24 channels (sampling frequency 10 Hz) was used to record the density of oxygenated hemoglobin (oxy hemoglobin) and deoxygenated hemoglobin (de oxy hemoglobin) in the frontal cortex area.

Driving movie for the experiment was recorded from a moving car, in which two T-junctions were included. In addition, there was a road sign with directions in the second scene. We used nine kinds of movies in about one minutes. Before showing the movie, subjects were taught directions turning to the right or left at the first T-junction. They were also taught the place which was on the road sign at the second T-junction. They had to decide the direction when they looked at the road sign. They were asked to push a button when they realized the direction in which they were to turn. Subjects took a rest during 10 seconds at least with their eyes close before movies were shown and they viewed the image after that. Finally, subjects took a rest again. The brain activity was recorded from the first eyes-closed rest to the last eyes-close rest.

Here, we defined Tasks A, B, and C; Tasks A and C were proposed as the same experiment tasks and subjects had to push the button. In tasks B, other operation was added. It was the operation that the steering wheel was turned in the direction of destination when subjects realized it.

For this experiment, driving movies were displayed on a HMD (Head Mounted Display). The PC emitted a trigger pulse at the start of the eyes-closed rest and driving movie. Then, NIRS was recorded the brain activity, the trigger pulse from PC and the pulse from the button pushed at the second T-junction. Figure 1 shows two T-junction of this experiment.

Subjects were seated in car seat. Then they were fitted with the NIRS probe and the HMD. They were covered with black cloth to shut out the light from outside.

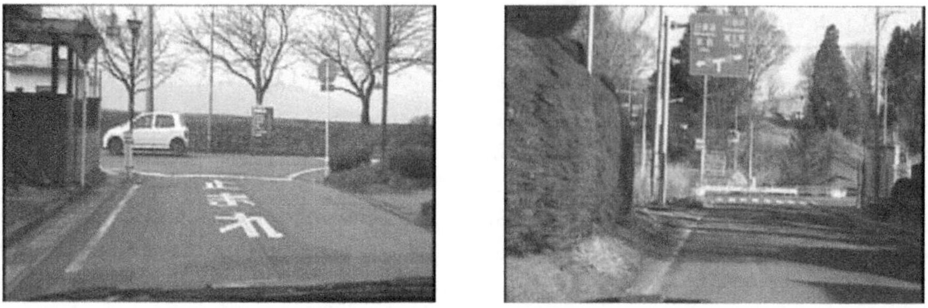

Fig. 1. Two T-junction included in driving movie

2.2 Brain Activity on Handling Motion

In this experiments, measurements were performed by f-NIRS (Functional Near Infrared Spectroscopy) made by SHIMADZE Co. Ltd with 44ch. Five subjects were a healthy male in their 20s, right handed with a good driving history. The subject was asked to perform simulated car driving, moving their hand in circles as if handling a steering wheel. A PC mouse on the table was used to simulate handling a wheel, and NIRS (near-infrared spectroscopy) was used to monitor oxygen density changes in the subjects' brain.

NIRS irradiation was performed to measure brain activities when the subject sitting on a chair drew a circle line of the right/left hand 1) clockwise, and 2) counterclockwise. The part of measurement was the frontal lobe. The subject was asked to draw on the table a circle 30 cm in diameter five times consecutively, spending four seconds per a circle. The time design was rest (10 seconds at least) –task (20 seconds) – rest (10 seconds).

2.3 Brain Activity on Car Driving

In general roads, experiments were performed by taking f-NIRS in the car, and measured the brain activity when subjects drove on designed road including intersections.

In this experiment, two kinds of measurements were performed. At first experiment, there were two intersections. And subjects were told to turn the right or left in first intersection. In addition, they were told to read the road map and judge the turning direction in the second intersection. And subjects were enlightened about turning direction before measurement. They were also taught the place on which the road sign was at the second T-junction. And, they were given the place where they have to go. So, they had to decide the direction when they looked at the road sign. Six subjects were a healthy male in their 20s, right handed with a good driving history. Subjects close their eyes for 10 seconds at least, and drove the car for 600 seconds. Three patterns were prepared for the task pattern.

Next, we performed second experiment to conduct verification about above experiment and increase number of subjects. We performed additional experiment which was achieved in a similar way. In this experiment, measuring and analyzing method was performed in same way, but experimental courses were different. Subjects were twelve males who were all right-handed.

3 Result of the Experiments

3.1 Brain Activity on Driving Movie Is Shown

For task A and C, the subjects were informed direction by suggested movie, and they let decided which way to turn under the road sign. After first T-junction, they were to push the button when they realized the direction at second direction. In task B, they performed other task, turning the steering wheel actually in concert with suggested movie. The hemoglobin variation was compared in the results of Tasks A and B, A and C to see the brain activity pertaining to spatial perception during the same movie.

Equation (1) was used to compare the data. τ1 was set the time as its length was 1 second before being pushed the button. Similarly, τ2 was set in a way similar to τ1. And xi (t) indicates variation of i channel oxy hemoglobin or deoxy hemoglobin. We then took a average of xi(t) through τ1 and τ2. In this situation, i of the defined c (i) was the channel for the brain activity. Because of the sampling frequency was set on 10 Hz, we calculated 10 times per sec.

$$c(i) = \overline{\sum_{\tau_2} x_i(\tau_2)} - \overline{\sum_{\tau_1} x_i(\tau_1)} \qquad (1)$$

A comparison was made between the situations in which the steering wheel was turned and when it was not. Figure 2 is the calculation result of oxy-Hb.

The next step was to calculate the average of all subjects. Figure 3 shows the results. Many upward tendencies could be found in Fig. 3. This might have occurred when they realized direction from a road sign. In addition, the results indicated a greater increase when the subjects turned the steering wheel. That indicated observation of brain activity has been made during movement based on spatial perceptions.

On the whole, the variation in de-oxy hemoglobin was smaller than in the oxy hemoglobin. However, there was a great increase in Channel 18. This might be the variation based on the spatial perceptions.

Next, differences were investigated concerning the subject's brain activity. The first case was when the vision was directed after having been told the direction. The Second case was when the vision was directed after having been told the direction gone to the direction which the subjects decided where to go from a road sign. d1 and d2 shown in Fig. 4 are defined as below. d1 is the variation of hemoglobin turning at the first T-junction. And d2 is variation of hemoglobin at the second one. From the measurement result, d1 and d2, all of the 269 times of each subject, there were significant differences in oxy hemoglobin 3ch. ($p < 0.02$: paired t test) and 20ch ($p < 0.03$) using NIRS.

Subjects pushed a button before turning at the second T-junction, so it influenced brain activities. The possibility of a correlation between d2 and the time until the movie was turned at the second T-junction after each subject pushed a button was investigated. Each correlation coefficient of hemoglobin channel was calculated. There was significant difference at only de-oxy hemoglobin 10ch. ($p < 0.07$) using paired t-test. In only this result, the relationship between pushing a button and d2 cannot be judged.

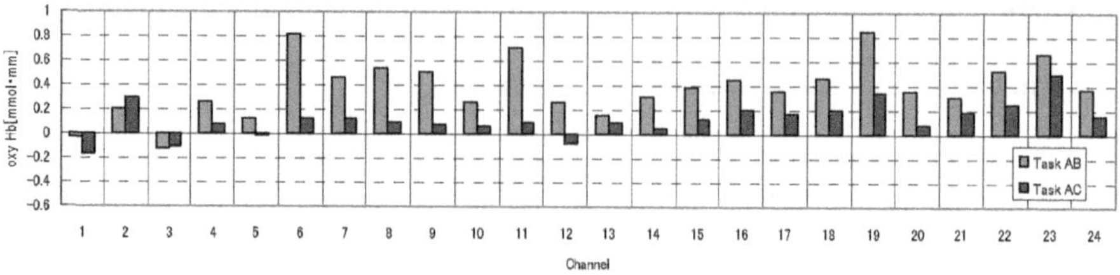

Fig. 2. Comparison between turning the steering wheel and not (oxy Hb of subject A)

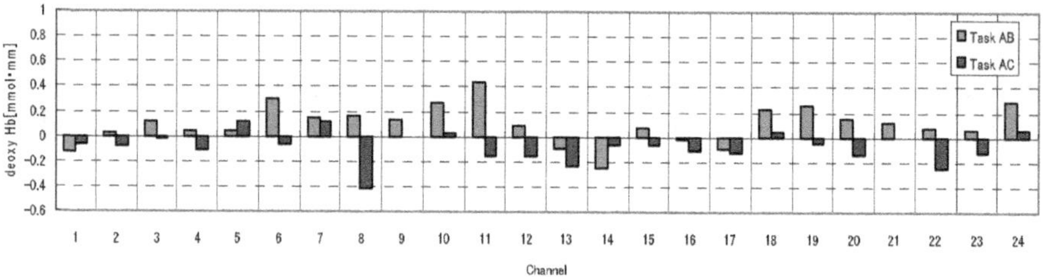

Fig. 3. Comparison between turning the steering wheel and not (oxy Hb of average)

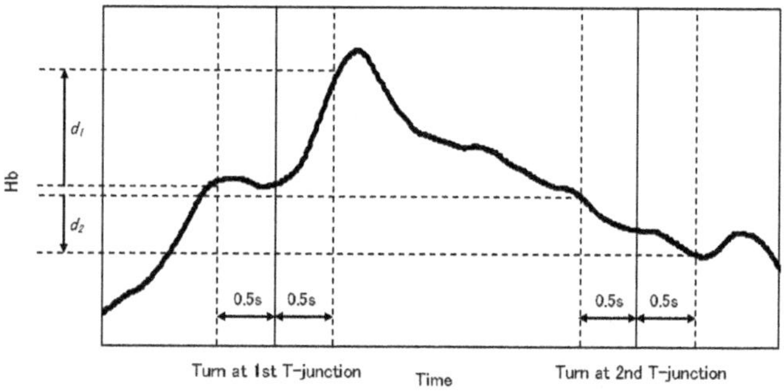

Fig. 4. Definition of variation of hemoglobin d1 and d2

3.2 Brain Activity on Handling Motion

During the motion, the increase of oxy hemoglobin density of the brain was found in all subjects. The different regions of the brain were observed to be active, depending on the individual. The subjects were to be observed 1) on starting, and 2) 3-5 seconds after starting moving their 3) right hand 4) left hand 5) clockwise 6) counterclockwise. Although some individual variation existed, the result showed the significant differences and some characteristic patterns.

The obtained patterns were shown as follows. Regardless of 1), 2), 3) and 4) above, the change in the oxy hemoglobin density of the brain was seen within the significant difference level 5% or less in the three individuals out of all five subjects. The part was the adjacent part both of left pre-motor area and of left prefrontal cortex. Especially, in the adjacent part of prefrontal cortex a number of significant differences were seen among in four out of five subjects.

Next more emphasis was put on the rotation direction: 5) clockwise or 6) counterclockwise. No large density change was found in the brain with all the subjects employing 6). But the significant difference was seen in four out of five subjects employing 5) (Fig. 5). It is well known that in the outside prefrontal cortex higher order processing is done such as of behavior control. It was inferred that the pre-motor area was activated when the subjects moved the hand in the way stated above because the pre-motor area was responsible for behavior control, for transforming visual information, and for generating neural impulses controlling.

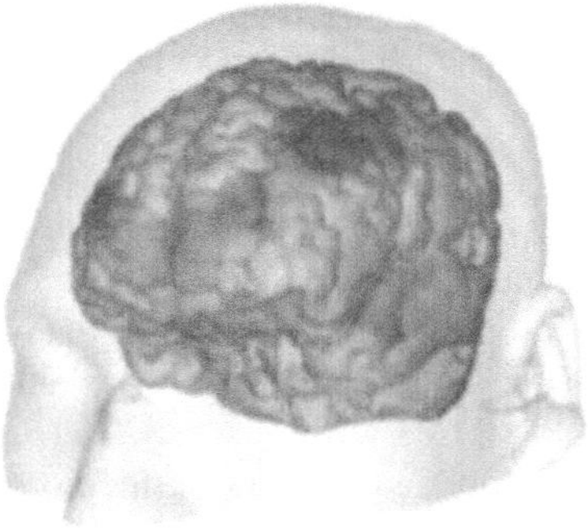

Fig. 5. Brain activity (clockwise)

3.3 Brain Activity on Car Driving

At the first, Hb-oxy was increased in overall frontal lobe after start of operation. This tendency was common among subjects. After that, Hb-oxy was decreased as subjects adjusted to driving the car. This meant that the brain activity changed from collective to local activities. Fig 6 shows one subject's brain activity.

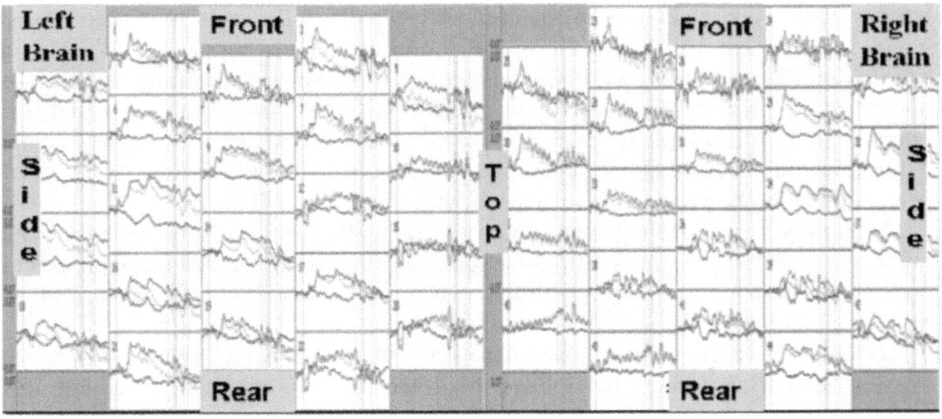

Fig. 6. The brain activity of some subject

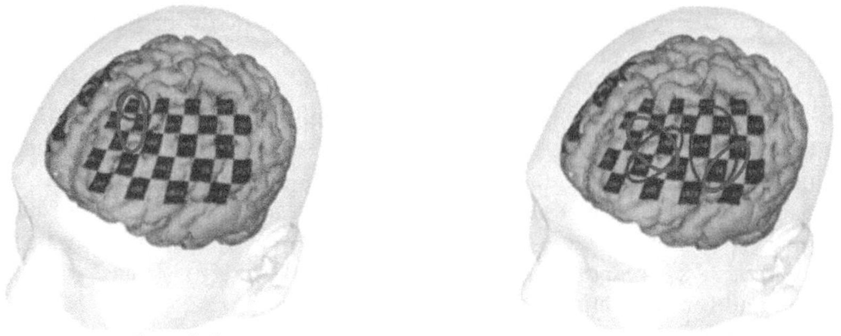

turning right turning left

Fig. 7. Significant differences at T-junctions

In this experiment, being considered time as zero when subjects turned a steering wheel. The analysis was performed one-sample t-test within the significant difference level 5% or less between zero and about four seconds after turning.As the results, there were significant differences around #46 area and #9 area of the dorsolateral prefrontal cortex and the premotor area of the left hemisphere brain at the turn left (Figure 7: red circles).

Around #46 area was corresponded to working memory. In additional experiment, analysis was conducted using same method, too. In this regard, we analyzed in both orders for confirming to be sequence-independent on the presence or absence of road sign (Figure 7: pink circles).

4 Conclusion

The hemoglobin density change of the human subjects' frontal lobe was partly observed in the experiments we designed, where three kinds of tasks were performed to analyze human brain activity from the view point of spatial perception.

The NIRS measures of hemoglobin variation in the channels suggested that human behavioral decision-making of different types could cause different brain activities as we saw in the tasks: 1) taking a given direction at the first T-junction, 2) taking a self-chosen direction on a road sign at the second T-junction and 3) turning the wheel or not. Some significant differences (paired t test) on NIRS's oxy-hemoglobin and less interrelated results between "pushing a button" and brain activity at the second T-junction are obtained. Researches into other human brain activities than spatial perception are to be necessary with accumulated data from fMRI, EEG, etc.

Furthermore, experimental results indicated that with the subjects moving their hand in circle, regardless of right or left, 1) the same response was observed in the prefrontal cortex and premotor area, and 2) different patterns of brain activities generated by moving either hand clockwise or counterclockwise.

The regions observed were only those with the 5% and less significance level. Possible extensions could be applied to other regions with the 10% and less significance level for the future study. With a larger number of subjects, brain activity patterns need to be made clear. In addition, it is thought to take particular note of participation concerning working memory when car is driven.

From results of these experiments, there was significant difference around working memory. So, experiments focusing on relationship turning wheel and working memory will be performed. In addition, we drew attention to differences on the basis of turning direction and dominant hand. We will plan the experiments in which subjects were narrowed down to left-handedness.

References

1. Kahana, M.J., Sekuler, R., Caplan, J.B., Kirschen, M., Madsen, J.R.: Human theta oscillations exhibit task dependence during virtual maze navigation. Nature 399, 781–784 (1999)
2. Nishiyama, N., Yamaguchi, Y.: Human EEG theta in the spatial recognition task. In: Proceedings of 5th World Multiconf. on Systemics, Cybernetics and Informatics (SCI 2001) (2001); Proc. 7th Int. Conf. on Information Systems, Analysis and Synthesis (ISAS 2001), pp. 497–500 (2001)
3. Maguire, E.A., Burgess, N., Donnett, J.G., Frackowiak, R.S.J., Frith, C.D., O' Keefe, J.: Knowing where and getting there: a human navigation network. Science 280 (May 8, 1998)
4. Shimizu, S., Hirai, N., Miwakeichi, F., et al.: Fundamental study for relationship between cognitive task and brain activity during car driving. In: Proc. 13th International Conference on Human-Computer Interaction, San Diego, CA, USA, pp. 434–440. Springer, Heidelberg (2009)
5. Takahashi, N., Shimizu, S., Hirata, Y., Nara, H., Miwakeichi, F., Hirai, N., Kikuchi, S., Watanabe, E., Kato, S.: Fundamental study for a new assistive system based on brain activity during car driving. In: Proc. International Conference on Robotics and Biomimetics, China (2010)
6. Takahashi, N., Shimizu, S., Hirata, Y., Nara, H., Miwakeichi, F., Hirai, N., Kikuchi, S., Watanabe, E., Kato, S.: Fundamental study for a new assistive system during car driving. In: The 28th Annual Conference of Robotics Society of Japan (2010)

ABSO: Advanced Bee Swarm Optimization Metaheuristic and Application to Weighted MAX-SAT Problem

Souhila Sadeg[1], Habiba Drias[2], Ouassim Ait El Hara[1], and Ania Kaci[1]

[1] Ecole Nationale Supérieure d'Informatique (ESI)
OuedSmar, Algiers, Algeria
[2] Computer Science Department, USTHB, LRIA
Algiers, Algeria

Abstract. We introduce an advanced version of Bee Swarm Optimization metaheuristic (BSO) which is inspired from the foraging behavior of real bees. The objective of this work is to enhance the performances of BSO by subdividing the set of variables into groups covering disjointed sub-regions in the search space. To each sub-region is assigned a bee that performs a local search, and the search process is guided by the intensification and diversification principles. The subdivision of the set of variables is strongly dependent on the considered problem and aims at both reducing the execution time and maximizing the coverage of the search space. Our new approach called ABSO for Advanced Bees Swarm Optimization was applied to the weighted MAX-SAT and the comparison of experimental results showed that it outperforms the BSO algorithm.

Keywords: Bio-inspired computing, Bees Swarm Optimization metaheuristic, Combinatorial optimization, Unsupervised classification, Weighted MAX-SAT problem.

1 Introduction

Among NP-Complete problems, the Boolean Satisfiability Problem (SAT) is one of the most important and extensively studied. Given a set of Boolean variables $X = \{x_1, x_2,...,x_n\}$, a Conjunctive Normal Formula (CNF) is a conjunction of clauses, each clause being a disjunction of literals, and each literal being a variable from X or its negation. A clause is satisfied if at least one of its literals is true. A formula is said satisfiable if an assignment of variables that satisfies all the clauses exists, and unsatisfiable if otherwise.

The SAT problem asks for an assignment of variables that satisfies a CNF. If such an assignment does not exist, the problem that consists in searching for an assignment that maximizes the number of the satisfied clauses is named MAXIMUM-SATISFIABILITY (or MAX-SAT for short). The generalization of the problem is to define a positive weight w_i for each clause C_i, and search for an assignment that makes the sum of the weights of the satisfied clauses as great as possible. This variant of the problem is named weighted MAX-SAT.

B. Hu et al. (Eds.): BI 2011, LNAI 6889, pp. 226–237, 2011.

Many algorithms have been proposed to tackle the weighted MAX-SAT problem, and we can divide them into two main classes:

- Exact or complete algorithms: they are used for solving instances of SAT problems such as [1, 2, 3, 4, 5] that are variants of the well-known Davis–Putnam–Logemann–Loveland procedure[6].
- Approximation or incomplete algorithms: They provide an alternative to exact methods and are generally nature inspired, and/or based on local search [7, 8, 9, 10, 11, 12, 13,14]. These approaches called heuristics or metaheuristics do not ensure to lead to the optimal solution, they are rather used to compute a good quality solution when the optimal one does not exist or the instance of the considered problem is very large.

In this paper, an advanced version of Bee Swarm Optimization (BSO) is proposed in order to enhance its performances in terms of the solution quality and the execution time. The BSO main steps that are; the determination of the search region; the local search, performed by the bees; and the determination of the reference solution were modified, and tests were carried out to compare the results of the two versions of the metaheuristic.

The article is organized as follows: Section 2 and 3 present respectively the general algorithms of BSO and ABSO metaheuristics. In section 4, we present an application of ABSO to weighted MAX-SAT problem. Experimental results of the performed tests are given in section 5 before we conclude.

2 Bee Swarm Optimization Metaheuristic

Many studies have investigated the foraging behavior of a real bee swarm [15, 16]. The foraging process of a bee starts with leaving the hive in order to search a food source to gather nectar. After finding a flower, the bee stores the nectar in her honey stomach and comes back to the hive. After the nectar is unloded, the forager bee which found a rich source communicates to the other bees its direction and distance in order to recruit them.

Inspired from the foraging behavior of real bees, the Bee Swarm Optimization metaheuristic proposed in [14] is based on a population of artificial bees cooperating together to solving an instance of an optimization problem. Firstly, an initial solution named initSol is generated randomly or via a method such as the local search or Johnson's algorithm. This solution will be the reference solution from which the searchRegion, is a set of candidate solutions, is determined using a certain strategy [14]. Each of these solutions is assigned to one bee and becomes the starting point of its local search in the search region. Once accomplished its search, each bee communicates its best found solution to the other bees through a table named Dance. One of the solutions in this table will be selected to be the new reference solution (refSol) in the next iteration of the search process. In order to avoid cycles, the reference solutions are stored in a taboo list.

To ensure both good quality of the solution and good search space coverage, the selection of the reference solution at the end of an iteration of the search process follows the intensification and diversification principles. The intensification principle allows to find good solutions by exploring a promising search region as long as it improves best global solution. If the solution is not improved after a certain number of iterations, which represents the number of chances granted to a search region. Hence, the reference solution of the iteration i+1 is the best solution found by the bees in the ith iteration, if this one is better than the best solution found hitherto, or if the area of research did not reach the maximum of granted chances. In the opposite case, the reference solution will be the solution among those found by the bees during the iteration i which is the most distant from all the solutions stored in the taboo list.

The algorithm stops when the optimal solution is found, or the maximum number of iterations is reached.

The BSO general algorithm is the following:

```
BSO general algorithm
begin
  refSol← initSol;
  While not condition of stop do
    Insert refSolin taboo list;
    Determine searchRegion from refSol;
    Assign a solution from searchRegion to each bee;
    For each Bee kdo
      Perform a local search;
      Store the result in the table Dance;
    EndFor
    Select the new reference solution RefSol;
  EndWhile
end
```

3 ABSO: Advanced Bee Swarm Optimization

In BSO, the search region is a set of candidate solutions that are obtained from the reference solution by inverting some bits, according to one of the methods described in [14]. In ABSO, we aim at making this first and very important step of the metaheuristic less “naïve” by making the bees search in disjointed subsets of the search region. Indeed, instead of generating the starting points of the bees by inverting some variables in the reference solution, we make the bees search in disjointed subsets of the search region by subdividing the set of variables into groups according to the characteristics of the considered problem. Consequently, each group of variables will point out at a sub-region of the search region to which a bee is assigned to performing a local search at each iteration. As the sub-regions are disjointed, the bees “visit” different candidate solutions. Besides reducing the run-time by allowing a collision-free search process, this modification improves the coverage of the search space.

Such as BSO algorithm, ABSO applies the intensification principle: At the end of an iteration, if among the solutions returned by the bees there is a solution that outperforms the best global solution, it is selected to be the reference solution in the next iteration of the search process. If such a solution does not exist, the diversification principle is integrated to escape local optima. Here is the general ABSO algorithm.

```
ABSO general algorithm
Begin
  Subdivide the set of variables into groups;
  Assign a number of bees to each group;
  Calculate initSol;
  refSol ← initSol;
  Assign refSol to all the groups as the starting point
  of their local search;
  While not condition of stop do
     For each group gi
        Perform a local search;
        Store the best found solution;
     EndFor
     For each group i
        Determine the new reference solution refSol;
     EndFor
  EndWhile
End
```

4 ABSO for Weighted MAX-SAT

Adapting ABSO to weighted MAX-SAT problem requires the definition of the following main elements: The search space, the fitness function, the initial solution generating method, the variable-set subdivision procedure, the local search procedure performed by each artificial bee, and the determination of the reference solution

Search space. According to the nature of the weighted MAX-SAT problem, a solution is a chain of n bits written as {0, 1} and corresponding to a truth assignment of Boolean variables. The search graph is constituted by all solutions whose total number is equal to 2^n. A move from one solution to another consists in inverting a bit from the current solution.

Fitness function. It is expressed in weighted MAX-SAT as the sum of the weights of the clauses that are satisfied simultaneously by the solution.

Initial solution. To generating the initial solution, the enhanced version of the Johnson algorithm called John2a[17] is used.

```
John2a algorithm
Begin
  Let C being the set of all the clauses and X the set
  of variables
  Assign a weight W(Ci)=2^-|Ci| to each clause Ci, |Ci|
  being the length of the clause;
  While X is not empty
   Select a variable xi from X having the greatest value
   of |positive - negative|, where positive (resp.
   negative) is the sum of the weights of clauses in C
```

```
    in which this variable appears positive (resp.
    negative).
    If (positive>negative) then xi← TRUE;
    Else xi← FALSE;
    EndIf
    Delete xi from X;
    For each clause Ci where xi appears
     If the assigned value satisfies Ci Then
     Delete Ci from C;
     Else W(Ci) ← 2 * W(Ci);
     EndIf
     CurrentSol ← found solution;
    EndFor
  EndWhile

  Return currentSol;
End
```

An improvement of the John2a algorithm consists to test if among the nearest neighbors of *currentSol*, there is better solution by executing the following instructions before returning *currentSol*.

```
  While (There exist a solution s so that
distance(s,Crrentsol)=1 and f(s)>f(CurrentSol))
  currentSol ← s;
  EndWhile
```

The following sections describe the main steps of the ABSO algorithm, namely, the determination of the groups of variables, the local search process performed by the bees and the determination of the reference solution.

4.1 Determination of the Groups of Variables

As the weighted MAX-SAT problem consists in maximizing the sum of the satisfied clauses in a CNF, we can subdivide the set of variables *X* into several groups such as a group contains variables that do not appear in the same clauses. Consequently, a group *g* of *n* variables "covers" (can satisfy) a subset of clauses *c* containing at least *n* clauses, and if X_i and X_j are the subsets of variables contained respectively into the groups g_i and g_j, then the subsets of the search regions $subRegion_i$ and $subRegion_j$ corresponding respectively to g_i and g_j are disjointed, ie., there is no candidate solution belonging to more than one sub-Region as no variable appears in more than one group of variables.

In this work, we propose a method called unsupervisedHMDIA (HMDIA for How Much Does It Add), inspired from the unsupervised clustering method, for classifying the variables into groups. UnsupervidesHMDIA aims to classify the variables of X into groups depending in whether they appear in the same clauses or not, and according to the number of clauses covered by these variables. Indeed, a variable is added to the group to which it brings the most part of the problem. A new group is created if the best value of the clauses added by a variable and that is called *bestVal* is less than a certain threshold. The algorithm stops when two successive iterations give the same results (the same groups) or the maximum number of iteration is reached.

```
UnsupervisedHMDIA
Begin
  Let nbGroups be the number of groups
  nbGroups ← 1;
  Assign the least occurring variable to the first group;
  Assign the variable with the least weighted difference
  between clauses in which it appears positive and those
  in which it appears negative, let this difference for a
  given variable v be called wpos-wneg;
  While (non condition of stop)
    Set the covered clauses of each group to be those in
    which its only variables appear;
    While it remains variables to be assigned
      V ← unassigned variable having the smallest wpos-
      wneg.
      bestG ← the group that covers the least weighted sum
      of clauses in which v appears;
      bestVal ← the weighted sum of clauses in which v
      appears and that are not covered by bestG;
      If (bestVal<((weighted sum of clauses in which v
      appears)*R)) R being a fixed ratio then
        Create a new group;
        nbGroups ← nbGroups +1;
      EndIf
      Update the covering of bestG to include the clauses
      in which v appears;
    EndWhile
    Empty the groups while leaving in each one the
    variable that appears in the most weighted clauses;
  EndWhile
Return the groups;
End
```

4.2 Local Search

After subdividing the search region into sub-regions, a bee is assigned to each sub-region in order to perform their iterative local search, starting from the reference solution. This one is initially computed using the Johnson algorithm, then determined at the end of each iteration as explained in section 4.3. The the local search algorithm is the following:

```
Local search
Begin
   d ← 0;
   While  (d  <  |gi|)  and  maximum  number  of
   iterations not reached)
     For each solution s in subRegioni
      If (distance (refSol, s) = d)
     evaluate s;
     EndIf
   EndFor
   d ← d+1;
   EndWhile
 Return the best solution found;
End.
```

Note that distance (refSol, s) = d if there is d different bits between refSol and s among those corresponding to the variables in g_i. For instance, if we consider that: $|X|=10$, $g_1 = (x_1, x_5, x_9)$, $s_1 = (0, 0, 1, 0, 0, 0, 1, 1, 1, 0)$, $s_2 = (1, 0, 1, 0, 1, 0, 1, 1, 1, 0)$ and $s_3 = (0, 0, 0, 1, 0, 0, 1, 0, 1, 0)$.Then, distance $(s_1, s_2) = 2$, and distance (s_1, s_3) cannot be calculated since s_1 and s_3 do not belong to the same search region.

4.3 The Determination of the Reference Solution

At the end of each iteration (each bee having searched into its corresponding region and returned the best found solution), the new reference solution is determined according to the results found in this iteration to be the starting point of the bees local search in the next iteration. This step is guided by the intensification and diversification principles; the diversification being carried out when a number of chances granted to a search region is exhausted.

The general idea is that at the end of each iteration, the best solution returned by the bees and called *bestSol* is compared to the best solution found hitherto by all the groups of bees and that is called *bestGlobalSol*. If *bestSol* is better than *bestGlobalSol*, this one is updated and become the reference solution of all the bees in the next iteration except for bees assigned to the group g_i which instead of searching pointlessly in the same region, will have as reference solution a solution returned by a function called *explore*. This one inverts alternatively in *bestSol* either all the variables of one group of variables among the other groups, or one variable per group. This alternation is done from an iteration to another to allowing a good coverage of the search space.

In case no bee has improved the global solution, and the chances granted to the search region are exhausted, a diversification is performed following the same algorithm than *explore* function. It determines the new reference solution for all the bees that will, thus, leave the current search region for another one.

The following algorithm explains the determination of the reference solution at the end of an iteration i:

```
solRefDetermination
Begin
  Let bestGlobalSol be the best solution so far and that
  is equal to init sol for the first iteration.
  Let bestSol be the best solution among those returned
  by all the bees at the iteration i, and bestBee the bee
  that has found it.
  Let nbChances be the number of chances remaining to the
  current search region, initially it is equal to
  nbGroups+1 (nbGroups being the number of the group of
  variables)
  Let intensification (resp. diversification) a Boolean
  variable that is set to true if an
  intensification(resp. diversification)must be performed

  If (f(bestSol)> f(bestGlobalSol))then
    bestGlobalSol ← bestSol;
    nbChances ← nbGroups+1;
    Intensification = true;
  Else
    nbChances ← nbchances-1;
    If(nbChances>0)then Intensification ← true;
    Else diversification ← true;
EndIf
End
```

4.4. ABSO for Weighted MAX-SAT

After describing the different steps of the ABSO applied to the weighted MAX-SAT problem, here is the overall algorithm:

```
ABSO for weighted MAX-SAT
Begin
   Calculate the initial solution
   Determine the search groups
   While (not condition of stop)
     For each group
       Perform a local search;
     Endfor
     refSolDetermination;
     if (intensification) then
       intensify;
     else
       if (diversification)then
       diversify;
     EndIf
   EndWhile
```

```
  End
Intensify
Begin
  For all the bees except bestBee
  refSol  ←bestSol;
  For bestBee
  refSol ← explore();
 End

Diversify
 Begin
  Calculate the new refSol of all the groups from bestSol
  by inverting either all the variables of one group or a
  variable per group;
 End
```

5 Computational Experiments

Before comparing the performances of ABSO to those of BSO [17], a series of tests were conducted on the Johnon's benchmark instances (http://www2.research.att.com/~mgcr/data/index.html) in order to determine the optimal values of the empirical parameters that are: The ratio (R), the maximum number of iterations in the local search algorithm (beeit) and the maximum number of chances granted to a search region (nbchances). A value is said better than another if it leads to either satisfying more instances, or minimizing the run-times The optimal values of the empirical parameters are illustrated in Table 1.

Table 1. Optimal values of BSO empirical parameters

Parameter	Aptimal value
R	0.5
beeit	92
nbchances	Nbg +1
nsteps	300000

BSO and ABSO algorithms were implemented in java and tests were conducted using a 2.3 GHZ dual core Pentium PC with 4 GO of RAM. The results showed that ABSO algorithm was able to satisfy 34 instances among 38, where BSO satisfied only 27 instances. We also observed that there is no instance satisfied by BSO and not satisfied by ABSO.

The algorithms were also compared in terms of run times on the 27 benchmarks satisfied by both. As BSO uses random functions in initial solution generating method and search region determination, the average times of several runs were compared with those of one ABSO run. The results showed that BSO times are broadly shortest even though ABSO times were butter for 12 instances among the 27.

Table 2. Comparison between the results of ABSO with those of BSO

Bench	Opt.Val	ABSO	*Time(s)*	BSO	**Time(s)**
Jnh 01	420925	420925	199,49	420925	13,48
Jnh 10	420840	420840	22,43	420840	33,81
Jnh 11	420753	420753	202,61	420728	38,36
Jnh 12	420925	420925	5,30	420925	3,24
Jnh 13	420816	420816	8,72	420816	38,87
Jnh 14	420824	420824	2,65	420824	36,94
Jnh 15	420719	420719	37,66	420719	35,51
Jnh 16	420919	420914	318,44	420914	38,64
Jnh 17	420925	420925	4,96	420925	1,96
Jnh 18	420795	420795	43,84	420795	33,30
Jnh 19	420759	420759	44,24	420759	34,12
Jnh 201	394238	394238	0,86	394238	0,97
Jnh 202	394170	394170	246,09	394029	30,53
Jnh 203	394199	394199	169,43	394199	35,41
Jnh 205	394238	394238	5,71	394238	2,19
Jnh 207	394238	394238	140,68	394238	5,36
Jnh 208	394159	394159	42,62	394159	36,36
Jnh 209	394238	394238	1,50	394238	18,97
Jnh 210	394238	394238	2,34	394238	4,19
Jnh 211	393979	393979	305,96	393979	34,15
Jnh 212	394238	394227	299,38	394227	38,08
Jnh 214	394163	394163	45,90	394163	37,93
Jnh 215	394150	394150	87,31	393951	37,10
Jnh 216	394226	394226	3,74	394226	37,08
Jnh 217	394238	394238	4,93	394238	1,01
Jnh 218	394238	394238	2,25	394238	11,32
Jnh 219	394156	394053	304,22	393942	38,50
Jnh 220	394238	394238	160,82	394155	36,85
Jnh 301	444854	444842	331,36	444842	42,58
Jnh 302	444459	444459	20,92	444459	41,73
Jnh 303	444503	444503	186,23	444503	42,94
Jnh 304	444533	444533	35,55	444472	40,81
Jnh 305	444112	444112	191,12	444112	41,92
Jnh 306	444838	444838	62,21	444838	42,43
Jnh 307	444314	444314	2,68	444314	41,78
Jnh 308	444724	444724	240,62	444568	43,34
Jnh 309	444578	444578	14,38	444578	41,46
Jnh 310	444391	444391	197,67	444353	43,23
Number of satisfied instances		34		27	

6 Discussion and Future Works

In this paper, an advanced version of BSO that modifies essentially the determination of search regions by subdividing the set of variables into groups covering disjointed regions in the search space is proposed. To apply the proposed metaheuristic to the weighted MAX-SAT problem an unsupervised classification problem is proposed that groups the variables according to their appearance in the same clauses or not, in order to maximize the search space coverage and reduce the runtime by avoiding collisions between the bees, as they explore different candidate solutions. This main modification induced other modifications in both the local search performed by the bees and the determination of the reference solution at the end of each iteration.

Tests were carried out on a series of benchmarks in order to evaluate ABSO performances by comparing the obtained solutions quality and run times with those of BSO. The analysis of the results showed that ABSO algorithm globally outperforms the BSO one. Moreover, as the research process of ABSO algorithm is deterministic and don't use random functions, thus gives good results at each execution.

In conclusion, we believe that the classification of combinatorial problem variables used in ABSO can be applied to other combinatorial problems and may lead to improved solutions. In our future works, we plan to apply ABSO to some of them.

References

1. Wallace, R., Freuder, E.: Comparative studies of constraint satisfaction and Davis-Putnam algorithms for maximum satisfiability problems. In: Johnson, D., Trick, M. (eds.) Cliques, Coloring and Satisfiability, vol. 26, pp. 587–615. American Mathematical Society, Providence (1996)
2. Borchers, B., Furman, J.: A two-phase exact algorithm for MAX-SAT and weighted MAXSAT problems. J. Combi. Opti. 2, 299–306 (1999)
3. Alsinet, T., Manyà, F., Planes, J.: Improved branch and bound algorithms for Max-SAT. In: Proceedings of the 6th International Conference on the Theory and Applications of Satisfiability Testing, S. Margherita Ligure, Portofino, Italy (2003)
4. Xing, Z., Zhang, W.: Efficient strategies for (weighted) maximum satisfiability. In: Proceedings of CP-2004, Toronto, Canada, pp. 690–705 (2004)
5. Alsinet, A., Manyà, F., Planes, J.: An efficient solver for weighted Max-SAT. Journal of Global Optimization 41(1), 61–73 (2008)
6. Davis, M., Logemann, G., Loveland, D.: A machine program for theorem-proving. Commun. ACM 5, 394–397 (1962)
7. Selman, B., Henry, A., Kautz, Z., Cohen, B.: Local Search Strategies for Satisfiability Testing. Presented at the second DIMACS Challenge on Cliques, Coloring, and Satisfiability (October 1993)
8. Frank, J.: A study of genetic algorithms to find approximate solutions to hard 3CNF problems. In: Proceedings of Golden West International Conference on Artificial Intelligence (1994)
9. Mazure, B., Sais, L., Greroire, E.: A Tabu search for Sat. In: Proceedings of AAAI (1997)
10. Resende, M., Pitsoulis, L., Pardalos, P.: Approximate solutions of weighted MAX-SAT problems using GRASP. In: Du, D.-Z., Gu, J., Pardalos, P. (eds.) Satisfiability Problem: Theory and Applications, pp. 393–405. American Mathematical Society, Providence (1997)
11. Drias, H.: Scatter search with random walk strategy for SAT and MAX-W-SAT problems. In: Monostori, L., Váncza, J., Ali, M. (eds.) IEA/AIE 2001. LNCS (LNAI), vol. 2070, pp. 35–44. Springer, Heidelberg (2001)
12. Drias, H., Taibi, A., Zekour, S.: Cooperative Ant Colonies for Solving the Maximum Weighted Satisfiability Problem. Springer, Heidelberg (2003)

13. Boughaci, D., Drias, H.: Solving Weighted Max-Sat Optimization Problems Using a Taboo Scatter Search Meta-heuristic. In: Proceedings of ACM SAC 2004, pp. 35–36 (2004)
14. Drias, H., Sadeg, S., Yahi, S.: Cooperative Bees Swarm for Solving the Maximum Weighted Satisfiability Problem. In: Cabestany, J., Prieto, A.G., Sandoval, F. (eds.) IWANN 2005. LNCS, vol. 3512, pp. 318–325. Springer, Heidelberg (2005)
15. Von Frisch, K., Lindauer, M.: The "language" and orientation of the honey bee. Annu. Rev. Entomol. 1, 45–58 (1956)
16. Seeley, T.: Honeybee ecology: a study of adaptation in social life. Princeton University Press, Princeton (1985)
17. Johnson, D.S.: Approximate Algorithmic for combinatorial Problems. Journal of Computer and System Sciences, 256–278 (1974)

Investigation into Stress of Mothers with Mental Retardation Children Based on EEG (Electroencephalography) and Psychology Instruments

Wen Zhao[1], Li Liu[1,*], Fang Zheng[1], Dangping Fan[1], Xuebin Chen[2], Yongxia Yang[3], and Qingcui Cai[3]

[1] The School of Information Science and Engineering, Lanzhou University, Lanzhou, China
[2] Department of Mental Health, The First Affiliated Hospital of Lanzhou University, Lanzhou, China
[3] The Special Education School, Lanzhou, China
liliu@lzu.edu.cn, wenzi4931@gmail.com, {zhengf05,fandp10}@lzu.cn, chenpsych@126.com, 916265735@qq.com, caiqingcui01@163.com

Abstract. This paper proposed a new method, combining EEG and psychology instruments, to detect stress which can contribute in prediction and intervention of major depression. Seven mothers with mental retardation children as stress group and four age-matched mothers with healthy children as normal controls are enlisted. Results showed that relative power in alpha rhythm of stress group is significantly less than normal controls, while relative power in theta rhythm is much larger than normal controls. Discrimination accuracy gets higher than only using psychology instruments for distinguishing the two groups in our experiment. Besides, combination of EEG linear and nonlinear features is better than using only linear ones. Combination of LZ-complexity, alpha relative power and PSQI achieves discrimination accuracy of 95.12%, which gains an improvement of 19.51% compared with accuracy by using only PSQI. As a result, the combination of EEG and psychology instruments will benefit the detection of stress.

Keywords: Stress, Major Depression, EEG, Psychology instruments, Naïve Bayes classifier.

1 Introduction

Special education for mental retardation children has gained real attention in China [1]. However, stress condition of mothers with mental retardation children has not got enough attention. In fact, pressure of mothers with mental retardation children comes from many directions, such as marriage status, children's state etc [2]. Normally, due to insufficient medical facilities, as well as lack of clinical psychiatrists, mothers' stress is not taken seriously until mental state develops into mental disorder (e.g., depression).

[*] Corresponding author.

B. Hu et al. (Eds.): BI 2011, LNAI 6889, pp. 238–249, 2011.

Detecting stress is crucial in prediction and intervention of major depression. Psychology instruments [3] and hormone as conventional assessment for stress have been widely used to detect stress due to their practicability and well-developed technology. Considering the variances of users' culture, language and subjectivity, psychology instruments may lose effectiveness in different populations. For example, when filling items of psychology instruments, participants from China prefer to select medium option due to the influences of Chinese culture. Therefore, assessing stress level completely based on the psychology instruments is partial. Besides, literature [4] proved that hormones are useful indicators of stress level. However, the invasion of hormones acquisition makes this method of narrow application.

EEG collected from scalp without invasions is precise and objective. EEG electrodes on scalp measure the field potentials originated from combined activity on neuronal cells [5]. The observed frequencies of EEG are divided into specific bands: delta (0-4Hz), theta (4-8Hz), alpha (8-13Hz), and beta (13-40Hz) for further analysis in different domains. EEG has been used in sleep disorder [6], epilepsy [7], personal identification [8], and etc. However, EEG is very sensitive owing to the fact that it is easily influenced by disturbance [5]. Therefore, EEG signals are always carrying noise such as EOG, EMG, etc. Thus, it may be better to combine psychology instruments and EEG for stress detection.

This paper presents a hybrid method to combine EEG and psychology instruments in order to detect stress of mothers with mental retardation children. Both objective EEG and conventional method psychology instruments are applied to distinguish stress group from normal controls. This new method takes advantage of EEG's objectivity and psychology instruments' practicability. De-noising and feature extraction are employed in this method. In this way, when stress is detected, intervene can be executed instead of letting stress develops into mental disorder.

2 Relative Research

Stress has been proposed associated with major depression disorder by many works. In [9], depression is proved significantly related to stress. Therefore, EEG is adopted to detect stress in this study. EEG has been widely studied in different domains [6-8]. Regarding to stress related mental disorder, depression is taken into consideration. C_0-complexity (C0) has been used on implication of brain or cognitive status, sleep staging and mental illness. C0 can not only get accurate results for small data sets, but also avoid time series reconstructed procedure which always takes long time to process. Prediction of eruption of epilepsy with second-order C_0-complexity has gained accuracy of 94.3% among 21 patients [10]. In [11], both major depression disorder (MDD) and post-traumatic stress disorder (PTSD) displayed more left than right-frontal activity. Meanwhile, MDD group were significantly right lateralized relative to controls. As to LZ-complexity (LZC), this value is higher for depression groups than the controls [12]. Both linear and nonlinear features of EEG are applied in this study.

3 EEG Recording

In our method, Fp1, Fp2, Fpz in pre-frontal areas according to international 10-20 standard (shown in Fig.1) are selected to record EEG based on the following two reasons. On the one hand, the frontal area of scalp, Fp1, Fp2, F7, F8, F3, F4 and Fpz has been proved particularly critical in emotional processing [13]. On the other hand, regarding the convenience of users, Fp1, Fp2 and Fpz is not covered by hair, which makes users more comfortable. Consequently, Fp1, Fp2, Fpz in pre-frontal areas are selected in our method. Meanwhile, M1 and M2 are used as reference potentials shown in Fig.1.

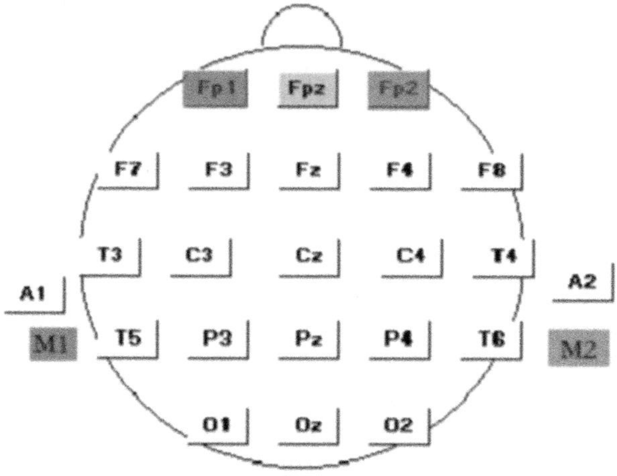

Fig. 1. EEG electrodes we used

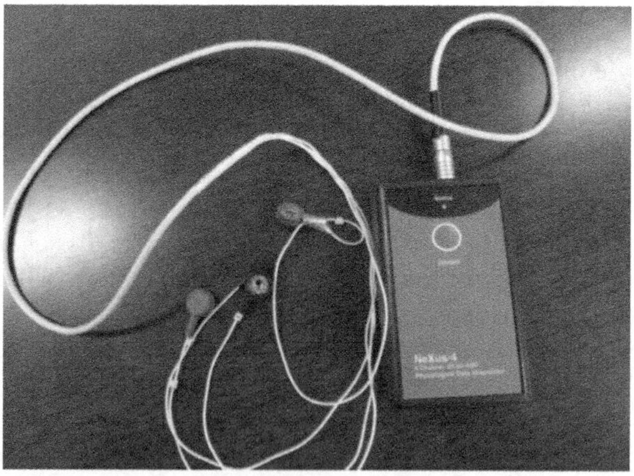

Fig. 2. A portable EEG collection device

A portable EEG collection device named Nexus-4 (shown in Fig.2) is applied to record EEG signal. Nexus-4 sends gathered EEG signal to computer via Bluetooth.

4 Methodology

This paper presents a solution for stress detection. The methodology of our approach (illustrated in Fig.3) which involves two main components: EEG processing and score acquisition of psychology instrument. In EEG processing, first of all, raw EEG data is acquired from the subjects. The de-noise procedure is necessary owing to the fact that there is usually a lot of noise in the raw data. After that, EEG features expected to characterize stress will be extracted from these signals. Regarding to psychology instruments, scales will be printed and fulfilled by participants and questionnaire results will be calculated. Finally, the EEG signals should be classified into their corresponding categories according to the EEG features and questionnaire results.

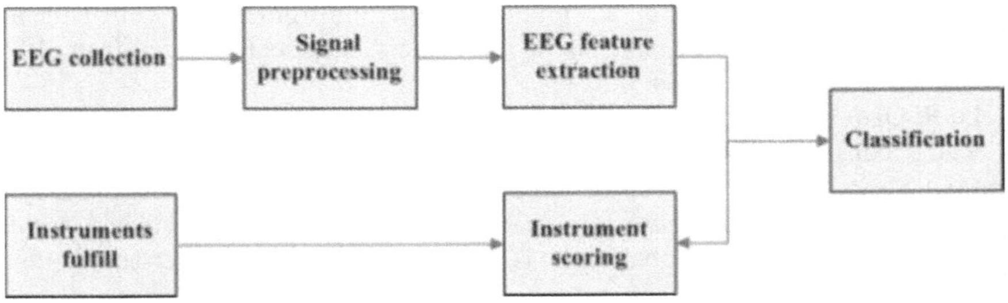

Fig. 3. The methodology of our hybrid method. The results of the classification are stress condition

5 Experiment

5.1 Participants

Seven stress subjects are recruited from mothers of mental retardation students. Four age matching mothers with health children were selected as control group. Participants' ages range from 34 to 41 years. For both groups, if one either has a personal history of depression/psychosis (acute & lifetime) or family history of depression/ psychosis in any first-degree relative (i.e. parents or children of the participant) or heavy drinking, heavy smoking, intake of any medications interfering with sleep are excluded.

5.2 Psychology Instruments

Psychology instruments are wildly used in psychology research. However after years' use, disadvantages of psychology instruments came to light. Usually, it takes quite a long time to complete the questionnaires. Besides, standardized questionnaires may lead some misinterpretation, while open-ended questions are hard to process and analysis. More importantly, after instrument data has been collected, it may not reflect participants' real state owing to misinterpretation or the truth that sometimes people are not capable of identifying their state objectively. Regardless of these drawbacks, in this study, BDI-II [3], K10 (10-item Kessler Psychological Distress Scale) [14], PSQI (Pittsburgh Sleep Quality Index) [15] which have got reliable results are adopted.

The BDI-II, 21-item BDI-II measuring the severity of self-reported depression in adolescents and adults is usually scored by summing its 21 symptom ratings to yield a single total score which addresses all nine of the symptom criteria listed in the American Psychiatric Association's Diagnostic and Statistical Manual of Mental Disorders for a major depressive episode. Each symptom is rated on a 4-point rating scale ranging from 0 to 3, consequently total scores range from 0 to 63. The time frame for the BDI-II ratings is for the "past 2 weeks, including today." According to [3], BDI-II total scores ranging from 0 to 13 represent normal to minimal depression, total scores from 14to 19 are mild, total scores from 20 to 28 are moderate, and total scores from 29 to 63 are severe.

K10 is a measure of non-specific psychological distress in the anxiety–depression spectrum. Item responses are on a 5-point scale ranging from 1 to 5, with 1 meaning none of the time and 5 meaning all of the time. Total score ranges from 10 (no distress) to 50 (severe distress).

The PSQI is a self-rating questionnaire resulting in a global score between 0 and 21, which consists of seven sub scores (Sleep quality, Sleep onset latency, Sleep duration, Sleep efficiency, Sleep disturbances, Use of sleeping medication, Daytime dysfunction). The questionnaire is easy to handle and can be completed within 5 minutes. The mean PSQI global score is also calculated. The higher score subjects get, the worse sleep quality is.

5.3 EEG Data Collection

EEG signals are recorded using a Nexus-4 device (see Fig.2). Fpz, Fp1, Fp2 according to 10-20 system [16] are selected. Simultaneously, M1 and M2 (the two ear lobes) are used as reference potentials. Fpz-M, Fp1-M1, and Fp2-M2, are monopole recording with M1, M2 used as reference potentials. In order to implement this goal, we collect EEG signal at twice, Fpz-M1 and Fp1-M1, Fp2-M2, with M2 and M1 used as ground respectively. Linear features and nonlinear features are calculated in the data from Fpz-M1. EEG data gathered from Fp1, and Fp2 is used to calculate alpha asymmetry.

Participants were lead to the empty laboratory one by one. One well-trained student assisted wearing EEG recording sensor, record EEG, and guide the procedure. After the participants settled themselves comfortably, they were told to breathe deeply to relax and then close their eyes, keep silent, try to minimize facial movements and eyeball movements and body movements during 85 seconds' recording. After EEG collecting, participants were asked to fulfill the questionnaires printed.

5.4 Signal Preprocessing

The raw EEG signals are notoriously noisy and difficult to analyze. Features extracted from these raw data would not be robust and reliable enough for further analysis.

Before the data can be used in our program, it has to be preprocessed. One important step of preprocessing is removing the noise from the signals. Because the electrical activity of the brain is produced in the order of micro volts and these signals are very weak, there must be a lot of noise contained. The presence of noise can be due to external and internal causes. The external causes include static electricity and electromagnetic field produced by surrounding devices. In addition to these external causes, the EEG signals are also heavily influenced by the internal causes, artifacts that originate from body movement or eye blinks included.

The noise present in the EEG signals could be de-noised using simple filters and wavelet transformation. In our study, four steps for EEG signal preprocessing were taken. First, remove the mean value of EEG signals. Second, bandpass filtering is used to eliminate EEG signal drifting and EMG disturbances by only keeping signals within the range of 2-45Hz. Third, Wavelet Algorithm (dp 7) is taken to eliminate EOG disturbances. Fourth, bandpass filtering is excuted again to extract certain frequency bands (theta, alpha, beta) for further analysis.

5.5 EEG Features Extraction

Both non-linear features including complexity and the largest Lyapunov exponent and relative power in linear aspect are calculated in this study.

C_0-complexity [17] is a description of time sequences randomness. Xu Jing-Hua et al. put forward C0 at practical analysis of EEG signal processing. The main idea of C_0-complexity is divided time sequences into regular part and random part. C_0-complexity is defined as the ratio of square between random part and time axis to square between the whole time sequences and time axis.

Lempel and Ziv [18] proposed an algorithm to generate a given sequence using two fundamental operations, namely: copy and insert by parsing it from left to right. The Lempel-Ziv complexity c(n) of a sequence of length n is given by the shortest sequence generated using the copy and insert operation that can generate the given sequence. In general, LZ-complexity measures the rate of generation of new patterns along a sequence and in the case of ergodic processes is closely related to the entropy rate of the source.

The largest Lyapunov exponent (marked as LLE) [19] is used to measure the exponential divergence of initially close state-space trajectories and estimate the amount of chaos in a system. The largest Lyapunov exponent is used to measure the exponential divergence of initially close state-space trajectories and estimate the amount of chaos in a system. If the largest lyapunov exponent λ <0, standing for two trajectories with nearby initial conditions contract; If λ >0, standing for two trajectories with nearby initial conditions diverge at an exponential rate and the system sensitivity to initial conditions, also indicating chaos.

Relative power is the ratio of the corresponding absolute power to total power of the signal. Alpha relative power equals the rate between alpha absolute power and total power of EEG. Theta relative power equals the rate between theta absolute power and total power of EEG.

5.6 Classification

Classification is one of the most important methods of data mining. Extracted EEG features and psychology instruments scores serve as the parameter input of the classifiers. The features extracted shall be computed and analyzed to find a tendency unveiling high stress population's stress level in contrast to normal controls. In our study, classification is trying to tell stress group from controls using both EEG signal features and psychology instruments results. Naïve Bayes classifier [20] based on applying Bayes' theorem is a simple probabilistic classifier. Still, Naive Bayes classifiers have worked quite well in many complex real-world situations, in spite of the naive design and apparently over-simplified assumptions. Also, Naïve Bayes classifier has been widely used in mental disorder research based on EEG and gain good results. The construction of naive Bayes classifier does not need any complicated iterative parameter estimation schemes. This mean it may be readily applied to huge data sets.

6 Experimental Results and Discussions

Each participant's EEG recording lasts 85 seconds. EEG recording was divided into 41 EEG epochs, each lasting 4 seconds, with an overlap of 50%. Consequently, there are 287 tuples in stress group, and 164 tuples in control group. Four persons' data in stress group and three in control group was randomly selected as training tuples. Left three persons' data in stress group and one person's data in normal group was assigned as test tuples.

Table 1. success rates of classification with Naïve Bayes classifier when using single feature

Features	Bayesian
C_0-complexity	61.58%
Alpha asymmetry	50%
LLE	70%
LZC	63.41%
Alpha relative power	71%
Theta relative power	70.12%
BDI-II	25%
K10	75%
PSQI total score	75.61%

According the discrimination rate shown in the Table 1, psychology instruments perform better than EEG features. Alpha relative power can tell stress group from normal controls with an accurate of 71%. In EEG spectral analysis, we can clearly see that alpha relative power of stress group is less than normal controls. And, theta relative power of stress group is much larger than normal controls. In general, resting EEG with eye closed, alpha rhyme appears. Fig.4 and Fig.5 show screen-capture of EEG spectral analysis, normal control and stressful female respectively.

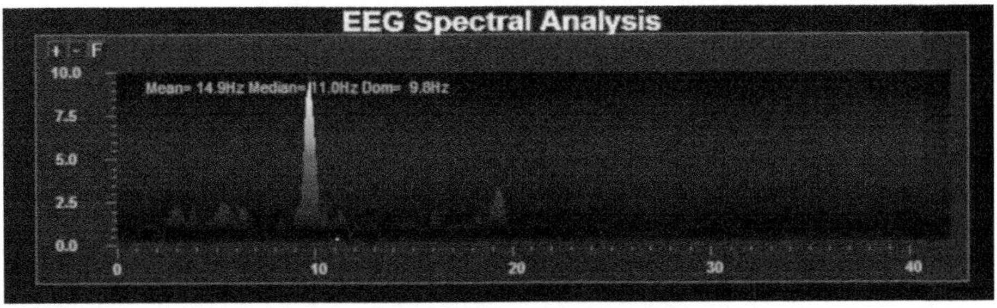

Fig. 4. screen-capture of a normal control

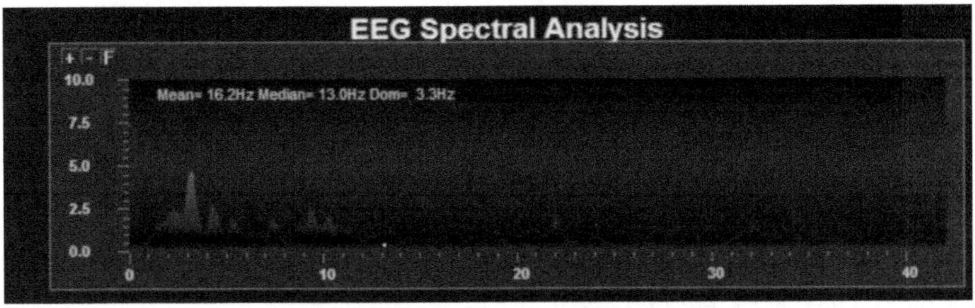

Fig. 5. screen-capture of a stressful female

As to alpha asymmetry, although alpha asymmetry has been focused in depression studies based on EEG, in our experiment, alpha asymmetry does not work well in discriminating two groups, which is inconsistent with many studies. This may be caused by the screening procedure. In screening samples, participants including stress group and normal controls have obvious depressive symptoms, or have a history of depression, or has a direct relative (father, mother, siblings) had been reported a history of depression are excluded. Alpha asymmetry is not a distinguished feature in this sample.

Nonlinear dynamics of EEG performs well in distinguishing two groups. It seems that complexity of EEG in stress group is higher than normal controls. It can be seen from Fig.4 and Fig.5 that alpha rhythm occupies most of the EEG power in normal controls, while, EEG power widely distributed in different bands (beta, alpha, theta). From this basic spectral analysis, complexity may be able to be explained.

With questionnaires we assessed, K10 gets a discrimination rate of 75%, and PSQI total score 75.61%. At the same time, BDI-II only gets a discrimination accuracy of 25%, which may be due to the fact that both two groups don't have obvious depression. All participants reported history of depression or direct relatives have a history of depression are excluded. It is obvious that using only EEG, accurate rate was not comparable to psychology instruments, with accurate ranging from 50% to 71%. However, according to the experiment, EEG seems to make up questionnaires' inadequate. For example, combination of C0 and K10 gains accuracy of 78.05%, which is larger than both using only C0 and using only K10. Combination of alpha relative power and PSQI total score reaches an accuracy of 93.29%, which gets arise of 22.29% comparing with alpha relative power, and 17.68% comparing with PSQI total score. To sum up, combination of one EEG feature and one psychology instrument result, shown in Table 2, gained accuracy higher than only using psychology instrument, with a raise range from 0 to 20.12% comparing with psychology instrument discriminating accuracy.

Table 2. Success rates of classification with Naïve Bayes classifierwhen using combined features

Features	accuracy
C0+K10	78.05 %
C0+ PSQI total score	89.02%
LLE+K10	81.71%
LLE+ PSQI total score	78.66%
LZC+K10	76.83%
LZC+ PSQI total score	92.07%
alpha relative power+K10	72.56%
alpha relative power+ PSQI total score	93.29%
theta relative power+ K10	75%
theta relative power+ PSQI total score	77.44%
LZC+ alpha relative power	68.29%
LZC+ alpha relative power+K10	85.98%
LZC+ alpha relative power+ PSQI total score	95.12%
Alpha relative power + theta relative power	71.34%
K10 + Alpha relative power + theta relative power	81.7%
Alpha relative power + theta relative power+ LLE	71.95%
Alpha relative power + theta relative power+ LLE +K10	83.54%

As to linear features, combination of alpha relative power and theta relative power has an accuracy of 71.34% higher than using only one of them. K10 has an accuracy of 75%. Combination of linear features and K10 gain an accuracy of 81.7%. At the same time, combination of LZC and alpha relative power reaches 95.12%, larger than combination of only linear features with psychology instrument, for example, K10, Alpha relative power, theta relative power gets 81.7%. Linear and nonlinear algorithms reflect information of EEG in different aspects. Combination of two performs better than using only one. However, it usually takes longer time to calculate a nonlinear feature. So combination of different nonlinear features is not taken into consideration.

Although EEG is always full of many kinds of noise and do perform fair, it may do make up the disadvantage of psychology instruments (i.e. subjectivity). The best accurate rate reaches 95.12%, with a combination of EEG nonlinear (LZC) and linear feature (alpha relative power) and psychology instrument (PSQI). If a new person comes, this system can tell whether he/she is in a condition of stress or not with an accurate of 95.12%.

7 Conclusion and Future Work

Detecting stress condition is critical at primary mental health care. When a stress is detected, therapist can guide him/her to cope with the current stressful events effectively. Despite of the fact that psychology instruments are commonly used in mental health research, they do have their inadequate, for example subjectivity. In this paper, we propose a new method using both psychology instruments and EEG features to detect the stress, which can contribute in prediction and intervention of major depression. Seven mother with mental retardation children and four mothers with age-matching healthy children are selected as participants in the experiment. Resting frontal EEG with eye closed and three psychology instruments selected serve as parameters input of Naïve Bayes classifier.

Combination of EEG and psychology instrument is better than using only EEG with arises range from 4.88% to 22.29% or only using psychology instrument with raises range from 0 to 20.12% Although, EEG features when used alone do not perform very well, when combined with psychology instruments they do make psychology instruments enhanced. This may be because EEG's objectivity and preciseness complement psychology instruments' disadvantages. At the same time, it is also found that combination of both linear and nonlinear methods perform better than only using linear ones. Combination of K10, alpha relative power and theta relative power gains accuracy of 81.7%. When LLE is added in, discrimination accuracy achieves 83.54%. This result is consistent with [6]. It is proved that using both methods is more effective than using only one, despite of different fields.

However, there are several disadvantages in this paper. We only have data of eleven subjects in the experiment. Afterwards, we are going to collect data of 25 or more persons under stress and 25 normal controls. Furthermore, different stressful events are taken into consideration, for example, students under the stress of examination and unemployed people. With more samples under different kind of stress, it will be much more persuasive and reliable than only using mothers with mental retardation children. Besides, in this paper, selecting and combination of EEG features and psychology instruments is done manually. In future work, it is planned that machine based rules that help to select and combine EEG features and psychology instruments, for example, ICA (independent component analysis) shall be used [21].

In summary, this paper indicates that EEG can be adopted as an assistant to psychology instruments in stress detecting. Alpha relative power of stress group is much less than normal controls. And, theta relative power of stress group is larger than normal controls. Results showed that discrimination accuracy gets higher than only using psychology instruments. Besides, combination of EEG linear and nonlinear features is better than using only linear ones for distinguishing the two groups in our experiment. It is concluded that using both EEG and psychology instruments is better in detecting stress than using only psychology instruments.

Acknowledgements. This work was supported by National Natural Science Foundation of China (grant no.60973138, 61003240), the EU's Seventh Framework Programme OPTIMI (grant no. 248544), National Basic Research Program of China

(973 Program) (No.2011CB711001) and Gansu Provincial Science & Technology Department (grant no. 1007RJYA010).

References

1. Yang, H., Wang, H.B.: Special Education in China. J. Spec. Educ. 28, 93–105 (Spring 1994)
2. Cate Miller, A., Gordon, R.M., Daniele, R.J., Diller, L.: Stress, Appraisal, and Coping in Mothers of Disabled and Nondisabled Children. J. Pediatr. Psychol. 17(5), 587–605 (1992)
3. Kumar, G., Steer, R.A., Karen, B., Teitelman, V.L.: Effectiveness of Beck Depression Inventory–II Subscales in Screening for Major DepressiveDisorders in Adolescent Psychiatric Inpatients. Assessment 9, 164–170 (2002)
4. van Praag, H.M.: Can Stress Cause Depression? Progress in Neuro-Psychopharmacology and Biological Psychiatry 28(5), 891–907 (2004)
5. Nunez, P.L.: Electric Fields of the Brain, 2nd edn. Oxford University Press, Oxford (2006)
6. Zhao, W., Yan, J., Hu, B., Ma, H., Liu, L.: Advanced Measure Selection in Automatic NREM Discrimination Based on EEG. In: The Fifth Pervasive Computing and Applications (ICPCA), pp. 26–31 (2010)
7. Kostopoulos, G., Gloor, P., Pellegrini, A., Siatitsas, I.: A Study of the Transition from Spindles to Spike and Wave Discharge in Feline Generalized Penicillin Epilepsy: EEG Features. Experimental Neurology 73(1), 43–54 (1981)
8. Peng, H., Hu, B., Liu, Q., Dong, Q., Zhao, Q., Moore, P.: User-centered Depression Prevention: An EEG approach to pervasive healthcare. In: Mindcare Workshop in Pervasive Health 2011, Dublin, Ireland (2011) (in print)
9. James, H., Johnson, I.G.: Sarason: Life stress, depression and anxiety: Internal- external control as a moderator variable. Journal of Psychosomatic Research 22(3), 205–208 (1978)
10. Bian, N.-y., Cao, Y., Wang, B., Gu, F.-j., Zhang, L.-m.: Prediction of Epileptic Seizures Based on Second-order c_0 complexity. Acta Biophysica Sinica 1 (2007)
11. Kemp, A.H., Griffiths, K., Felmingham, K.L., Shankman, S.A., Drinkenburg, W., Arns, M., Clark, C.R., Bryant, R.A.: Disorder Specificity Despite Comorbidity: Resting EEG Alpha Asymmetry in Major Depressive Disorder and Post-traumatic Stress Disorder. Biological Psychology 85(2), 350–354 (2010)
12. Li, Y., Tong, S., Liu, D., Gai, Y., Wang, X., Wang, J., Qiu, Y., Zhu, Y.: Abnormal EEG Complexity in Patients with Schizophrenia and Depression. Clinical Neurophysiology 119(6), 1232–1241 (2008)
13. Tucker, D.M.: Later Brain Function, Emotion, and Conceptualization. Psychological Bulletin 89, 19–46 (1981)
14. Andrews, G.: Tim Slade: Interpreting scores on the Kessler Psychological Distress Scale (K10). Australian and New Zealand Journal of Public Health 25(6), 494–497 (2007)
15. Backhaus, J., Junghanns, K., Broocks, A., Riemann, D., Hohagen, F.: Test-retest Reliability and Validity of the Pittsburgh Sleep Quality Index in Primary Insomnia. Journal of Psychosomatic Research 53, 737–740 (2002)
16. Jasper, H.: The Ten Twenty Electrode System of the International Federation. Electroencephalography and Clinical Neurophysiology 10, 371–375 (1958)
17. Chen, F., Gu, F., Xu, J., Liu, Z., Liu, R.: A New Measurement of Complexity for Studying EEG Mutual Information. In: The Fifth International Conference on Neural Information Processing, ICONIP R98, pp. 435–437. IOA Press, Kitakyushu (1998)

18. Nagarajan, R., Szczepanski, J., Wajnryb, E.: Interpreting Non-random Signatures in Biomedical Signals with Lempel–Ziv Complexity. Physica D: Nonlinear Phenomena 237(3), 359–364 (2008)
19. Rosenstein, M.T., Collins, J.J., Luca, C.J.D.: A Practical Method for Calculating Largest Lyapunov Exponents from Small Data Sets. Physica D: Nonlinear Phenomena 65(1-2), 117–134 (1993)
20. Domingos, P., Pazzani, M.: On the Optimality of the Simple Bayesian Classifier under Zero-one Loss. Machine Learning 29, 103–130 (1997)
21. Ekenel, H.K., Sankur, B.: Feature Selection in the Independent Component Subspace for Face Recognition. Pattern Recognition Letters 25(12), 1377–1388 (2004)

Evaluation and Recommendation Methods Based on Graph Model

Yongli Li, Jizhou Sun, Kunsheng Wang and Aihua Zheng

Beijing Institute of Information and Control, Beijing 100037, China

Abstract. Evaluation and recommendation are different actions, but they are consistent in mining and using information efficiently and effectively to improve their persuasiveness and accuracy. From the view of information processing, the paper builds a two-dimensional graph model which expresses the relationships between evaluators and objects. This graph model reflects the original information of evaluation or recommendation systems and has its equivalent matrix form. Next, the principle of matrix projection can be applied to get the evaluation or recommendation vector by solving the matrix maximization problems. What's more, a rating data set of online move is selected to verify the model and method. In conclusion, from the example analysis, it is found that the proposed evaluation method is reasonable, and from the numerical experimental comparison, the proposed recommendation method is proved to be time-saving and more accurate than the generally adopted recommendation methods.

Keywords: Data Mining, Evaluation, Recommendation System, Graph Model.

1 Introduction

Evaluation and recommendation are two common actions for almost everyone and everyday. For example, many people who shop online often participate in the evaluation of the purchased items with scores and words. This phenomenon attracts various researchers to study the scores and words, which are the key information to evaluate and recommend, as such in the above example, researchers have confirmed that these online scores and words will influence the purchase of other buyers[1-4].

However, there are two issues that need to be discussed further. The first one is whether the widely applied rating method for evaluation is scientific. The averaging score of an item, which was widely used, was adopted by some big online shopping websites[5-6], that is, the score of an item for evaluation was the average of all the rated scores. If the score is an important variable in the purchase decision as confirmed in the above literatures, the method of obtaining the score is very important. Therefore, it is necessary to know whether the existing method of simply average score is scientific and rational. Is there a better way to get the rated score? The second issue is whether the existing score

B. Hu et al. (Eds.): BI 2011, LNAI 6889, pp. 250–259, 2011.

information has been fully utilized to give an effective recommendation. Some literatures pointed that few websites implemented an effective recommendation mechanism[7-9]. In fact, There have been mainly two recommendation methods currently used in the above websites[10-16], which are either based on the similarity between items, or based on the similarity between people. In the former condition, when a person buys a certain item, he or she would therefore be recommended the items with relatively high similarity to the item that he or she buys; In the latter condition, if two buyers have a relatively high degree of similarity, when a certain item is purchased by one of them, the item will be recommended to the other. Is there a better way to utilize the given information for effective recommendations?

The above two questions is different, so they may have different ways to be solved. However, in this paper we will point that the two issues are essentially consistent from the view of the information utilization. They are consistent in establishing the information processing approach to reflect the available information. Take example of the above evaluation and recommendation methods which are currently widely used. For the evaluation method of average scores, the information is processed in an isolated manner with the whole scores from the solo item, without noticing the connection between items and the evaluators. And, for the recommendation methods, though both of the existing recommendation methods consider the connection between items or people, the people-item-people connection is not established in the comprehensive perspective of the issue. Therefore, some information is destined to be left out from the beginning in the above existing information processing methods. In this paper, the information processing methods are approached as a foundation to avoid the above flaws, reserving as much information as possible and reflecting the connection between items and people. The evaluation and recommendation methods are discussed on such basis, and are compared with the existing methods.

2 Model

The online evaluation and recommendation systems are described as the following model: there are M individuals (numbered from No.1 to No.M) and N kinds of items (numbered from No.1 to No.N), and the individuals evaluate some of the items α-point scale is adopted in the system and usually a 5-point scale is adopted on the websites. The evaluators are asked to give integer scores, and according to the rating scores on these items, $v^m_{\alpha N\times 1}$ by individual No.m is defined as follows:

$$\left.\begin{array}{l}
\text{When individual No.}m\text{ does not evaluate item No.}k\text{:}\\
\qquad v^m_{l\times 1}=0, l\in\{\alpha k-\alpha+1,\alpha k-\alpha+2,\cdots,\alpha k\}\\
\text{When individual No.}m\text{ evaluates item No.}k\text{ with the score }z\text{:}\\
\begin{cases} v^m_{l\times 1}=1, l=\alpha k-z+1\\ v^m_{l\times 1}=0, l\in\{\alpha k-\alpha+1,\alpha k-\alpha+2,\cdots,\alpha k\}\backslash\{\alpha k-z+1\}\end{cases}\\
\text{Among which, }m\in\{1,2,\cdots,M\}, k\in\{1,2,\cdots,N\}, z\in\{1,2,\cdots,\alpha\}
\end{array}\right\}\quad(1)$$

The rating matrix $A^m_{\alpha N\times\alpha N}$ of individual No.m is defined as follows:

$$A^m_{\alpha N\times\alpha N} = \frac{v^m_{\alpha N\times 1}(v^m_{\alpha N\times 1})^T - diag(v^m_{\alpha N\times 1})}{n^m - 1} \tag{2}$$

where n^m represents the total number of items that individual No.m has evaluated, and $diag(v^m_{\alpha N\times 1})$ represents the diagonal matrix with the diagonal as $v^m_{\alpha N\times 1}$. It is specified that when the numerator is zero matrix, the division formula will be zero matrix. Then sum all the individuals' rating matrixes to get the system rating matrix $A_{\alpha N\times\alpha N}$:

$$A_{\alpha N\times\alpha N} = \sum_{m=1}^{M} A^m_{\alpha N\times\alpha N} = \sum_{m=1}^{M} \frac{v^m_{\alpha N\times 1}(v^m_{\alpha N\times 1})^T - diag(v^m_{\alpha N\times 1})}{n^m - 1} \tag{3}$$

Matrix $A_{\alpha N\times\alpha N}$ is the result of information processing of rating system in this paper. The information of rating system is transformed into mathematical expression by the matrix based on the Graph Model, where an item is regarded as a point and the evaluation is regarded as a side, which constitute the form of a graph. Take a 2-point rating system for example, individual No.m_1 evaluates three items, namely item No.1, item No.2 and item No.3, with the scores shown in Fig.1 below, and individual No.m_2 evaluates two items, namely item No.1 and item No.2, with the scores shown in Fig.2 below.

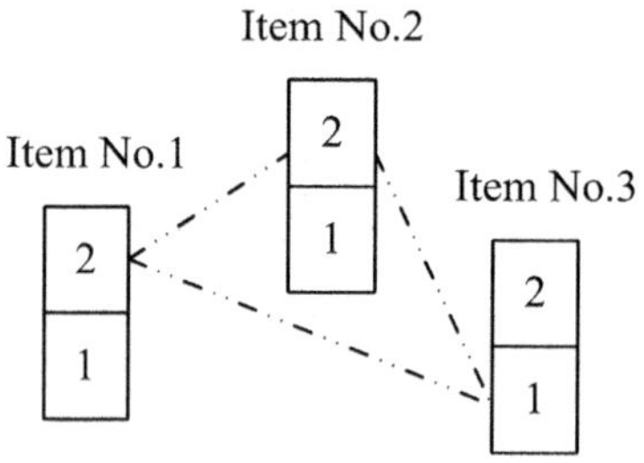

Fig. 1. Rating Graph by Individual m_1

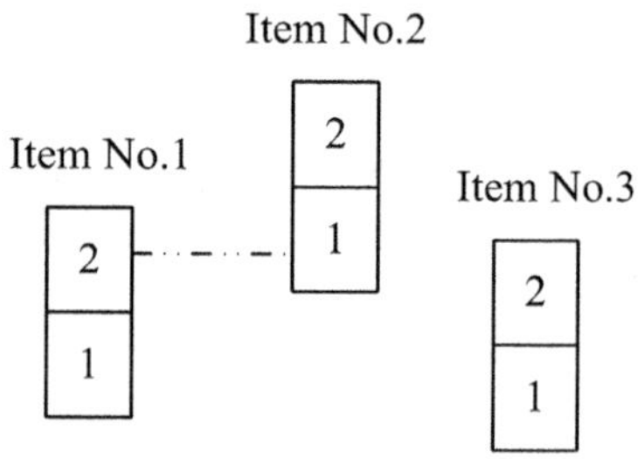

Fig. 2. Rating Graph by Individual m_2

According to the definition of the rating vector defined by (1), the rating vector of individual No.m_1 is $v^{m_1}_{6\times 1} = (1\ 0\ 1\ 0\ 0\ 1)'$, and the rating vector of individual No.m_2 is $v^{m_2}_{6\times 1} = (1\ 0\ 0\ 1\ 0\ 0)'$, therefore it can be calculated according to (2):

$$\begin{array}{c} \\ \\ A^{m_1}_{6\times 6} = \end{array} \begin{array}{c} \begin{array}{cccccc} \text{item1} & & \text{item2} & & \text{item3} & \\ 2p & 1p & 2p & 1p & 2p & 1p \end{array} \\ \left[\begin{array}{cc:cc:cc} 0 & 0 & 1/2 & 0 & 0 & 1/2 \\ 0 & 0 & 0 & 0 & 0 & 0 \\ \hdashline 1/2 & 0 & 0 & 0 & 0 & 1/2 \\ 0 & 0 & 0 & 0 & 0 & 0 \\ \hdashline 0 & 0 & 0 & 0 & 0 & 0 \\ 1/2 & 0 & 1/2 & 0 & 0 & 0 \end{array}\right] \end{array} \begin{array}{ll} 2p & \text{item1} \\ 1p & \\ 2p & \text{item2} \\ 1p & \\ 2p & \text{item3} \\ 1p & \end{array}$$

Here, 'p' means point. Similarly, $v^{m_2}_{6\times 6}$ and $v_{6\times 6}$ can be obtained. The matrix blocks correspond to the category of items, such as 1/2 in the first row and the third column means that item No.1 is rated as 2 points, and item No.2 is rated as 2 points, corresponding to the connection between item No.1 and item No.2 in Fig.1. Other numbers have the similar explanations.

In this example, it is found that the definition of $A^m_{\alpha N\times\alpha N}$ is the matrix expression of the rating graph of individual No.m, with the matrix and graph expressing the same information, and the scores and quantity (denominator of the rated value in matrix plus 1) of the items evaluated by the individual can be obtained. The rating graph is the characterization showed by the individual in the system, without losing any information during the modeling process.

As for the averaging method and similarity approach between items or between individuals, the system information is not utilized on such a comprehensive connection perspective. The averaging method only focuses on all the evaluation information of one item and ignores the connection between the item and other items established through the evaluation process. The similarity approach between items ignores the connection between individuals, and the similarity approach between individuals ignores the connection between items, failing to represent all the relationships in the rating system. It can be seen that information processing method in this paper retains more raw information compared with the existing evaluation and recommendation methods.

When $A^m_{\alpha N\times\alpha N}$ of all individuals is summed, the rating matrix $A_{\alpha N\times\alpha N}$ of the entire system will be obtained. The matrix depicts the connection between items and persons in the system, containing the information of both the evaluators and the evaluated items. The connection, namely the side of the graph, is generated through the evaluation action of each individual.

Following are some of the properties of these two matrixes, which are useful for the methodological analysis later.

(1) $A^m_{\alpha N\times\alpha N}$ is a symmetric matrix, with the sum of rows being 1 or 0. When the sum is 1, it means individual No.m scores the item corresponding to the row. When the sum is 0, it means the corresponding evaluation point properties are not supported by the individual. The sum of columns means the same due to the symmetry of the matrix.

(2) The sum of rows of $A^m_{\alpha N\times\alpha N}$, which can be derived from the formula (3), is the value representing the number of people who are in favor of the score of an item.

3 Method

3.1 Description of the Evaluation Method

Matrix $A_{\alpha N\times\alpha N}$ of the entire system is obtained through the above method. In order to reflect the main information of matrix $A_{\alpha N\times\alpha N}$ through the column vector $X_{\alpha N\times 1}$, it means reaching the maximum value of the following formula:

$$\max_{X_{\alpha N\times 1}} \frac{(A_{\alpha N\times\alpha N}X_{\alpha N\times 1}, X_{\alpha N\times 1})}{(X_{\alpha N\times 1}, X_{\alpha N\times 1})} \tag{4}$$

Explanation of the maximization formula: the maximization problem is equivalent to the projection value of matrix $A_{\alpha N\times\alpha N}$ on the direction of vector $X_{\alpha N\times 1}$. The larger the value of the above formula is, the more information will be reflected in vector $X_{\alpha N\times 1}$ containing $A_{\alpha N\times\alpha N}$. In fact, the solution of equation(4) leads to the largest eigenvalue of matrix $A_{\alpha N\times\alpha N}$ and the corresponding eigenvector[17]. Obviously, $A_{\alpha N\times\alpha N}$ is a non-negative irreducible matrix. According to Perron-Frobinus Theorem[18], when the sum of columns of $X_{\alpha N\times 1}$ is limited to 1, there exists the only solution for the above optimization problem.

The *ith* Element of $X_{\alpha N\times 1}$ is defined as x_i. The vector elements of each item will be normalized:

$$\hat{x}_i = \frac{x_i}{\sum\limits_{j=1}^{\alpha} x_{(\lceil \frac{i}{\alpha}\rceil - 1)\times\alpha + j}} \tag{5}$$

$\lceil \frac{i}{\alpha}\rceil$ means ceiling of $\frac{i}{\alpha}$. Then the score of individual No.n is as follows:

$$g_n = \sum_{i=1}^{\alpha} \hat{x}_{\alpha(n-1)+i} \times (\alpha + 1 - i) \tag{6}$$

3.2 Description of the Recommendation Method

In order to infer the personalized recommendation method, it is necessary to process the original $A_{\alpha N\times\alpha N}$ by deleting the inconsistent evaluation information of individual No.m, resulting in $\tilde{A}^m_{\alpha N\times\alpha N}$, which is defined as follows:

Let v_i^m as *ith* element of rating vector $v^m_{\alpha N\times 1}$ by individual No.m.

If individual No.m doesn't evaluate the item No.j, then $\tilde{A}^m_{i,:} = A_{i,:}$, where $i \in \{(j-1)\alpha+1, (j-1)\alpha+2, \cdots, j\alpha\}$.

If individual No.m evaluates the item No.j by score z ($z \in \{1, 2, \cdots, \alpha\}$), then $\tilde{A}^m_{i,:} = A_{i,:}$, where $i = \alpha j + 1 - z$ and $\tilde{A}^m_{i,:} = 0$, where $i \in \{(j-1)\alpha+1, (j-1)\alpha+2, \cdots, j\alpha\}\backslash\{\alpha j + 1 - z\}$.

In the definition above, the ratings which are inconsistent with individual No.m are deleted in $A_{\alpha N\times\alpha N}$ and the evaluation information of the items that the individual does not evaluate or which is consistent with the individual No.m is retained. The algorithm can be done by copying the evaluation methods in 3.1, by just replacing $A_{\alpha N\times\alpha N}$ with $\tilde{A}^m_{\alpha N\times\alpha N}$ to obtain the rating g_n^m by the individual No.m.

The mathematical approach is applied in both of the methods above on the basis of matrix projection, and the solution process is basically the same.

4 Comparisons between the Evaluation Methods

The 2-point scale rating system with 3 items and 34 individuals involved is presented here, obtaining the overall rating matrix as:

$$A = \left[\begin{array}{cc:cc:cc} 0 & 0 & 0 & 1 & 23/2 & 3/2 \\ 0 & 0 & 1 & 0 & 3/2 & 23/2 \\ \hdashline 0 & 1 & 0 & 0 & 7/2 & 1/2 \\ 1 & 0 & 0 & 0 & 7/2 & 1/2 \\ \hdashline 23/2 & 3/2 & 7/2 & 7/2 & 0 & 0 \\ 3/2 & 23/2 & 1/2 & 1/2 & 0 & 0 \end{array}\right]$$

According to the method and matrix characteristics expressed in Part 2 of this paper, it can be inferred through summing up the columns of the matrix that 14 persons rate 2 points for item No.1 and 14 persons rate 1 point for item No.1, 5 persons rate 2 points for item No.2 and 5 persons rate 1 point for item No.2, and 20 persons rate 2 points for item No.3 and 14 persons rate 1 point for item No.3.

According to the evaluation method in Part 3 of this paper, the following can be obtained with the maximization of the formula:

$$X = (0.2300, 0.01774; 0.0814, 0.0851; 0.2496, 0.1764).$$

The result of each item after normalization is:

$$\hat{X} = (0.5645, 0.4355; 0.4887, 0.5113; 0.5860, 0.4140).$$

According to formula g_n, the ratings of three items can be obtained as 1.565, 1.489 and 1.586 respectively. However, based on the averaging method, 14 persons rate 2 points for item No.1 and 14 persons rate 1 point, so it can be inferred that the average score is 1.50. Similarly, the score of item No.2 is 1.50, and the score of item No.3 is 1.59.

Now, we can find that the results of these two methods are different. In the method proposed in this paper, the ratings are: item No.3 $\succ$ item No.1 $\succ$ item No.2, where $\succ$ means "better than". While in the averaging method commonly used, the ratings are: item No.3 $\succ$ item No.1 $=$ item No.2. Which result is more reasonable? In the segmental matrix containing 23/2 and 3/2, it can be inferred that large amounts of data support the idea that item No.3 and item No.1 are the same good or the same bad. However, when item No.3 is compared with No.2, it can be determined that the front should be better than the latter. And while the property of item 1 worse than item 2 is supported by only a small amount of data from the segmental matrix containing 7/2 and 1/2. If the size of the data quantity is an important indicator of the results' credibility, and then based on the analysis above, it can be inferred that item No.3 is not disadvantage compared to item No.1 or item No.2, and it is significantly better than item No.2, inferring that item No.3 is the best. At the same time, there is more data in favor of the consistency between item No.3 and item No.1. So it is regarded that the evaluation results of item No.1 and item No.3 should be more close compared to item No.2, while item No.2 is not dominant compared to the other two items, and it is significantly worse than item No.3, inferring that item No.2 is the worst. The analysis results are consistent with the results with the method in this paper and different from the results with the averaging method.

5 Numerical Results

5.1 Sources of Data

The rating data sets of online movie are selected, including the rating data of the movie by each reviewer in the collection. It is rated from 1 to 5 points, with 1 as the worst and 5 as the best. The website of the data sets is `www.gruoplens.org` , providing two rating data sets of different sizes. There are the rating data of 1,682 films by 943 participants in the selected data set with the total evaluation score of about 100000. Based on the Graph Model, the data are read as a sparse rating matrix.

5.2 Numerical Results of Recommendation

In order to verify the validity and accuracy of the recommendation algorithm, the original data sets are divided randomly, 80% as the sample set and 20% as the test set. Recommendation algorithm will be applied in the sample set, and then we will obtain the corresponding scores of the films appeared in the test set to compare the calculated score with the recommendation algorithm with the actual scores in the test set. Index MAE selected for comparison is defined as follows:

$$MAE = \frac{\sum_{n=1}^{N} |v_{i,\alpha}^{n} - round(\hat{v}_{i,\alpha}^{n})|}{N} \tag{7}$$

N is the total number of score data in the test set, among which $v_{i,\alpha}^{n}$ expresses data No.n, reflecting the score on film No.α by individual No.i. $\hat{v}_{i,\alpha}^{n}$ expresses the predicted value on film No.α by individual No.i by the recommendation method in this paper, $round()$ indicates rounding.

Meanwhile, the recommendation accuracy D is defined as:

$$D = \frac{\aleph(|v_{i,\alpha}^{n} - round(\hat{v}_{i,\alpha}^{n})| = 0)}{N} \tag{8}$$

The numerator $\aleph(|v_{i,\alpha}^{n} - round(\hat{v}_{i,\alpha}^{n})| = 0)$ expresses the number of accurate recommendations in the test set.

Methods of the similarity between items or individuals are adopted in the experiment for the comparison, which are the same with Herlocker(2002) [12], besides the method of random recommendation which means giving a score randomly to each items on the test sets is also adopted. It is noted that the result in the Table 1 has gotten by averaging the results which has been calculated

Table 1. Comparisons of Four Recommendation Methods

Method	MAE	D
Method of graph model in this paper	0.78	37.1%
Method of the similarity between items	0.88	31.6%
Method of the similarity between individuals	0.86	32.3%
Method of random recommendation	1.38	21.7%

based on randomly divided sets of the original data five times. MAE and D of the four recommendation methods mentioned above are listed in Table 1.

Meanwhile, the pie chart of $|v_{i,\alpha}^n - round(\hat{v}_{i,\alpha}^n)|$ is as follows:

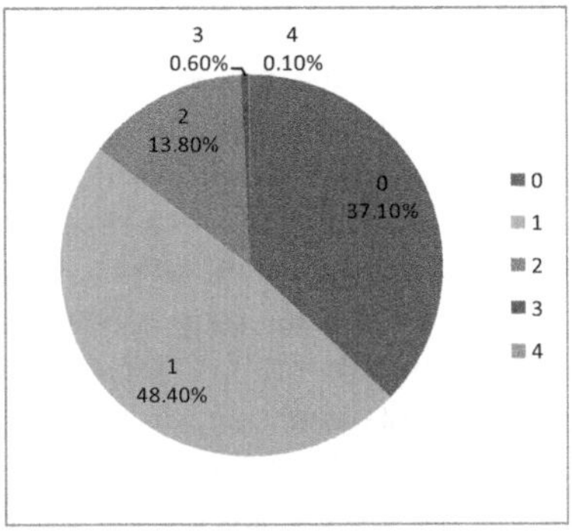

Method in this paper

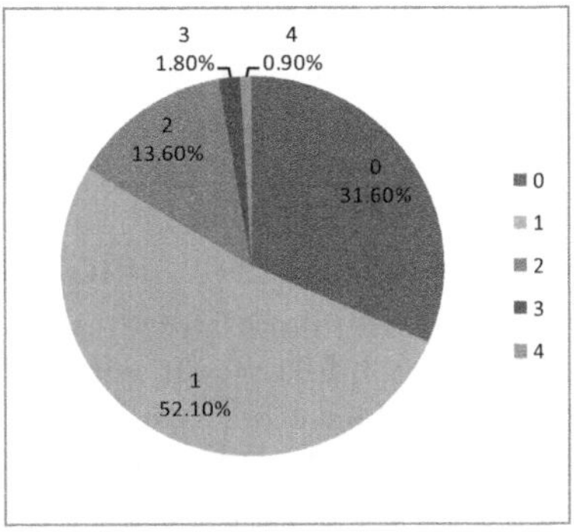

Method of similarity between items

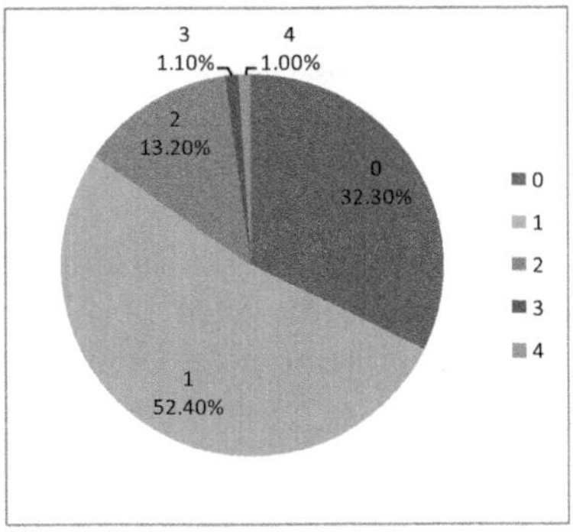

Method of similarity between individuals

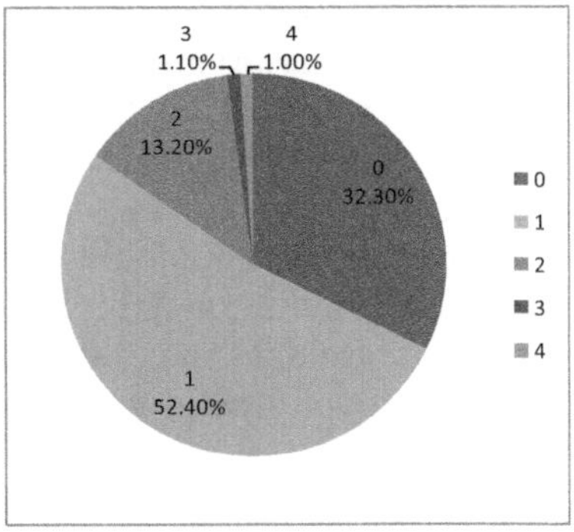

Method of random recommendations

Fig. 3. Pie Chart of Four Different Methods of Recommendation

Form these figures, the method based on graph model in this paper has the highest currency rate in all the methods, and meanwhile the lowest rate of more than 2-point variance with the actual score. Obviously, random recommendation is worse than the others, which tells us that these three methods are useful.

Computing time of the four recommendation methods is showed respectively: Based on the data set containing 100000 comments and PC of 2G memory, the average time is 8.8 seconds by the method proposed in this paper, compared to it, 6.5 seconds by the method of similarity between items and 4.9 seconds by that of similarity between individuals. For random recommendation method, that is less than 1 second. From the above results, we can find that the method of this paper is in the same level with the two similar methods in computing time, so it is efficient and available for on-line and real-time recommendations.

6 Conclusions and Future Work

In the principle of Graph Model, the evaluation information given by the evaluators will be transformed into a graph representation, which retains the original evaluation information, laying the foundation for further comprehensive evaluations and personalized recommendations. According to the corresponding expression between graph and matrix, it is more convenient to process information with mathematical methods. The principle of matrix projection is applied in this paper, maximizing the retention of the matrix information, and therefore working on evaluations and recommendations. The numerical results show that according to the method in this paper, the designed algorithm is practical and efficient, taking short time to obtain the result and giving more accurate recommendation information compared to the existing recommendation method based on similarity between items and similarity between people, with the accuracy rate of 37.1%, and an average error of 0.78, resulting in improvement by about 5% in terms of accuracy and reduction by approximately 0.10 in average errors than the two methods above.

It is noted that only the form of numerical evaluation is presented in this paper. It can be further progressed in two ways: 1. expand the commentary methods which can be evaluated, such as including text comments, etc.; 2. further mine the customer information – the connection between customers is built up with item rating in this paper, and there can also be more connections, such as the gender, occupations, hobbies, etc., so that the graph can be multi-dimensional and the corresponding matrix would become the matroid. Such problems can be considered based on the evaluation and recommendation approaches of maximizing information utilization in this paper.

References

1. Sulin, B., Paul, A.P.: Evidence of the Effect of Trust Building Technology in Electronic Markets: Price Premiums and Buyer Behavior. MIS Quarterly 26(3), 243–268 (2002)
2. Paul, A.P., David, G.: Building Effective Online Marketplaces with institution-Based Trust. Information Systems Research 15(1), 37–59 (2004)
3. Paul, A.P., Liang, H., Xue, Y.J.: Understanding and mitigating uncertainty in online exchange relationships: A principal-agent perspective. MIS Quarterly 31(1), 105–136 (2007)

4. Park, D.H., Kim, S.: The effects of consumer knowledge on message processing of electronic word-of-mouth via online consumer reviews. Electronic Commerce Research and Applications 7(4), 399–410 (2008)
5. Linden, G., Smith, B., York, J.: Amazon.com recommendations: item-to-item collaborative filtering. IEEE Internet Computing 7(1), 76–80 (2003)
6. Asela, G., Guy, S.: A Survey of Accuracy Evaluation Metrics of Recommenda- tion Tasks. The Journal of Machine Learning Research 10(12), 2935–2962 (2009)
7. Zhang, Z.K., Zhou, T., Zhang, Y.C.: Personalized recommendation via integrated diffusion on user-item-tag tripartite graphs. Physica A: Statistical Mechanics and its Applications 389(1), 179–186 (2010)
8. Zhang, Y.C., Medo, M., Ren, J.: Recommendation model based on opinion diffusion. Europhysics Letters 80(6), 68003 (2007)
9. Azene, Z., Anthony, F.N.: Representation, similarity measures and aggregation methods using fuzzy sets for content-based recommender systems. Fuzzy Sets and Systems 160(1), 76–94 (2009)
10. Liu, R.R., Jia, C.X., Zhou, T.: Personal recommendation via modified collaborative filtering. Physica A: Statistical Mechanics and its Applications 388(4), 462–468 (2009)
11. Panagiotis, S., Alexandros, N., Apostolos, N.P.: Nearest-balusters' collaborative filtering based on constant and coherent values. Information Retrieval 11(1), 51–75 (2008)
12. Herlocker, J.L., Konstan, J.A., Riedl, J.: An Empirical Analysis of Design Choices in Neighborhood-based Collaborative Filtering Algorithms. Information Retrieval 5, 287–310 (2002)
13. Shang, M.S., Lü, L., Zeng, W.: Relevance is more significant than correlation: Information filtering on sparse data. Europhysics Letters 88(6), 68008 (2009)
14. Zhou, T., Su, R.Q., Liu, R.R.: Accurate and diverse recommendations via eliminating redundant correlations. New Journal of Physics 11(12), 123008 (2009)
15. Liu, J.G., Zhou, T., Wang, B.H.: Degree Correlation of Bipartite Network on Personalized Recommendation. International Journal of Modern Physics C 21(1), 137–147 (2010)
16. Pan, X., Deng, G.S., Liu, J.G.: Information Filtering via Improved Similarity Definition. Chin. Phys. Lett. 27(6), 068903 (2010)
17. Richard, B.: Introduction to matrix analysis. McGraw-Hill Book Company, New York (1970)
18. David, G.L.: Introduction to Dynamic Systems: Theory, Models and Applications. John Wiley & Sons, Chichester (1979)

An Improved EDP Algorithm to Privacy Protection in Data Mining

Mingzheng Wang and Na Ge

Institute of Systems Engineering, Dalian University of Technology,
Dalian, 116024, People's Republic of China
mzhwang@dlut.edu.cn, genajyc@126.com

Abstract. In this paper, we propose an improved pruning algorithm with memory, which we call improved EDP algorithm. This method provides the better trade-off between data quality and privacy protection against classification attacks. The proposed algorithm reduces the time complexity degree significantly, especially in the case of the complete binary tree of which worst-case time complexity is of order $O(M \log M)$, where M is the number of internal nodes of the complete tree. The experiments also show that the proposed algorithm is feasible and more efficient especially in the case of large and more complex tree structure with more internal nodes, etc. From a practical point of view, the improved EDP algorithm is more applicable and easy to implement.

Keywords: decision tree pruning, privacy protection, complexity.

1 Introduction

On September 9, 2010, the American Civil Liberties Union of Northern California, Lambda Legal and the AIDS Legal Services Alliance sent a letter to officials at the California Department of Health Care Services accusing the agency of violating state privacy laws because state health officials sent names, addresses and telephone numbers of about 5,000 HIV-positive residents to the foundation over the past 24 months, see reference [1]. Although data mining techniques are used to help enterprises to find the useful and common information about customers from large data, there are growing concerns on privacy disclosure [2]. Sweeney [3] reported that 87% Americans can be uniquely identified with gender, birthday and zip code.These three attributes are normally included in the deidentified data distributed by health-care organizations and also accessible from data sources with identity attributes such as voter registration lists. If data collectors and owners can't protect personal privacy when release data, they will face plenty of problems such as legal sanctions, honor loss, etc. How to adopt the appropriate safety measures to protect privacy is a big problem for them. As a result, more and more organizations will not publish the survey data, while questionnaire recipients increasingly refuse to give their personal information or lie when asked about their personal habits and preference. To a certain extent, these actions protect individual privacy. However, it deteriorates data resource

B. Hu et al. (Eds.): BI 2011, LNAI 6889, pp. 260–271, 2011.

and quality, and ultimately prevents science and technology development and social progress.

Data mining experts increasingly do research on high disclosure risk problem in data mining [4,5,6]. Their works aim at protecting privacy while carrying out useful data mining. Reiss [7] proposed a data-swapping method to approximately preserve the distribution of t-order statistics while swapping data. This method can preserve relationships between attributes under the condition of protecting confidential attribute values. The method is, however, just applicable for categorical data. When numeric data are present, they need be conversed into categorical data, which leads to information loss. Estivill-Castro and Brankovic [8] proposed a data-swapping method based on decision tree, which attempts to maintain the same decision rules while swapping data. Their basic idea is to swap class values (the records with different confidential attribute values) in the same leaves. Their method, however, has a bad effect on pure or higher classification accuracy leaves in which there are higher disclosure risk records in the dataset. At the same time, it also faces the information loss problem for type conversion. Agrawal & Srikant [9] proposed a fixed value perturbed method called EM (expectation maximization) algorithm, which can approximately preserve summary statistics when conversion single data. The method randomly generates Y from the same distribution. Then by using Z=X+Y, the method only provides perturbed values of X rather than the original data X. Agrawal & Aggarwal [10] proved that the EM algorithm converges to the maximum likelihood estimate of the original distribution based on the perturbed data. Another problem is that the EM algorithm can't deal with categorical data. Even to numeric data, there is also information loss problem. The above researches just deal with a single type data, numeric data or categorical data. From a data miner's standpoint, they discussed how to protect privacy while preserving data utility. There is, however, a lack of study on whether and how a data-mining technique can be directly used to disclose personal privacy.

Different from the above studies, Li & Sarkar [11] from data owner standpoint firstly discussed that there is serious classification attacks problem in decision tree which can be an effective tool for malicious invaders. To solve this problem, they proposed EDP(Error Divergence Pruning) algorithm. The EDP algorithm based on classification attacks can identify records with high disclosure risk and effectively deal with mixed numeric and categorical data, but would spend amounts of time when meet large data which will greatly influence the application scope of the algorithm.

With the rapid development of computer hardware technology, huge storage space can be used. In this paper, we propose an improved algorithm with storage memory, which we call improved EDP algorithm. Through storing initial error-divergence values of all internal nodes of the tree, the improved EDP algorithm avoids repeating computations effectively.

The rest of this paper is organized as follow: In Section 2, we propose the improved EDP algorithm with storage memory. In Section 3, we analyze the worst-time complexity of the complete binary tree and prove that the proposed algorithm reduce time complexity significantly. In Section 4, using experiment results from 3 datasets, we further show the improved EDP algorithm is feasible and effective. In the last section, we make a brief conclusion.

2 The Improved EDP Algorithm

In this section, we will introduce the improved algorithm, and then use the improved EDP algorithm to solve an example from the real life. The idea of the improved EDP algorithm is to balance disclosure risk and data utility. It aims at identifying the nodes with records that have the highest disclosure risk, and thus is subject to mask, so it can get the tree with the best trade-off between disclosure risk and data utility. Now we introduce some related definitions and symbols.

- The error-divergence is denoted by R_t, the significance level is denoted by α, the swapping rate is denoted by p, etc. Here, α measures the disclosure risk of leaves, p measures the extent of privacy protection, etc.

- Let C be the number of classes of the confidential attribute. Let F_k and f_k be the frequency distributions of the class values in a node t and in the full dataset, respectively. The node divergence of t is defined as

$$D(t) = \sum_{k=1}^{c} f_k \log \frac{f_k}{F_k} .$$

  $D(t)$ follows asymptotically χ^2 distribution with $C - 1$ degrees of freedom. Algorithm introduces p-value in statistics inference, that is $P[\chi(c-1) > D(t)]$, to measure whether f and F distributions are significantly different.

- The branch B_t is a subtree whose root node is an internal node t but non-root node in a tree. Let n_t be the number of records in B_t. Let B_t have m leaves $(L_1, \cdots, L_m)$and let $n_1^t, \cdots, n_m^t$ be the number of records in each of its leaves. The divergence of subtree B_t is defined as

$$D(B_t) = \sum_{i=1}^{m} \frac{n_i^t}{n_t} D(L_i) .$$

- Let $E(t)$be the error rate of the node t, which is the ratio of minority records over all records in the node t. Let $E(B_t)$ be the error rate of the subtree B_t and is defined by $E(B_t) = \sum_{i=1}^{m} \frac{n_i^t}{n_t} * E(L_i)$. The error-divergence of the internal node t is defined as

$$R_t = \frac{D(B_t) - D(t)}{E(t) - E(B_t)} .$$

  Here, the divergence measures disclosure risk, the error rate measures data utility, and error-divergence of t is the value that balance disclosure risk and data utility.

The EDP algorithm (see appendix 1) computes R_t of all internal nodes in every iteration. However, in fact, only the values R_t of the father nodes of the pruned internal nodes would change in the tree and others are the same as before. Based on this idea, we propose the improved algorithm: store initial R_t of the all internal nodes of the complete tree, just update changed R_t (the father nodes of the pruned internal nodes) in new tree if continuing the algorithm, delete the values R_t of the children nodes of the pruned internal nodes. The detailed algorithm is provided as follow.

The Improved EDP algorithm

---

0. Let N be the number of records in the data set and C be the number of the classes. Let p and α be the values specified.
1. Calculate initial R_t of the all internal nodes in the complete tree and store these values.
2. Select the largest R_t, prune this corresponding internal node t into be a leaf .
3. Count the total number of records available for swapping, P_s. Select the maximum leaf divergence $D(L_*)$. If $P_s \geq p$ or $P\left[\chi(c-1) > D(L_*)\right] > \alpha$, stop; otherwise, go to the next step.
4. Update: recalculate R_t of all the father nodes of the pruned internal nodes, delete the values R_t of the child nodes of the pruned internal nodes. Go to Step 2.

Now, we illustrate the advantages of the improved EDP algorithm. A health-care organization owns a regional database of patient records regarding a sensitive, contagious disease. The data is available for related experts for medical and health-care research purpose. Based on protecting privacy, the identifying attributes such as name and phone number in the database have been deleted. The other attributes are nonconfidential attributes such as age, gender, zip code, and a confidential attribute, the diagnostic result. Figure 1 shows a subtree of the built decision tree based on the released database. Under the circumstance, Li & Sarkar have proved that each patient of the released database still faces disclosure risk, especially ones in the purer leaves. The improved EDP algorithm can find high disclosure-risk patients. It is helpful for data owners to preferably mask these patients' confidential attribute values. In this sense, it reaches the goal of protecting privacy while maintaining the structure of decision tree as far as possible.

Based on the illustrative example, we analyze and compare the improved EDP algorithm with the EDP algorithm. Let swapping rate p be 0.5, significant level α be 0.9 and follow the pruning procedure. At first, calculate all error-divergence of internal nodes of the tree: R_1,R_2,R_3,R_4,R_6,R_9,R_{13}. Select the maximum error-divergence R_6, prune node 6 to be a leaf. We find the stopping criterion is not satisfied. Recalculate all the father nodes of the pruned internal nodes 6: R_1,R_2. Go to step 2 and continue to iterate until the algorithm stops. However, the EDP algorithm, after the first pruning, need to recalculate all error-divergences of internal nodes of the new tree: R_1,R_2,R_3,R_4,R_9,R_{13}. Because data in real-world life is large scale, the EDP algorithm need recalculate all R_t in every iteration which will increase the running time. Overcoming this disadvantage,

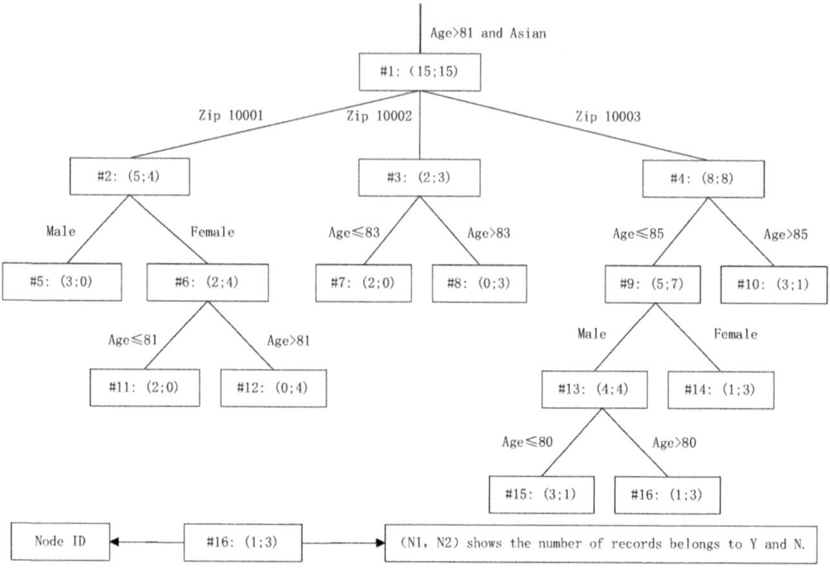

Fig. 1. An illustrative example

the improve EDP takes full advantage of unused storage space to improve the high efficiency of the algorithm.

2.1 Analysis of Computation Complexity

In this section, we analyze the worst-time complexity of the improved EDP algorithm. And by comparing with the EDP algorithm, we further demonstrate that the improved EDP algorithm how to avoids computing a large number of unnecessary values R_t.

The proposed algorithm aims at disposing decision tree protection privacy problem in the real life. Now we introduce some related definitions. Consider a decision tree K where at least an internal node has k branches ($k \geq 2$, and k value also can't be too big for considering balancing accuracy and simple [12]), Let the depth of decision tree K be $n+1$, and let M and m_i be the number of internal nodes in the decision tree K and $i-$th depth ($i = 1, 2, \cdots, n$), respectively. Thus, one has that

$$m_1 + m_2 + m_3 + \ldots + m_{n-1} + m_n = 1 + \sum_{i=2}^{n} m_i = M . \quad (1)$$

We suppose $m_1 = 1, m_i \geq 2, i = 2, \ldots n; n \geq 4$. Then we can know $M \geq 7$. In the following, we give the worst-case time of the improved EDP algorithm.

Theorem 1. *To the improved EDP algorithm, the worst-case time iterations is* $M + 1 + \sum_{i=2}^{n} (i-1) * m_i$.

To determine the node to be pruned, the algorithm must find the maximum R_t value in each loop. At first, the algorithm visits all internal node, computes the values of the error-divergence measure R_t and stores them. Then it just recalculates the changed values of R_t after pruning the tree. The procedure continues until a stopping criterion is met or the root node is reached. In the worst-scenario case, each iteration just prunes one internal node which is the deepest one. Therefore, the total number of R_t evaluations for the entire process is

$$M+1+(2-1)*m_2+(3-1)*m_3+\cdots+(n-1)*m_n = M+1+\sum_{i=2}^{n}(i-1)*m_i\ . \quad (2)$$

Theorem 2. *Comparing with the EDP algorithm, the worst-case iterations of the improved EDP algorithm is at least reduced* $\frac{M}{2}+\sum_{i=2}^{n}(i-2)*m_i-\frac{3}{2}$.

PROOF. The worst-case iterations of the EDP algorithm is $\frac{M(M+1)}{2}$, see [11]. By applying (2), one has that

$$\frac{M(M+1)}{2}-(M+1+\sum_{i=2}^{n}(i-1)m_i)=\frac{M}{2}+\frac{(\sum_{i=2}^{n}m_i)^2-2\sum_{i=2}^{n}(i-1)m_i}{2}-\frac{3}{2}. \quad (3)$$

Using mathematical induction, we only need to prove that the following relationship holds:

$$(\sum_{i=2}^{n}m_i)^2-2*\sum_{i=2}^{n}(i-1)*m_i \ge \sum_{i=2}^{n}(2i-4)*m_i\ . \quad (4)$$

When $n=2$, one has that $m_2^2-2m_2=m_2(m_2-2)\ge 0$. Suppose it holds for $n=k$, that is, the following conclusion holds:

$$(\sum_{i=2}^{k}m_i)^2-2*\sum_{i=2}^{k}(i-1)*m_i \ge \sum_{i=2}^{k}(2i-4)*m_i\ .$$

Then for $n=k+1$, one has that

$$\begin{aligned}&(\sum_{i=2}^{k+1}m_i)^2-2*\sum_{i=2}^{k+1}(i-1)*m_i\\ &=(\sum_{i=2}^{k}m_i)^2-2*\sum_{i=2}^{k}(i-1)*m_i+m_{k+1}*(2\sum_{i=2}^{k}m_i+m_{k+1}-2k+2). \quad (5)\end{aligned}$$

One has further that

$$2\sum_{i=2}^{k}m_i+m_{k+1}-2k+2\ge 2*2*k+2-2k+2=2k+4>2k-2. \quad (6)$$

$$\sum_{i=2}^{k+1}(2i-4)*m_i=\sum_{i=2}^{k}(2i-4)*m_i+m_{k+1}*[2k-2)]. \quad (7)$$

Applying (6) and (7) to (5), one has that

$$(\sum_{i=2}^{k+1} m_i)^2 - 2 * \sum_{i=2}^{k+1}(i-1) * m_i$$
$$\geq \sum_{i=2}^{k}(2i-4) * m_i + m_{k+1} * [2k-2)]$$
$$= \sum_{i=2}^{k+1}(2i-4) * m_i \ .$$

Thus, we proved that the conclusion (4) held.

Applying (4) to (3), we finally get the reduced iterations of the improved EDP algorithm is

$$\frac{M(M+1)}{2} - (M+1+\sum_{i=2}^{n}(i-1) * m_i) \geq \frac{M}{2} + (\sum_{i=2}^{n}(i-2) * m_i) - \frac{3}{2} \ .$$

That is, comparing with EDP algorithm, the worst-case time iterations of the improved EDP algorithm is at least reduced $\frac{M}{2} + \sum_{i=2}^{n}(i-2) * m_i - \frac{3}{2}$. □

Remark 1. When there are more complex tree structure with more internal nodes, the more values R_t in the decision do not change in each loop of the improved EDP algorithm. In particular, in the case of the complete binary decision tree, the worst-case time complexity can be lowed to of order $O(M \log M)$, where M is the number of internal nodes of the complete tree. To programmers, the basic idea of the proposed algorithm is simple and easy to realization. To computers, the proposed algorithm makes the best use of unused storage. After above all, it is not difficult to find that the improved EDP algorithm is more efficient for the real-life problem.

3 Time Complexity Analysis of the Complete Binary Tree

Now by analyzing the complete binary tree, we furthermore show that the improved EDP algorithm is efficient. In the complete binary tree, the improved EDP algorithm can reduce time complexity to be of order $O(M \log M)$, where M is the number of internal nodes of the complete tree. We firstly define the complete binary tree. Let T be the complete binary tree. Based on (1), the complete binary tree T has the following relations:

$$m_i = 2^{i-1} \ . \tag{8}$$

$$M = \sum_{i=1}^{n} 2^{i-1} = 2^n - 1 \ . \tag{9}$$

Theorem 3. *To the complete binary tree T, the time complexity of the improved EDP algorithm is of order $O(M \log M)$, where M is the number of internal nodes of the complete tree.*

To a complete binary tree T, the algorithm needs to compute the values of R_t for all internal nodes of the tree and store them firstly. Then it just recalculates the changed values of R_t after pruning the tree. The process continues until a stopping criterion is met or the root node is reached. In a worst-scenario, each iteration just prunes one internal node, and the pruned node is the deepest one.

Applying (1) and (8) to (2):

$$\begin{aligned} M+1+\sum_{i=2}^{n}(i-1)*m_i &= M+1+\sum_{i=2}^{n}(i-1)*2^{i-1}. \\ &= M+2^n(n-2)+3\,. \end{aligned} \tag{10}$$

Substituting (9) into (10):

$$M+1+\sum_{i=2}^{n}(i-1)*m_i = (M+1)\log(M+1)-M+1\,.$$

Thus, the time complexity of the improved EDP algorithm is of order $\mathrm{O}(M \log M)$.

Remark 2. The time complexity ($\mathrm{O}(M \log M)$) of the improved EDP algorithm is much better than one ($\mathrm{O}(M^2)$) of the EDP algorithm. The time complexity is of order $\mathrm{O}(M \log_3 M)$ when it is the complete trigeminal tree. To a decision tree has triangle shape, the improved EDP algorithm is able to radically avoid the unnecessary computations. With the scale of the decision tree increasing, the superiority of the improved algorithm will be more obvious.

4 Experiments

To show the effectiveness of the improved EDP algorithm, we use 3 datasets which usually be used to grow decision trees in UCI Machine Learning Repository[1]. We first build the decision trees based on CART algorithm, then use the improved EDP algorithm and the EDP algorithm to prune the tree, respectively. Trough comparing the running time, it shows that the proposed algorithm is computationally quite efficient, as formally described before. The details of datasets are shown as table 1:

[1] Datasets can be attained electronically by the following web sites:
`http://archive.ics.uci.edu/ml/datasets/Balance+Scale`
`http://archive.ics.uci.edu/ml/datasets/Tic-Tac-Toe+Endgame`
`http://archive.ics.uci.edu/ml/datasets/Car+Evaluation`

Table 1. Datasets

Dataset ID	Number of Records (n)	Number of Internal Nodes of the Complete Tree
1	625	34
2	958	66
3	1728	48

The trade-off between disclosure risk and data utility can be examined by specifying different values for the swapping proportion p, or the significance level α, or both. However, changing significance α value hardly affects the pruning results. So the swapping proportion p was used to primary control parameter for disclosure risk, whereas let the significance level α be 0.9. Our code was implemented in MatlabR2007b and we conducted our experiments on a PC running windows XP operating system on Intel Pentium Core-2 Processor, 4G Memory. Because a slight change of computer operation external conditions will affect experiment results, we run the algorithm ten times. The average results are reported and compared.

Experiment results are shown in from figure 2 to 4. When the swapping proportion is small, the decision tree is not pruned. When the swapping proportion is overly large, the pruning algorithm can fail to produce a meaningful classifier (e.g., the resulting tree may contain only one root node). Our experiments focus on the ranges of p where the trade-offs between disclosure risk and data quality are meaningful. By adjusting values of the parameter p, we obtain figure 2 and 3 corresponding to dataset 1 and 2, respectively, where the horizontal axis represents swapping proportion $p(\%)$ and the vertical axis represents time $t(s)$. By adjusting the parameter p in dataset 3, we got the pruned trees which are very close to each other.So we don't generate the corresponding figure. By randomly pruning each of the three complete trees based on dataset 1, 2 and 3, respectively,

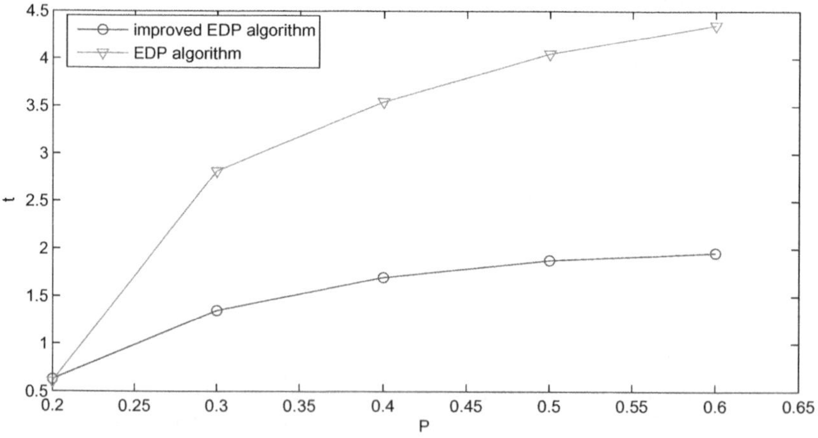

Fig. 2. Running time of pruning the decision tree based on dataset 1

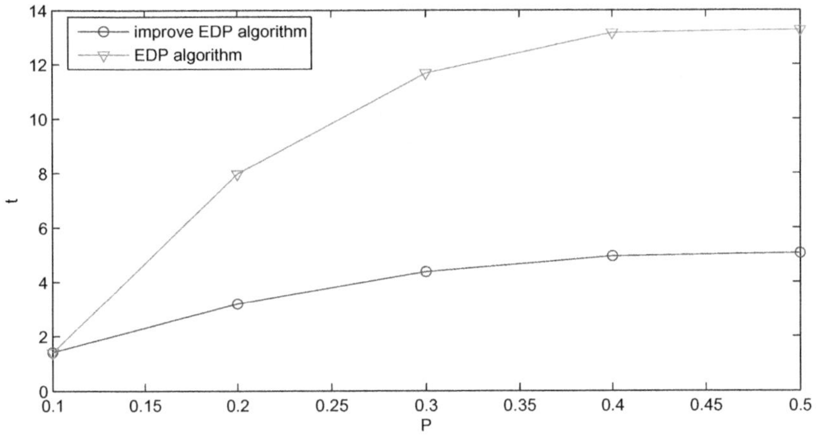

Fig. 3. Running time of pruning the decision tree based on dataset 2

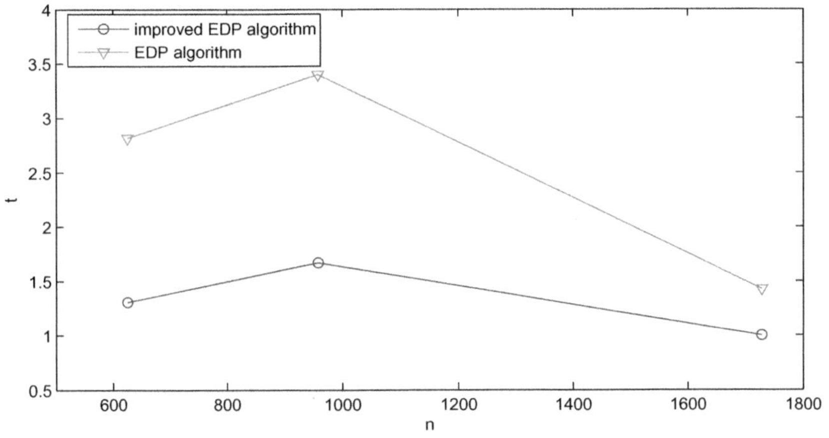

Fig. 4. Running time of pruning the decision tree with the same internal nodes

we obtain three decision tree with 34 internal nodes. Let p be 0.4. Then using the improved EDP algorithm and the EDP algorithm respectively to prune the three trees, we obtain figure 4. In figure 4, the horizontal axis represents dataset records (n) and the vertical axis represents time $t(s)$.

We find from Figure 1-3 that the improved EDP algorithm clearly outperform the EDP algorithm. The first points in figure 2 and 3 are very close, because value of parameter p is very small and both of the algorithms don't prune the trees. So the times of both algorithms spent are the same because both algorithms need to compute R_t for all the internal nodes of the complete trees. With the increase of the swapping proportion, the decision trees begin to be pruned. We see from figure 2 and 3 that the running time of the improved EDP algorithm is distinctly less than the one of the EDP algorithm and the reduced running time in figure 3 is much more than that in figure 2 when the swapping proportions are the same. For example, when the swapping proportion p is 0.2, the reduced running time in figure 2 is 1.47s while it is 7.30s in figure 3, which shows the improved EDP algorithm is better for the decision tree with large records and more internal nodes. As we expected, the larger the swapping proportion p is, the more reduced running time of the improved EDP algorithm comparing with the EDP algorithm is. We observe that when the swapping proportion is relatively large, the improved EDP algorithm performs better than the EDP algorithm. In figure 4, the reduced running time is significantly more in dataset 2 than that in dataset 1. That is to say, when the decision trees have the same internal nodes and similar structure, the more the records are, the better the improved EDP algorithm will be. However, the performance is worse in dataset 3 which records are much more than dataset 1 and 2. It suggests that the tree structure will also affect the performance of the algorithm.

5 Conclusions

Based on balancing disclosure risk and data utility, we proposed an improved EDP algorithm. The improved EDP algorithm can reduce time complexity by using the storage. The worst-case time iterations of the improved EDP algorithm is $(M + 1 + \sum_{i=2}^{n}(i-1) * m_i)$, where M is the number of internal nodes of the complete tree, n is the depth of the internal node and m_i is the number of internal nodes in i–th depth. Comparing with the EDP algorithm, the worst-case time iterations of the improved EDP algorithm is at least reduced $(\frac{M}{2} + \sum_{i=2}^{n}(i-2) * m_i - \frac{3}{2})$. Especially for the complete binary tree, the improved EDP algorithm can reduce the time complexity from $O(M^2)$ to $O(M \log M)$. When a better time complexity is required, it may worse the space complexity, namely occupy more storage space; conversely, when a better space complexity is required, it may worse the time complexity, namely occupy more running time. Based on trade-off between storage space and running time, the improved EDP algorithm reduces computation complexity by using unused storage spaces. At present, the number of the internal nodes of the decision tree in common is mainly under10000. Even when M is 10000, it only needs additional 40K memory to store values. Hence, in practical application, the improved EDP algorithm is much better than the EDP algorithm.

Acknowledgements. This work was partly supported by National Natural Science Foundation of China (No. 71031002), National Science Fund for Distinguished Young Scholars (No. 70725004) and Basic Foundation for Research of Central Universities (No. DUT11SX11).

References

1. Groups accuse DHCS of improperly sharing data on patients with HIV (September 2010), http://www.californiahealthline.org/articles/2010/9/10/groups-accuse-state-agency-of-sharing-data-on-patients-with-hiv.aspx
2. Greengard, S.: Privacy: Entitlement or illusion? Personnel Journal 75(5), 74–88 (1996)
3. Sweeney, L.: K-anonymity: a model for protecting privacy. International Journal of Uncertainty, Fuzziness and Knowledge-Based Systems 10(5), 557–570 (2002)
4. Verykios, V.S., Elmagarmid, A.K., Bertino, E., Saygin, Y., Dasseni, E.: Association rule hiding. IEEE Transactions on Knowledge and Data Engineering 16(4), 434–447 (2004)
5. Li, X.B., Sarkar, S.: Privacy protection in data mining: A perturbation approach for categorical data. Information Systems Research 17(3), 254–270 (2006)
6. Li, X.B., Sarkar, S.: A tree-based data perturbation approach for privacy-preserving data mining. IEEE Transactions on Knowledge and Data Engineering 18(6), 1278–1283 (2006)
7. Reiss, S.P.: Practical data-swapping: the first steps. ACM Transactions on Database Systems 9(1), 20–37 (1984)
8. Estivill-Castro, V., Brankovic, L.: Data swapping: Balancing privacy against precision in mining for logic rules. In: Mohania, M., Tjoa, A.M. (eds.) DaWaK 1999. LNCS, vol. 1676, pp. 389–398. Springer, Heidelberg (1999)
9. Agrawal, R., Srikant, R.: Privacy-preserving data mining. In: The 2000 ACM SIGMOD International Conference on Management Of Data, New York, NY, USA, pp. 439–450 (2000)
10. Agrawal, D., Aggarwal, C.C.: On the design and quantification of privacy preserving data mining algorithms. In: The 20th ACM SIGMOD-SIGACT-SIGART Symposium on Principles of Database Systems, New York, NY, USA, pp. 247–255 (2001)
11. Li, X.B., Sarkar, S.: Against classification attacks: A decision tree pruning approach to privacy protection in data mining. Operation Research 57(6), 1496–1509 (2009)
12. Bohanec, M., Bratko, I.: Trading accuracy for simplicity in decision trees. Machine Learning 15(3), 223–250 (1994)

Appendix:1

The EDP algorithm is introduced as follow:

The EDP algorithm

---

0. Let N be the number of records in the data set and C be the number of the classes. Let p and α be the values specified.
1. Calculate R_t of the all internal nodes in the tree and store.
2. Select the largest R_t, prune internal node t into be a leaf.
3. Count the total number of records available for swapping, P_s. Select the maximum divergence $D(L_*)$. If $P_s \geq p$ or $P\ [\chi(c-1) > D(L_*)] > \alpha$, stop; otherwise, go to Step 1.

A Hybrid Multiple Attributes Two-Sided Matching Decision Making Method with Incomplete Weight Information

Zhen Zhang and Chong-Hui Guo*

Institute of Systems Engineering, Dalian University of Technology, Dalian, 116024, People's Republic of China
zhangzhen@mail.dlut.edu.cn, guochonghui@tsinghua.org.cn

Abstract. For multiple attributes two-sided decision making problems with different evaluation attributes of both matching objects, this paper takes into account different formats of evaluation information of the matching objects and proposes a method for dealing with such two-sided matching decision making problems with incomplete weight information. Based on the ideal solution principle, the proposed method calculates the weight of attributes by solving quadratic programming models, and gets the best matching for the matching objects by solving a binary integer programming problem. The illustrative examples show the feasibility and effectiveness of the proposed method.

Keywords: decision analysis, two-sided matching, optimization model, incomplete weight information.

1 Introduction

There are many two-sided matching decision making problems in socio-economic and management areas, such as marriage matching[1], matching between employees and job positions[2–7] and exchange matching between buyers and sellers [8–11]. These problems are of great practical significance, and there is a need to develop analysis methods to deal with such problems.

The two-sided matching problem initially originates from college admissions and the matching of marriage[1]. Due to the wide existence, two-sided matching problems have received more and more attention from researchers in recent years. Drigas et al. [2] presented an expert system for the matching between an unemployed with an offered job based on the analysis of a corporate database of unemployed and enterprises profile data using Neuro-Fuzzy techniques. In order to solve military personnel assignment problems, Korkmaz et al. [4] established a two-sided matching based decision support system to assist the decision makers. The system could generate positions' preferences from position requirement profiles and personnel competence profiles by using analytic hierarchy process and match personnel to positions by using two-sided matching.

* Corresponding author.

B. Hu et al. (Eds.): BI 2011, LNAI 6889, pp. 272–283, 2011.

For personnel assignment problem, Huang et al.[6] proposed a bi-objective binary integer programming-based approach with a feedback mechanism, in which the interdependencies among positions and the differences among the selected employees were considered simultaneously. Chen and Fan [7] considered different formats of evaluation information for the employees and positions and proposed a decision making method based on binary integer programming. For multi-objective trade matching problems, Wang [8] established a multi-objective assignment model and designed a multi-nutrient colony location algorithm to solve the model. Besides, Jiang et al. [9] presented an approach to optimize the matching of one-shot multi-attribute exchanges with quantity discounts in E-brokerage based on the conception and definition of matching degree and quantity discount. In order to solve matching problem between ventures and venture capitalists through an intermediary, Li et al. [12] established a multi-objective optimization model and gave the corresponding solution to the model.

Prior studies have significantly advanced the area of two-sided matching. Due to the lack of knowledge, for actual two-sided matching problems, there may be cases that the weight information of attributes for matching objects is not given accurately. For instance, for a matching problem between employees and positions, the employees may consider that the attribute "developing space" is twice as important as the attribute "salary level". However, most of the existing approaches aim to deal with two-sided matching problems with perfect weight information of evaluation attributes, and studies for two-sided matching problems with incomplete weight information have seldom been addressed. Although Jiang et al.[11] proposed an analysis method for trade matching problem with incomplete attribute weight in consumer to consumer e-commerce environment, the method couldn't deal with two-sided matching problems with different attribute sets for the two sides. In addition, the evaluation information given by the matching objects is usually diverse, which is also an issue that needs to be considered for actual two-sided matching problems. Due to the wide existence of such problems in the real world, it is necessary to develop new analysis method to deal with two-sided matching problems with incomplete weight information and different formats of evaluation information, which is also the motivation of this paper.

The rest of this paper is organized as follows. In Section 2, we give the formal description of two-sided matching problem with different evaluation attributes for the two sides. After that, we present a decision analysis method to deal with the problem through establishing some optimization models in Section 3. In section 4, two illustrative examples are given to illustrate the feasibility and effectiveness of the proposed method. Finally, we conclude this paper in Section 5.

2 Description of the Decision Making Problem

For the convenience of analysis, in this section, we give the formal description of the two-sided matching decision making problem considered in this paper.

Let $E = \{E_1, E_2, \ldots, E_n\}$ and $P = \{P_1, P_2, \ldots, P_m\}$ be the set of matching objects, where E_i and P_j denote the ith matching object in E and the jth matching object in P, respectively. The matching object E_i $(i = 1, 2, \ldots, n)$ evaluates the matching object in P according to attribute set $C = \{c_1, c_2, \ldots, c_q\}$, and the weight vector is denoted as $w_i = (w_{i1}, w_{i2}, \ldots, w_{iq})$, where $i = 1, 2, \ldots, n$, $0 \leq w_{ik} \leq 1$, $\sum_{k=1}^{q} w_{ik} = 1$. In addition, the matching object P_j $(j = 1, 2, \ldots, m)$ also gives his evaluation on the matching object in P with regard to attribute set $I = \{i_1, i_2, \ldots, i_p\}$, and the corresponding weight vector is denoted as $\mu_j = (\mu_{j1}, \mu_{j2}, \ldots, \mu_{jp})$, where $j = 1, 2, \ldots, m$, $0 \leq \mu_{jl} \leq 1$, $\sum_{l=1}^{p} \mu_{jl} = 1$.

For different types of evaluation attributes, the matching objects may express their assessment using different formats of information. In this paper, we consider the following six formats of evaluation information, namely utility value, interval utility value, binary value, linguistic value, ordinal value and ordinal interval value. In the rest of this section, we give a brief introduction of some types of attributes.

(1) Binary value

This type of attribute value is usually used to denote whether a matching object possesses an attribute. Without loss of generality, if a matching object possesses an attribute, the value is 1, else the attribute value will be set to 0.

(2) Linguistic value

Due to the lack of knowledge and people's limited expertise related with problem domain, people sometimes tend to express their preference using linguistic information[13].

Let $S = \{s_0, s_1, \ldots, s_T\}$ denote a pre-defined linguistic term set with odd cardinality, the element s_h of which represents the hth linguistic variable, and $T + 1$ is the cardinality of the linguistic term set S. For instance, a typical linguistic term set with seven terms can be expressed as S=\{s_0: Very Poor, s_1: Poor, s_2: Slightly Poor, s_3: Fair, s_4: Slightly Good, s_5: Good and s_6: Very Good\}.

(3) Ordinal value

Ordinal value[14] is used to denote the ranking of a matching object. It is obvious that the smaller the ranking of a matching object, the better the matching object. If there are N matching objects to be ranked, the ranking value of a matching object is an integer number between 1 and N.

(4) Ordinal interval value

Due to the lack of knowledge, the ranking of a matching object sometimes may be given as an ordinal interval value[15]. For example, the ranking of an object may be given as [1,3], i.e. the ranking of the object may be 1, 2 or 3. Similar to ordinal number, if there are N matching objects to be ranked, both the lower boundary and upper boundary of an ordinal interval value will be integer numbers between 1 and N.

As mentioned above, it is difficult for a matching object to give a clear judgment on the attribute weight. Thus the weight information given by the matching objects is incomplete in most cases. Taking the weight vector w_i as an example, the attribute weight information satisfies the following five forms[16]:

(1) $w_{ik_1} - w_{ik_2} \geq \varepsilon_{ik_1}$;
(2) $w_{ik_1} \geq \beta_{ik_1} w_{ik_2}$;
(3) $w_{ik_1} - w_{ik_2} \geq w_{ik_3} - w_{ik_4}, k_1 \neq k_2 \neq k_3 \neq k_4$;
(4) $\gamma^-_{ik_1} \leq w_{ik_1} \leq \gamma^+_{ik_1}$;
(5) $\rho^-_{ik_1} w_{ik_2} \leq w_{ik_1} \leq \rho^+_{ik_1} w_{ik_2}$, or $\rho^-_{ik_1} \leq w_{ik_1}/w_{ik_2} \leq \rho^+_{ik_1}, w_{ik_2} \neq 0$.

where $k_1, k_2, k_3, k_4 \in \{1, 2, \ldots, q\}$ and for any k_1, we have $\varepsilon_{ik_1}, \gamma^-_{ik_1}, \gamma^+_{ik_1} \in [0, 1]$, and $\beta_{ik_1}, \rho^-_{ik_1}, \rho^+_{ik_1}$ are positive real numbers.

These forms of incomplete weight information can construct a weight vector space Ω_i, which means that the weight vector of the ith matching object $w_i = (w_{i1}, w_{i2}, \ldots, w_{iq}) \in \Omega_i$, $i = 1, 2, \ldots, n$.

The two-sided matching decision making problem to be solved in this paper is to calculate the weight information of all the matching objects and obtain an optimal matching for the matching objects with regard to the provided information.

3 Decision Making Method

3.1 Data Preprocessing

In order to aggregate different formats of evaluation information, it is essential to carry out preprocessing for the initial evaluation data. For convenience, we take the preprocessing for the evaluation information given by matching objects in E on each matching object in P as an example.

First of all, we denote the evaluation value given by the ith matching object in E on P_j with regard to the kth attribute by x_{ijk}, $i = 1, 2, \ldots, n$, $j = 1, 2, \ldots, m$, $k = 1, 2, \ldots, q$, and an evaluation matrix given by E_i can be obtained as $X_i = (x_{ijk})_{m\times q}$, $i = 1, 2, \ldots, n$, $j = 1, 2, \ldots, m$, $k = 1, 2, \ldots, q$.

According to the difference between attributes, the attributes set $C = \{c_1, c_2, \ldots, c_q\}$ can be divided into six subsets, i.e. $C = \{C_1, C_2, \ldots, C_6\}$, where $C_1, C_2, \ldots, C_6$ are attributes subsets in which the attribute values are expressed with utility values, interval utility values, binary values, linguistic values, ordinal values and ordinal interval values, respectively. And $C_t \cap C_r = \phi$, $t, r = 1, 2, \ldots, 6$, $t \neq r$, $\bigcup_{t=1}^{6} C_t = C$, where ϕ is an empty set. In addition, we denote the cardinality of C_t by $|C_t|$, $t = 1, 2, \ldots, 6$.

Then the evaluation value x_{ijk} can be denoted specifically as

$$x_{ijk} = \begin{cases} a_{ijk} \in R^+ & \text{if } c_k \in C_1 \\ \left[a_{ijk}^L, a_{ijk}^U\right] & \text{if } c_k \in C_2 \\ a_{ijk} \in \{0,1\} & \text{if } c_k \in C_3 \\ a_{ijk} \in S_i & \text{if } c_k \in C_4 \\ a_{ijk} \in \{1,2,\ldots,m\} & \text{if } c_k \in C_5 \\ \left[a_{ijk}^L, a_{ijk}^U\right] \in \{[x,y]\,|x \le y,\ x,y\ \in \{1,2,\ldots,m\}\} & \text{if } c_k \in C_6 \end{cases} \quad (1)$$

where S_i $(i = 1,2,\ldots,n)$ denotes the linguistic terms set for the ith matching object in E.

For $c_k \in C_1$ and $c_k \in C_2$, we carry out normalization by Formulae (2) and (3), respectively.

$$v_{ijk} = \frac{a_{ijk}}{\max\limits_{1 \le j \le m} \{a_{ijk}\}} \quad i = 1,2,\ldots,n,\ j = 1,2,\ldots,m,\ k = 1,2,\ldots,|C_1| \quad (2)$$

$$v_{ijk} = \left[v_{ijk}^L, v_{ijk}^U\right] = \left[\frac{a_{ijk}^L}{a_{ik}^*}, \frac{a_{ijk}^U}{a_{ik}^*}\right] \quad i = 1,2,\ldots,n,\ j = 1,2,\ldots,m,\ k = 1,2,\ldots,|C_2| \quad (3)$$

where $a_{ik}^* = \max\limits_{1 \le j \le m} \left\{a_{ijk}^U\right\},\ i = 1,2,\ldots,n,\ k = 1,2,\ldots,|C_2|$.

After that, we transform linguistic attribute values into triangle fuzzy numbers. The hth linguistic term s_h in linguistic term set $S = \{s_0, s_1, \ldots, s_T\}$ can be denoted by

$$\hat{r}_h = (r_h^1, r_h^2, r_h^3) = \left\{\max(\frac{h-1}{T}, 0), \frac{h}{T}, \min(\frac{h+1}{T}, 1)\right\}, \text{for all } h = 0,1,\ldots,T. \quad (4)$$

Therefore the linguistic evaluation value in X_i $(i = 1,2,\ldots,n)$ can be denoted as $v_{ijk} = (v_{ijk}^1, v_{ijk}^2, v_{ijk}^3)$, $i = 1,2,\ldots,n,\ j = 1,2,\ldots,m,\ k = 1,2,\ldots,|C_4|$.

For $c_k \in C_3$, C_5 and C_6, let $v_{ijk} = x_{ijk}$. Then a new evaluation information can be obtained as $V_i = (v_{ijk})_{m \times q}$, $i = 1,2,\ldots,n, j = 1,2,\ldots,m, k = 1,2,\ldots,q$.

Since the preprocessing procedure for the evaluation information given by matching objects in P on each matching object in E is similar, we will not illustrate it in detail.

3.2 Weight Determining for the Matching Objects

Since weight information is incomplete for the decision making problem, it is the key issue to determine attribute weight for all the matching objects. In this paper, weight vectors are obtained based on the ideal solution principle[17].

First of all, we determine the attribute weight vector given by matching object E_i, $i = 1, 2, \ldots, n$. Let v_k^+ denote the ideal solution for the kth attribute, $k = 1, 2, \ldots, q$. Specifically, the notations and values of the ideal solutions for different formats of attributes are shown in Table 1.

Table 1. Notations and values of ideal solution for different formats of attributes

attribute type	notation	value
binary value, benefit utility value and ordinal value	v_k^+	1
cost utility value	v_k^+	0
benefit interval value and ordinal interval value	$[v_k^{+L}, v_k^{+U}]$	[1,1]
cost interval value	$[v_k^{+L}, v_k^{+U}]$	[0,0]
linguistic value	$(v_k^{+1}, v_k^{+2}, v_k^{+3})$	(1,1,1)

Then the distance between the jth matching object ($j = 1, 2, \ldots, m$) and the ideal solution with regard to the kth attribute ($k = 1, 2, \ldots, q$) can be calculated by

$$D(v_{ijk}, v_k^+) = \begin{cases} \left|v_{ijk} - v_k^+\right| & \text{forbinary and utility value} \\ \left|v_{ijk} - v_k^+\right|/m & \text{for ordinal value} \\ \sqrt{\dfrac{\left(v_{ijk}^L - v_k^{+L}\right)^2 + \left(v_{ijk}^U - v_k^{+U}\right)^2}{2}} & \text{for interval value} \\ \dfrac{1}{m}\sqrt{\dfrac{\left(v_{ijk}^L - v_k^{+L}\right)^2 + \left(v_{ijk}^U - v_k^{+L}\right)^2}{2}} & \text{for ordinal interval value} \\ \sqrt{\dfrac{1}{3}\sum_{c=1}^{3}\left(v_{ijk}^c - v_k^{+c}\right)^2} & \text{for linguistic value.} \end{cases} \tag{5}$$

According to the ideal solution principle, the optimal weight vector should be the one that minimizes the deviation from all the matching objects evaluated by E_i to the ideal solution. Therefore, a deviation function can be established as $D(w_i) = \sum_{j=1}^{m} \sum_{k=1}^{q} D^2(v_{ijk}, v_k^+) w_{ik}^2$, $i = 1, 2, \ldots, n$.

For each matching object E_i, $i = 1, 2, \ldots, n$, an optimization model can be established as

$$\begin{aligned} \min \quad & D(w_i) = \sum_{j=1}^{m} \sum_{k=1}^{q} D^2(v_{ijk}, v_k^+) w_{ik}^2 \\ \text{s.t.} \quad & w_i \in \Omega_i, \\ & \sum_{k=1}^{q} w_{ik} = 1, \\ & w_{ik} \geq 0, \ k = 1, 2, \ldots, q. \end{aligned} \tag{M-1}$$

It is obvious that model (M-1) has optimal solution(s). With the use of some optimization software packages, such as Lingo, WinQSB, the weight vector for E_i can be obtained as $w_i = (w_{i1}, w_{i2}, \ldots, w_{iq})$, $i = 1, 2, \ldots, n$.

Based on the previous analysis, the weight vector for the jth matching object in P can also be obtained as $\mu_j = (\mu_{j1}, \mu_{j2}, \ldots, \mu_{jp})$, $j = 1, 2, \ldots, m$.

3.3 Establishment of the Two-Sided Matching Model

Based on the weight vector calculated in the previous subsection, the matching satisfaction degree (MSD) of the two sides can be obtained. Specifically, the MSD for matching object E_i $(i = 1, 2, \ldots, n)$ on P_j $(j = 1, 2, \ldots, m)$ can be denoted as

$$\alpha_{ij} = 1 - \sqrt{\sum_{k=1}^{q} D^2(v_{ijk}, v_k^+) w_{ik}^2}, \quad \text{for all } i = 1, 2, \ldots, n, j = 1, 2, \ldots, m. \tag{6}$$

And the MSD matrix for matching objects in E on matching objects in P can be obtained as $\mathrm{A} = (\alpha_{ij})_{n \times m}$, $i = 1, 2, \ldots, n$, $j = 1, 2, \ldots, m$.

In the same way, the MSD matrix for matching objects in P on matching objects in E can also be denoted as $\mathrm{B} = (\beta_{ji})_{m \times n}$, $i = 1, 2, \ldots, n$, $j = 1, 2, \ldots, m$, where β_{ji} denotes the MSD for matching object P_j on matching object E_i, $i = 1, 2, \ldots, n$, $j = 1, 2, \ldots, m$.

Let x_{ij} ($i = 1, 2, \ldots, n$, $j = 1, 2, \ldots, m$) be a binary decision variable that denotes whether E_i $(i = 1, 2, \ldots, n)$ matches P_j $(j = 1, 2, \ldots, m)$ or not, i.e. if E_i $(i = 1, 2, \ldots, n)$ matches P_j $(j = 1, 2, \ldots, m)$, then $x_{ij} = 1$, else $x_{ij} = 0$.

It is obvious that the matching is optimal when the matching satisfaction degree of the two sides is the maximum. Thus, based on the MSD matrices, a multi-objective optimization model which aims to maximize the matching satisfaction degree of all the matching objects can be established as

$$
\begin{aligned}
\max \quad & Z_1 = \sum_{i=1}^{n}\sum_{j=1}^{m} \alpha_{ij} x_{ij} \\
\max \quad & Z_2 = \sum_{i=1}^{n}\sum_{j=1}^{m} \beta_{ij} x_{ij} \\
\text{s.t.} \quad & \sum_{j=1}^{m} x_{ij} \le \mu_i, \; i = 1, 2, \ldots, n \\
& \sum_{i=1}^{n} x_{ij} \le \theta_j, \; j = 1, 2, \ldots, m \\
& x_{ij} \in \{0, 1\}, \; i = 1, 2, \ldots, n, j = 1, 2, \ldots, m.
\end{aligned} \tag{M-2}
$$

where μ_i and θ_j denote the maximum number of matching objects for E_i and P_j $(i = 1, 2, \ldots, n, \; j = 1, 2, \ldots, m)$, respectively.

Given a weight coefficient ω, model (M-2) can be transformed into a single objective model by the linear weighted method, i.e.

$$
\begin{aligned}
\max \quad & Z = \omega \sum_{i=1}^{n}\sum_{j=1}^{m} \alpha_{ij} x_{ij} + (1 - \omega) \sum_{i=1}^{n}\sum_{j=1}^{m} \beta_{ij} x_{ij} \\
\text{s.t.} \quad & \sum_{j=1}^{m} x_{ij} \le \mu_i, \; i = 1, 2, \ldots, n \\
& \sum_{i=1}^{n} x_{ij} \le \theta_j, \; j = 1, 2, \ldots, m \\
& x_{ij} \in \{0, 1\}, \; i = 1, 2, \ldots, n, j = 1, 2, \ldots, m.
\end{aligned} \tag{M-3}
$$

Model (M-3) is a simple linear binary programming problem which can be solved using optimization software packages. According to the value of the decision variables, the optimal matching can be obtained.

4 Illustrative Examples

In this section, we take the matching problem between employees and job positions as an example to illustrate the feasibility and effectiveness of the proposed method.

Example 1. BS company intends to recruit staff for four job positions (P_1, P_2, P_3, P_4) and eight candidates ($E_1, E_2, \ldots, E_8$) apply for the four positions (adapted from [7]). The eight candidates give their evaluation on the four positions and the criteria are developing space (c_1), working environment (c_2), industry potentiality (c_3), salary and welfare level (c_4). All the evaluation information is given by linguistic terms. The incomplete weight information given by the candidates is $w_{i2} \leq 0.4w_{i1}$; $w_{i1} \leq 0.8w_{i3}$; $w_{i4} \leq 0.35$, $i = 1, 2, \ldots, 8$. The company also assesses the candidates with regard to eight criteria, i.e. work experience (i_1), whether the employee masters two foreign languages (i_2), expected salary (i_3), professional knowledge (i_4), English proficiency (i_5), computer skills (i_6), cooperation skills (i_7) and honesty (i_8). Among the eight criteria, i_1 and i_2 are binary value criteria, i_3 is a cost criterion with interval utility value, i_4 and i_5 are ordinal value and ordinal interval value criteria, respectively, and i_6, i_7 and i_8 are linguistic value criteria. The incomplete weight information given by the company for the positions is as follows: $\mu_{j1} - 0.6\mu_{j3} \geq 0$; $\mu_{j4} - \mu_{j3} \geq \mu_{j5} - \mu_{j1}$; $\mu_{j6} \leq 0.8\mu_{j7}$; $\mu_{j2} \geq 0.15$, $j = 1, 2, \ldots, 4$. Here the linguistic terms set for the company and the candidates are the same, i.e. $S=\{s_0 = AL$: Absolutely Low, $s_1 = VL$: Very Low, $s_2 = L$: Low, $s_3 = M$: Middle, $s_4 = H$: High, $s_5 = VH$: Very High, $s_6 = AH$: Absolutely High$\}$.

The evaluation information provided by the candidates and the company is shown in Table 2-3. We also assume that a position can only recruit one candidate, and a candidate can only be selected for one position.

Table 2. Candidates' evaluation information on the positions

E_i	P_1				P_2				P_3				P_4			
	C_1	C_2	C_3	C_4	C_1	C_2	C_3	C_4	C_1	C_2	C_3	C_4	C_1	C_2	C_3	C_4
E_1	VH	H	VH	H	AH	H	H	H	H	M	H	M	M	L	H	H
E_2	H	H	H	VH	AH	H	VH	VH	VH	H	M	H	H	M	M	H
E_3	H	H	H	M	H	M	H	H	VH	M	M	M	H	M	H	M
E_4	M	VH	H	H	M	H	H	VH	H	H	M	H	H	H	H	H
E_5	M	M	H	VH	H	M	M	VH	H	M	M	H	H	M	M	H
E_6	H	M	H	M	H	M	M	H	H	M	L	M	M	L	L	M
E_7	M	H	M	AH	M	H	M	VH	M	M	M	H	L	L	L	H
E_8	H	H	H	VH	VH	H	M	VH	H	M	M	H	H	L	M	M

In the rest of this section, we will utilize the proposed method to find the optimal matching.

By solving model (M-1) for the candidates, the optimal weight vector for each candidate can be obtained as $w_1 = (0.2948, 0.1179, 0.3685, 0.2188)$; $w_2 = w_4 = w_5 = w_7 = w_8 = (0.2453, 0.0981, 0.3066, 0.3500)$; $w_3 = (0.3030, 0.1212, 0.3787, 0.1971)$; $w_6 = (0.2610, 0.1043, 0.3262, 0.3085)$.

Then the matching satisfaction degree matrix for the candidates on the positions can be calculated as

$$A = \begin{bmatrix} 0.8647 & 0.8360 & 0.7931 & 0.7887 & 0.8087 & 0.7740 & 0.7908 & 0.8360 \\ 0.8375 & 0.8912 & 0.8013 & 0.8122 & 0.7968 & 0.7705 & 0.7802 & 0.8131 \\ 0.7868 & 0.7875 & 0.7610 & 0.7760 & 0.7731 & 0.7058 & 0.7553 & 0.7731 \\ 0.7685 & 0.7731 & 0.7882 & 0.8074 & 0.7731 & 0.6867 & 0.6972 & 0.7347 \end{bmatrix}^T.$$

Table 3. Positions' evaluation information on the candidates

E_i	P_1								P_2							
	I_1	I_2	I_3	I_4	I_5	I_6	I_7	I_8	I_1	I2	I_3	I_4	I_5	I_6	I_7	I_8
E_1	1	0	[3000, 4000]	8	[1, 3]	H	VH	H	1	0	[4000, 5000]	7	[4, 6]	VH	H	H
E_2	1	0	[2000, 3000]	7	[3, 5]	H	M	H	1	0	[3000, 4000]	1	[2, 4]	H	M	H
E_3	1	1	[4000, 5000]	6	[4, 7]	M	H	H	1	1	[4000, 5000]	8	[1, 2]	M	H	H
E_4	0	1	[3000, 4000]	3	[2, 4]	VH	H	H	0	1	[4000, 5000]	4	[3, 5]	VH	H	H
E_5	0	0	[2000, 3000]	4	[5, 7]	H	VH	VH	0	0	[3000, 4000]	2	[2, 3]	H	VH	H
E_6	1	1	[4000, 5000]	5	[6, 8]	AH	M	H	1	1	[4000, 5000]	5	[6, 8]	AH	M	H
E_7	0	0	[2000, 3000]	1	[2, 3]	H	H	VH	0	0	[3000, 4000]	6	[5, 7]	H	H	H
E_8	0	1	[3000, 4000]	2	[7, 8]	H	VH	H	0	1	[3000, 4000]	3	[6, 8]	H	H	H
E_i	P_3								P_4							
	I_1	I_2	I_3	I_4	I_5	I_6	I_7	I_8	I_1	I2	I_3	I_4	I_5	I_6	I_7	I_8
E_1	1	0	[4000, 5000]	8	[5, 6]	M	H	H	1	0	[3000, 4000]	1	[2, 3]	H	H	H
E_2	1	0	[2000, 3000]	6	[4, 7]	M	L	H	1	0	[3000, 4000]	8	[6, 8]	H	M	H
E_3	1	1	[3000, 4000]	4	[1, 3]	L	H	H	1	1	[4000, 5000]	7	[4, 6]	M	M	M
E_4	0	1	[3000, 4000]	7	[3, 5]	H	H	M	0	1	[3000, 4000]	6	[3, 5]	VH	M	M
E_5	0	0	[3000, 4000]	2	[2, 4]	M	VH	H	0	0	[2000, 3000]	4	[2, 4]	H	VH	H
E_6	1	1	[4000, 5000]	5	[7, 8]	VH	L	H	1	1	[4000, 5000]	2	[5, 6]	AH	M	M
E_7	0	0	[2000, 3000]	1	[2, 4]	M	M	VH	0	0	[2000, 3000]	5	[7, 8]	H	H	H
E_8	0	1	[3000, 4000]	3	[6, 8]	M	H	H	0	1	[3000, 4000]	3	[1, 3]	H	H	H

In the same way, the optimal weight vector for the positions can also be calculated as $\mu_1 = (0.0476, 0.1500, 0.0486, 0.0870, 0.0825, 0.1625, 0.2031, 0.2187)$; $\mu_2 = (0.0514, 0.1500, 0.0389, 0.0940, 0.0975, 0.1644, 0.2055, 0.1983)$; μ_3=$(0.0629, 0.1500, 0.0605, 0.1151, 0.1115, 0.1198, 0.1497, 0.2305)$; μ_4=$(0.0587, 0.1500, 0.0563, 0.1074, 0.1098, 0.1584, 0.1981, 0.1613)$.

Then the matching satisfaction degree matrix for the positions on the candidates can also be obtained as

$$\mathrm{B} = \begin{bmatrix} 0.7970 & 0.7783 & 0.8390 & 0.8688 & 0.8083 & 0.8410 & 0.8086 & 0.8599 \\ 0.7925 & 0.7904 & 0.8390 & 0.8642 & 0.8077 & 0.8399 & 0.7825 & 0.8466 \\ 0.7692 & 0.7674 & 0.8568 & 0.8150 & 0.7969 & 0.8197 & 0.7982 & 0.8343 \\ 0.8096 & 0.7612 & 0.8088 & 0.8265 & 0.8056 & 0.8438 & 0.7778 & 0.8664 \end{bmatrix}.$$

Let ω=0.5. By solving the optimization model (M-3), we can get $x_{22} = x_{33} = x_{44} = x_{81} = 1$ and the values of other decision variables are 0. According to the solution of the optimization model, we can conclude that the optimal matching for the candidates and the positions is (E_8, P_1), (E_2, P_2), (E_3, P_3) and (E_4, P_4), and there is no position that can match E_1, E_5, E_6 and E_7.

Example 2. In the following, we utilize the data given by [7] to show the effectiveness of the proposed method.

In [7], the weight information is given in advance, i.e. $w_i = (0.3, 0.25, 0.2, 0.25)$, $i = 1, 2, \ldots, 4$; $\mu_j = (0.12, 0.08, 0.08, 0.2, 0.16, 0.16, 0.1, 0.1)$, $j = 1, 2, \ldots, 8$. By their method, we can get the optimal matching as follows: (E_1, P_1), (E_2, P_2), (E_3, P_3) and (E_4, P_4).

Let the weight information be the incomplete case as the first example, i.e. $w_{i2} \leq 0.4w_{i1}$; $w_{i1} \leq 0.8w_{i3}$; $w_{i4} \leq 0.35$, $i = 1, 2, \ldots, 8$; $\mu_{j1} - 0.6\mu_{j3} \geq 0$; $\mu_{j4} - \mu_{j3} \geq \mu_{j5} - \mu_{j1}$; $\mu_{j6} \leq 0.8\mu_{j7}$; $\mu_{j2} \geq 0.15$, $j = 1, 2, \ldots, 4$. By the proposed method, the weight vector for each candidate can be obtained $w_1 = (0.2948, 0.1179, 0.3685, 0.2188)$; $w_2 = w_4 = w_5 = w_7 = w_8 = (0.2453, 0.0981, 0.3066, 0.3500)$; $w_3 = (0.3030, 0.1212, 0.3787, 0.1971)$; $w_6 = (0.2610, 0.1043, 0.3262, 0.3085)$. Meanwhile, the optimal weight vector for the positions can also be calculated as $\mu_1 = (0.0413, 0.1500, 0.0422, 0.1342, 0.1248, 0.1411, 0.1764, 0.1899)$; $\mu_2 = (0.0477, 0.1500, 0.0361, 0.1176, 0.1218, 0.1525, 0.1906, 0.1838)$; $\mu_3 = (0.0633, 0.1500, 0.0607, 0.1107, 0.1132, 0.1203, 0.1504, 0.2315)$; $\mu_4 = (0.0540, 0.1500, 0.0519, 0.1405, 0.1268, 0.1459, 0.1824, 0.1486)$.

Let $\omega = 0.5$. By solving the optimization model (M-3), we can get the optimal matching for the candidates and the positions are (E_8, P_1), (E_2, P_2), (E_3, P_3) and (E_4, P_4), which is slightly different to the result obtained by the method in [7]. However, our method takes into account the case when the attribute weight information of the matching objects is incomplete, which can describe the actual situation. Besides that, the proposed method incorporates other two types of evaluation information, i.e. ordinal value and ordinal interval value, which may appear in actual two-sided matching decision making problems.

5 Conclusions

Due to the wide existence of two-sided matching problems, it is necessary for us to develop analysis method to solve such problems. In this paper, we take into account six formats of evaluation information for the matching objects and propose an analysis method for two-sided matching problems. The proposed method can deal with the situation that the evaluation attributes for the two sides are different and the weight information for the matching objects is incomplete. The proposed method is simple and easy to implement on the computer. Although the illustrative examples shown in this paper are for the matching of employees and positions, the method can also be extended to other areas, such as marriage matching and trades matching between buyers and sellers.

Acknowledgements. This work was partly supported by National Natural Science Foundation of China (No. 70871015), the Key Program of National Natural Science Foundation of China (No. 71031002) and the Fundamental Research Funds for the Central Universities of China (DUT11SX04).

References

1. Gale, D., Shapley, L.S.: College admissions and the stability of marriage. The American Mathematical Monthly 69(1), 9–15 (1962)
2. Drigas, A., Kouremenos, S., Vrettos, S., Vrettaros, J., Kouremenos, D.: An expert system for job matching of the unemployed. Expert Systems with Applications 26(2), 217–224 (2004)
3. Golec, A., Kahya, E.: A fuzzy model for competency-based employee evaluation and selection. Computers & Industrial Engineering 52(1), 143–161 (2007)
4. Korkmaz, I., Gken, H., Etinyokus, T.: An analytic hierarchy process and two-sided matching based decision support system for military personnel assignment. Information Sciences 178(14), 2915–2927 (2008)
5. Lin, H.T.: A job placement intervention using fuzzy approach for two-way choice. Expert Systems with Applications 36(2, Part 1), 2543–2553 (2009)
6. Huang, D.K., Chiu, H.N., Yeh, R.H., Chang, J.H.: A fuzzy multi-criteria decision making approach for solving a bi-objective personnel assignment problem. Computers & Industrial Engineering 56(1), 1–10 (2009)
7. Chen, X., Fan, Z.P.: Research on two-sided matching problem between employees and positions based on multiple format information. Operational Research and Management Science 18(6), 103–109 (2009)
8. Wang, D.W.: Multi-objective trade matching problem and optimization method of E-Brokerage. China Journal of Information Systems 1(1), 102–109 (2007)
9. Jiang, Z.Z., Ip, W.H., Lau, H.C.W., Fan, Z.P.: Multi-objective optimization matching for one-shot multi-attribute exchanges with quantity discounts in e-brokerage. Expert Systems with Applications 38(4), 4169–4180 (2011)
10. Kameshwaran, S., Narahari, Y., Rosa, C.H., Kulkarni, D.M., Tew, J.D.: Multi-attribute electronic procurement using goal programming. European Journal of Operational Research 179(2), 518–536 (2007)
11. Jiang, Z.Z., Sheng, Y., Fan, Z.P., Yuan, Y.: Research on multi-objective decision model for bipartite matching with incomplete information on attribute weights. Operational Research and Management Science 17(4), 138–142 (2008)
12. Li, Y.H., Fan, Z.P., Chen, X., Kang, F.: A multi-objective optimization model for matching ventures and venture capitalists. In: 4th International Conference on Wireless Communications, Networking and Mobile Computing. IEEE Press, New York (2008)
13. Herrera, F., Herrera-Viedma, E.: Linguistic decision analysis: steps for solving decision problems under linguistic information. Fuzzy Sets and Systems 115(1), 67–82 (2000)
14. González-Pachón, J., Romero, C.: Aggregation of partial ordinal rankings: an interval goal programming approach. Computers & Operations Research 28(8), 827–834 (2001)
15. Gardenfors, P.: Assignment problem based on ordinal preferences. Computers & Operations Research 20(3), 331–340 (1973)
16. Kim, S.H., Choi, S.H., Kim, J.K.: An interactive procedure for multiple attribute group decision making with incomplete information: Range-based approach. European Journal of Operational Research 118(1), 139–152 (1999)
17. Hwang, C.L., Yoon, K.: Multiple Attribute Decision Making: Methods and Applications. Springer, Heidelberg (1981)

A New Linguistic Aggregation Operator and Its Application

Cuiping Wei*, Xia Liang, and Lili Han

Management School, Qufu Normal University,
Rizhao 276826, P.R. China
wei_cuiping@yahoo.com.cn

Abstract. In this paper, we define a new function, the generalized linguistic weighted OWA (GLWOWA) operator, to aggregate linguistic information. The proposed operator combines the advantages of the linguistic weighted arithmetic averaging (LWAA) operator and the extended OWA (EOWA) operator, and improves the linguistic weighted OWA (LWOWA) operator. We study some of its properties and compare it with the linguistic hybrid arithmetic averaging (LHAA) operator. Based on the LWAA operator and the GLWOWA operator, we develop an approach to multi-attribute group decision making with linguistic information.

Keywords: multi-attribute group decision making, linguistic information aggregation, GLWOWA operator.

1 Introduction

In multi-attribute decision making (MADM) problems, due to the complexity and uncertainty of the objective things, as well as the fuzziness of the human mind, decision makers usually confront with some qualitative attributes, which are suitable to be evaluated in the form of language [1–7]. Such as evaluating the qualities of the students, the decision makers prefer to use "excellent", "good" and "poor" to give an evaluation. Herrera [2–4] introduced a finite and totally ordered discrete linguistic label set. Xu [5] defined a finite and totally ordered discrete linguistic label set with zero as the symmetrical center and a continuous linguistic label set.

For MADM problem with linguistic information, the key work is to aggregate linguistic satisfactions, expressed by linguistic labels, of individual attributes to obtain an overall evaluation value for an alternative, which can then be used to rank alternatives. Authors defined many operators to aggregate linguistic

* Corresponding author. This research was supported by the National Natural Science Foundation of China (No.11071142), Humanities and Social Sciences Project of Ministry of Education under Grant No.10YJC630269 and A Project of Shandong Province Higher Educational Science and Technology Program No.J09LA14,J10LG04.

B. Hu et al. (Eds.): BI 2011, LNAI 6889, pp. 284–294, 2011.

information, which were concluded in [8]. Among these operators, the linguistic weighted arithmetic averaging (LWAA) operator and the extended OWA (EOWA) operator were proposed by Xu in [5]. The LWAA operator weights linguistic arguments themselves, while the EOWA operator weights the ordered position of linguistic arguments. Therefore, in the LWAA and EOWA operators, weights represent different aspects. In order to combine the advantages of the two operators, Xu [6] and Torra [9] defined the linguistic hybrid arithmetic averaging (LHAA) operator and the linguistic weighted OWA (LWOWA) operator, respectively.

The LWOWA operator is an averaging operator, it satisfies idempotency and monotonicity. But in the aggregation process of the LWOWA operator, the round operation is repeatedly used to deal with the aggregated value of linguistic labels, which leads to the loss of decision information. Compared with the LWOWA operator, the LHAA operator can be used in the same decision making situation as the LWOWA operator and can preserve more decision information, but it is not an averaging operator.

Motivated by the above-mentioned work, we define an averaging operator, generalized linguistic weighted OWA (GLWOWA) operator, to improve the the LWOWA operator, and propose a practical approach to handle multi-attribute group decision making problem with linguistic information. To do that, this paper is organized as follows. In section 2, we review the basic concepts and analyze the drawback of the LWOWA operator. In section 3, we define a GLWOWA operator and study its properties. Then we compare it with the LHAA operator. In section 4, we provide an approach to solve multi-attribute group decision making problem with linguistic information. A practical example is used to illustrate the proposed approach in section 5. The paper is concluded in section 6.

2 Basic Concepts

For MADM problems with qualitative attributes, we need to use a linguistic label set to describe the decision information. Herrera [2–4] introduced a linguistic label set $S_1 = \{s_\alpha | \alpha = 0, 1, \cdots, \tau\}$, where s_α represents a possible value for a linguistic variable and τ is even. Xu [5] introduced a finite and totally ordered discrete linguistic label set $S_2 = \{s_\alpha | \alpha = -\tau, \cdots, -1, 0, 1, \cdots, \tau\}$, where zero is the symmetrical center and τ is a positive integer. Any label s_α in S_2 must have the following characteristics:

(1) The set is ordered: $s_\alpha > s_\beta$ if $\alpha > \beta$.
(2) There is the negative operator: $neg(s_\alpha) = s_{-\alpha}$.

To preserve all the given information, Xu [5] extended the discrete linguistic label set S_2 to a continuous linguistic label set $\overline{S}_2 = \{s_\alpha | \alpha \in [-q, q]\}$ where $q (q > \tau)$ is a sufficiently large positive integer.

Let $s_\alpha, s_\beta \in \overline{S}_2$ and $\lambda \in [0, 1]$, then two operational laws of linguistic variables are given as follows [5]:

(1) $s_\alpha \oplus s_\beta = s_\beta \oplus s_\alpha = s_{\alpha+\beta}$.
(2) $\lambda s_\alpha = s_{\lambda\alpha}$.

Definition 1 [5]. Let $(s_{\alpha_1}, s_{\alpha_2}, \cdots, s_{\alpha_n})$ be a collection of linguistic variables. A linguistic weighted arithmetic averaging (LWAA) operator is a mapping: $(\overline{S}_2)^n \to \overline{S}_2$, such that

$$LWAA(s_{\alpha_1}, s_{\alpha_2}, \cdots, s_{\alpha_n}) = w_1 s_{\alpha_1} \oplus w_2 s_{\alpha_2} \oplus \cdots \oplus w_n s_{\alpha_n} = s_{\overline{\alpha}}, \quad (1)$$

where $\overline{\alpha} = \sum_{j=1}^{n} w_j \alpha_j$ and $w = (w_1, w_2, \cdots, w_n)^T$ is the weighting vector of $s_{\alpha_i}(i = 1, 2, \cdots, n)$ with $w_j \in [0, 1]$ and $\sum_{j=1}^{n} w_j = 1$.

Definition 2 [5]. Let $(s_{\alpha_1}, s_{\alpha_2}, \cdots, s_{\alpha_n})$ be a collection of linguistic variables. An extended OWA (EOWA) operator is a mapping: $(\overline{S}_2)^n \to \overline{S}_2$, such that

$$EOWA(s_{\alpha_1}, s_{\alpha_2}, \cdots, s_{\alpha_n}) = w_1 s_{\beta_1} \oplus w_2 s_{\beta_2} \oplus \cdots \oplus w_n s_{\beta_n} = s_{\overline{\beta}}, \quad (2)$$

where $\overline{\beta} = \sum_{j=1}^{n} w_j \beta_j$, s_{β_j} is the jth largest of $s_{\alpha_j}(j = 1, 2, \cdots, n)$, and $w = (w_1, w_2, \cdots, w_n)^T$ is an associated vector of the operator with $w_j \in [0, 1]$ and $\sum_{j=1}^{n} w_j = 1$.

From Definition 1 and Definition 2, we can see the LWAA operator weights only the linguistic arguments s_{α_j} of the jth information source (or attribute, expert) according to the weight w_j. On the other hand, in the EOWA operator, each w_j is attached to the jth argument s_{β_j} in decreasing order without considering which information source it comes from. In order to combine the advantages of the two operators, Xu [6] and Torra [9] proposed the linguistic hybrid arithmetic (LHAA) operator and the linguistic weighted OWA (LWOWA) operator, respectively.

Definition 3 [6]. Let $(s_{\alpha_1}, s_{\alpha_2}, \cdots, s_{\alpha_n})$ be a collection of linguistic variables. An linguistic hybrid arithmetic (LHAA) operator is a mapping: $(\overline{S}_2)^n \to \overline{S}_2$, such that

$$LHAA(s_{\alpha_1}, s_{\alpha_2}, \cdots, s_{\alpha_n}) = w_1 s_{\beta_1} \oplus w_2 s_{\beta_2} \oplus \cdots \oplus w_n s_{\beta_n}, \quad (3)$$

where s_{β_j} is the jth largest of the linguistic weighted arguments $\overline{s}_{\alpha_j}(\overline{s}_{\alpha_i} = np_i s_{\alpha_i}, i = 1, 2, \cdots, n)$; $p = (p_1, p_2, \cdots, p_n)^T$ be the weighting vector of $s_{\alpha_j}(j = 1, 2, \cdots, n)$ with $p_j \in [0, 1]$ and $\sum_{j=1}^{n} p_j = 1$; $w = (w_1, w_2, \cdots, w_n)^T$ be an associated vector of the operator with $w_j \in [0, 1]$ and $\sum_{j=1}^{n} w_j = 1$, and n is the balancing coefficient.

The LWOWA operator is defined by Torra [9] on linguistic label set S_1. In order to compare it with the LHAA operator, it is defined on linguistic label set S_2 as follows.

Definition 4 [9]. Let $(a_1, a_2, \cdots, a_n)$ be a collection of linguistic variables. Let $w = (w_1, w_2, \cdots, w_n)^T$ be a weighting vector of dimension n with $w_j \in [0,1]$ and $\sum_{j=1}^{n} w_j = 1$, and $p = (p_1, p_2, \cdots, p_n)^T$ be the weighting vector of $a_j (j = 1, 2, \cdots, n)$ with $p_j \in [0,1]$ and $\sum_{j=1}^{n} p_j = 1$. A linguistic weighted OWA (LWOWA) operator is a mapping: $(S_2)^n \to S_2$, such that

$$LWOWA(a_1, a_2, \cdots, a_n) = C^n \{v_k, b_k, k = 1, 2, \cdots, n\}$$

$$= v_1 \odot b_1 \oplus_1 (1 - v_1) \odot C^{n-1} \left\{ v_h / \sum_{k=2}^{n} v_k, b_h, h = 2, 3, \cdots, n \right\}, \qquad (4)$$

where $(b_1, b_2, \cdots, b_n) = (a_{\sigma(1)}, a_{\sigma(2)}, \cdots, a_{\sigma(n)})$ is a permutation of $(a_1, a_2, \cdots, a_n)$ such that $a_{\sigma(i)} \geq a_{\sigma(j)}$ for all $i \leq j$, and the weight v_i is defined as $v_i = W^*(\sum_{j \leq i} p_{\sigma(j)}) - W^*(\sum_{j<i} p_{\sigma(j)})$ with W^* a monotone increasing function that interpolates the points $(\frac{i}{n}, \sum_{j \leq i} w_j)$ together with the point $(0,0)$. W^* is required to be a straight line when the points can be interpolated in this way. C^n is the convex combination operator [10] of n terms and if $n = 2$, it is defined as $C^2 \{v_i, b_i, i = 1, 2\} = v_1 \odot s_j \oplus_1 (1 - v_1) \odot s_i = s_k$, with $s_j = \max\{b_1, b_2\}$, $s_i = \min\{b_1, b_2\}$, and $k = \min\{\tau, i + round(v_1 \times (j - i))\}$, "round" is the usual round operation.

From Definition 4, for the weighting vector $w = (w_1, w_2, \cdots, w_n)^T$, we can obtain the piecewise linear function W^*, which is monotone increasing and interpolates the points $(\frac{i}{n}, \sum_{j \leq i} w_j)$ together with the point $(0,0)$:

$$W^*(x) = \sum_{k=1}^{j-1} w_k + w_j(nx - (j-1)), \quad \frac{j-1}{n} \leq x \leq \frac{j}{n}. \qquad (5)$$

So the associated weighting vector $v = (v_1, v_2, \cdots, v_n)^T$ of the LWOWA operator can be obtained, where

$$v_i = W^*(\sum_{j \leq i} p_{\sigma(j)}) - W^*(\sum_{j<i} p_{\sigma(j)}), \ i = 1, 2, \cdots, n. \qquad (6)$$

Example 1. Suppose x_1, x_2, x_3 are three alternatives which are evaluated using the label set

$$S_2 = \{s_{-3} = extremely\ poor, s_{-2} = very\ poor, s_{-1} = poor, s_0 = fair, \\ s_1 = good, s_2 = very\ good, s_3 = extremely\ good\}$$

under four attributes u_1, u_2, u_3, u_4. We assume that $p = (0.1, 0.3, 0.2, 0.4)^T$ is the weighting vector of the attributes, $w = (\frac{1}{6}, \frac{1}{3}, \frac{1}{3}, \frac{1}{6})^T$ is a weighting vector, and decision making matrix R is given as follows:

$$R = \begin{array}{c} \\ x_1 \\ x_2 \\ x_3 \end{array} \begin{array}{c} \begin{array}{cccc} u_1 & u_2 & u_3 & u_4 \end{array} \\ \begin{pmatrix} s_1 & s_0 & s_2 & s_{-1} \\ s_0 & s_2 & s_{-1} & s_1 \\ s_2 & s_1 & s_{-1} & s_0 \end{pmatrix} \end{array}.$$

Now we utilize the LWOWA operator to derive the overall aggregated values $z_i(i = 1, 2, 3)$ of the alternatives $x_i(i = 1, 2, 3)$. By formula (5), we obtain the function

$$W^*(x) = \begin{cases} \frac{2}{3}x, & 0 \le x \le \frac{1}{4}; \\ \frac{4}{3}x - \frac{1}{6}, & \frac{1}{4} < x < \frac{3}{4}; \\ \frac{2}{3}x + \frac{1}{3}, & \frac{3}{4} \le x \le 1. \end{cases}$$

By formula (6), we obtain the associated weighting vector $v^{(1)} = (0.13, 0.1, 0.4, 0.37)^T$ of the LWOWA operator for alternative x_1. Let $(a_1, a_2, a_3, a_4) = (s_1, s_0, s_2, s_{-1})$, b_j be the jth largest argument of $a_i(i = 1, 2, 3, 4)$.

Then

$$z_1 = LWOWA(s_1, s_0, s_2, s_{-1}) = C^4 \left\{ v_k^{(1)}, b_k, k = 1, 2, 3, 4 \right\}$$
$$= 0.13 \odot s_2 \oplus_1 (1 - 0.13) \odot C^3 \left\{ v_h^{(1)} / \sum_{k=2}^{4} v_k^{(1)}, h = 2, 3, 4 \right\}.$$

Let $\gamma_h = v_h^{(1)} \Big/ \sum\limits_{k=2}^{4} v_h^{(1)}, h = 2, 3, 4$. Then $\gamma_2 = 0.11, \gamma_3 = 0.46, \gamma_4 = 0.43$. Thus

$$C^3 \{\gamma_h, b_h, h = 2, 3, 4\} = 0.11 \odot s_1 \oplus_1 0.89 \odot C^2 \{\gamma_h', b_h, h = 3, 4\}.$$

Let $\gamma_h' = \gamma_h \Big/ \sum\limits_{k=3}^{4} \gamma_h, h = 3, 4$. Then $\gamma_3' = 0.52, \gamma_4' = 0.48$. Thus

$$C^2 \{\gamma_h', b_h, h = 3, 4\} = 0.52 \odot s_0 \oplus_1 0.48 \odot s_{-1} = s_k.$$

Since $k = \min\{3, -1 + round(0.52 \times (0 + 1))\} = 0$, $C^2 \{\gamma_h', b_h, h = 3, 4\} = s_0$. Therefore, $C^3 \{\gamma_h, b_h, h = 2, 3, 4\} = s_0$, $C^4 \{v_k, b_k, k = 1, 2, 3, 4\} = s_0$, that is $z_1 = s_0$.

By formula (6), we obtain the associated weighting vectors $v^{(2)} = (0.23, 0.54, 0.1, 0.13)^T$ and $v^{(3)} = (0.07, 0.3, 0.5, 0.13)^T$ for alternatives x_2 and x_3, respectively. So we get

$$z_2 = LWOWA(s_0, s_2, s_{-1}, s_1) = s_0 \text{ and } z_3 = LWOWA(s_2, s_1, s_{-1}, s_0) = s_0.$$

Comparing the overall aggregated values $z_i(i = 1, 2, 3)$, we have the ranking of the alternatives is: $x_1 \sim x_2 \sim x_3$.

From the aggregated process of the LWOWA operator, we can see that the round operation is repeatedly used to deal with the aggregated value of linguistic labels. The computational techniques used present a common drawback, the "loss of information", that implies a lack of precision in the final results [3]. In the following section, we will improve the LWOWA operator.

3 The GLWOWA Operator and Its Properties

Definition 5. Let $(a_1, a_2, \cdots, a_n)$ be a collection of linguistic variables, $w = (w_1, w_2, \cdots, w_n)^T$ be a weighting vector of dimension n with $w_j \in [0,1]$ and $\sum_{j=1}^{n} w_j = 1$, $p = (p_1, p_2, \cdots, p_n)^T$ be a weighting vector of $a_j (j = 1, 2, \cdots, n)$ with $p_j \in [0,1]$ and $\sum_{j=1}^{n} p_j = 1$. A generalized linguistic weighted OWA (GLWOWA) operator is a mapping: $(\overline{S}_2)^n \to \overline{S}_2$, such that

$$GLWOWA(a_1, a_2, \cdots, a_n) = v_1 b_1 \oplus v_2 b_2 \oplus \cdots \oplus v_n b_n, \tag{7}$$

where the linguistic variables $b_i (i = 1, 2, \cdots n)$ and the weights $v_i (i = 1, 2, \cdots n)$ are defined according to Definition 4.

We can easily prove the following proposition.

Proposition 1. Let $(s_{\alpha_1}, s_{\alpha_2}, \cdots, s_{\alpha_n})$ be a collection of linguistic variables, $w = (w_1, w_2, \cdots, w_n)^T$ be a weighting vector with $w_j \in [0,1]$ and $\sum_{j=1}^{n} w_j = 1$, and $p = (p_1, p_2, \cdots, p_n)^T$ be the weighting vector of $s_{\alpha_j} (j = 1, 2, \cdots, n)$ with $p_j \in [0,1]$ and $\sum_{j=1}^{n} p_j = 1$. Then the GLWOWA operator satisfies the following properties:

(1) (Boundary): $\min_i \{s_{\alpha_i}\} \leq GLWOWA(s_{\alpha_1}, s_{\alpha_2}, \cdots, s_{\alpha_n}) \leq \max_i \{s_{\alpha_i}\}$.

(2) (Monotonicity): Let $(s_{\beta_1}, s_{\beta_2}, \cdots, s_{\beta_n})$ and $(s_{\alpha_1}, s_{\alpha_2}, \cdots, s_{\alpha_n})$ be any two collections of linguistic labels such that $s_{\alpha_i} \leq s_{\beta_i}$ for all i. Then

$$GLWOWA(s_{\alpha_1}, s_{\alpha_2}, \cdots, s_{\alpha_n}) \leq GLWOWA(s_{\beta_1}, s_{\beta_2}, \cdots, s_{\beta_n}).$$

(3) (Commutativity): Let $(s_{\beta_1}, s_{\beta_2}, \cdots, s_{\beta_n})$ be a permutation of $(s_{\alpha_1}, s_{\alpha_2}, \cdots, s_{\alpha_n})$. Then $GLWOWA(s_{\alpha_1}, s_{\alpha_2}, \cdots, s_{\alpha_n}) = GLWOWA(s_{\beta_1}, s_{\beta_2}, \cdots, s_{\beta_n})$ if and only if $p_i = \frac{1}{n} (i = 1, 2, \cdots, n)$.

(4) (Idempotency): If $s_{\alpha_j} = s_\alpha$ for all j, then $GLWOWA(s_\alpha, s_\alpha, \cdots, s_\alpha) = s_\alpha$.

(5) If $p = (\frac{1}{n}, \frac{1}{n}, \cdots, \frac{1}{n})^T$, then the GLWOWA operator is reduced to the EOWA operator.

Proof: If $p_i = \frac{1}{n}$ for all i, we have

$$v_i = W^*(\sum_{j \leq i} p_{\sigma(j)}) - W^*(\sum_{j < i} p_{\sigma(j)}) = W^*(\frac{i}{n}) - W^*(\frac{i-1}{n}) = \sum_{j \leq i} w_j - \sum_{j \leq i-1} w_j = w_i.$$

Thus, $GLWOWA(s_{\alpha_1}, s_{\alpha_2}, \cdots, s_{\alpha_n}) = EOWA(s_{\alpha_1}, s_{\alpha_2}, \cdots, s_{\alpha_n})$.

(6) If $w = (\frac{1}{n}, \frac{1}{n}, \cdots, \frac{1}{n})^T$, then the GLWOWA operator is reduced to the LWAA operator.

Proof: If $w_i = \frac{1}{n}$ for all i, then $W^*(x) = x$ and $v_i = p_{\sigma(i)}$. This conclusion is proved in [9]. Thus, $GLWOWA(s_{\alpha_1}, s_{\alpha_2}, \cdots, s_{\alpha_n}) = LWAA(s_{\alpha_1}, s_{\alpha_2}, \cdots, s_{\alpha_n})$.

Now we utilize the GLWOWA operator to aggregate the information in Example 1. For the given weighting vector $p = (0.1, 0.3, 0.2, 0.4)^T$ of the attributes and the weighting vector $w = (\frac{1}{6}, \frac{1}{3}, \frac{1}{3}, \frac{1}{6})^T$, we can obtain the associated vectors $v^{(i)}(i = 1, 2, 3)$ of the GLWOWA operator for alternatives $x_i(i = 1, 2, 3)$, which are the same as the ones of the LWOWA operator. So we derive the overall aggregated values $z_i(i = 1, 2, 3)$ of the alternatives $x_i(i = 1, 2, 3)$:

$$\begin{aligned} z_1 &= GLWOWA(s_1, s_0, s_2, s_{-1}) = v_1^{(1)} s_2 \oplus v_2^{(1)} s_1 \oplus v_3^{(1)} s_0 \oplus v_4^{(1)} s_{-1} \\ &= 0.13 s_2 \oplus 0.10 s_1 \oplus 0.40 s_0 \oplus 0.37 s_{-1} = s_{-0.01}, \end{aligned}$$

$$\begin{aligned} z_2 &= GLWOWA(s_0, s_2, s_{-1}, s_1) = v_1^{(2)} s_2 \oplus v_2^{(2)} s_1 \oplus v_3^{(2)} s_0 \oplus v_4^{(2)} s_{-1} \\ &= 0.23 s_2 \oplus 0.54 s_1 \oplus 0.10 s_0 \oplus 0.13 s_{-1} = s_{0.87}, \end{aligned}$$

$$\begin{aligned} z_3 &= GLWOWA(s_2, s_1, s_{-1}, s_0) = v_1^{(3)} s_2 \oplus v_2^{(3)} s_1 \oplus v_3^{(3)} s_0 \oplus v_4^{(3)} s_{-1} \\ &= 0.07 s_2 \oplus 0.30 s_1 \oplus 0.50 s_0 \oplus 0.13 s_{-1} = s_{0.31}. \end{aligned}$$

Comparing the overall aggregated values $z_i(i = 1, 2, 3)$, we have the ranking of the alternatives is: $x_2 \succ x_3 \succ x_1$.

From the aggregation process of the GLWOWA operator, we know that the GLWOWA operator uses the operation between indexes of linguistic labels, and allows a continuous representation of the linguistic information. Hence it can aggregate linguistic information without loss of information. So the GLWOWA operator overcomes the limitation of the LWOWA operator which could not distinguish alternatives precisely.

Yager [11] introduced concepts of an averaging operator and a scoring operator. He point out that an aggregation operator is called a scoring operator if it satisfies monotonicity, and an aggregation operator is called an averaging operator if it not only is monotonic and idempotent but also remains between the minimum and maximum of the arguments. From Proposition 1, we know that the GLWOWA operator generalizes the LWAA operator and the EOWA operator and is an averaging operator. As another generalized form of the LWAA operator and the EOWA operator, the LHAA operator is only a scoring operator which dose not remain between the minimum and the maximum of the arguments and does not satisfy the idempotency.

4 The Application of the GLWOWA Operator in Multi-attribute Group Decision Making

In this section, we develop an approach, based on the LWAA operator and the GLWOWA operator, to multi-attribute group decision making with linguistic information. The multi-attribute group decision making problem which is considered in this paper can be represented as follows.

We suppose $X = \{x_1, x_2, \cdots, x_n\}$ is a set of evaluation alternatives, $U = \{u_1, u_2, \cdots, u_m\}$ is an attribute set, and $w = (w_1, w_2, \cdots, w_m)^T$ is the weighting vector of attributes such that $w_j \geq 0$ and $\sum_{j=1}^{m} w_j = 1$. Let $D = \{d_1, d_2, \cdots, d_s\}$ be the set of decision makers and $\lambda = (\lambda_1, \lambda_2, \cdots, \lambda_s)^T$ be the weighting vector of decision makers such that $\lambda_k \geq 0$ and $\sum_{k=1}^{s} \lambda_k = 1$. Let $R_k = \left(r_{ij}^{(k)}\right)_{n \times m}$ be a linguistic decision matrix, where $r_{ij}^{(k)} \in S$ is the linguistic assessment provided by the decision maker $d_k \in D$ for the alternative $x_i \in X$ with respect to the attribute $u_j \in U$.

We rank the alternatives $x_i (i = 1, 2, \cdots, n)$ by the following steps:

Step 1. Utilize the LWAA operator to derive the individual overall aggregated values $z_i^{(k)} (i = 1, 2, \cdots, n)$ of alternatives $x_i (i = 1, 2, \cdots, n)$, where

$$z_i^{(k)} = LWAA(r_{i1}^{(k)}, r_{i2}^{(k)}, \cdots, r_{im}^{(k)}) = w_1 r_{i1}^{(k)} \oplus w_2 r_{i2}^{(k)} \oplus \cdots \oplus w_m r_{im}^{(k)}.$$

Step 2. Utilize the GLWOWA operator to derive the overall aggregated values $z_i (i = 1, 2, \cdots, n)$ of alternatives $x_i (i = 1, 2, \cdots, n)$, where

$$z_i = GLWOWA(z_i^{(1)}, z_i^{(2)}, \cdots, z_i^{(s)}) = v_1 z_i^{\sigma(1)} \oplus v_2 z_i^{\sigma(2)} \oplus \cdots \oplus v_s z_i^{\sigma(s)},$$

where $v = (v_1, v_2, \cdots, v_s)^T$ is calculated by formulas (5) and (6) using the weighting vector $w' = (w'_1, w'_2, \cdots, w'_s)^T$ with $w'_j \in [0, 1]$ and $\sum_{j=1}^{s} w'_j = 1$ and the weighting vector of decision makers $\lambda = (\lambda_1, \lambda_2, \cdots, \lambda_s)^T$ with $\lambda_k \in [0, 1]$ and $\sum_{k=1}^{s} \lambda_k = 1$.

Step 3. Utilize the overall aggregated values $z_i (i = 1, 2, \cdots, n)$ to rank the alternatives $x_i (i = 1, 2, \cdots, n)$ and then to select the best one(s).

5 Illustrative Example

We adopt the example which is used in [12] and [6] to illustrate the proposed approach.

A practical use of the proposed approach involves the evaluation of university faculty for tenure and promotion. The attributes used at some universities are teaching (u_1), research (u_2) and service (u_3) whose weighting vector is $w = (0.14, 0.26, 0.60)^T$. Five faculties $x_i (i = 1, 2, 3, 4, 5)$ are to evaluated using the label set

$$S_2 = \{s_{-3} = none, s_{-2} = very\ low, s_{-1} = low, s_0 = medium,$$
$$s_1 = high, s_2 = very\ high, s_3 = perfect\}$$

by three decision makers $d_k(k = 1,2,3)$ (whose weighting vector $\lambda = (0.2, 0.5, 0.3)^T$) under these three attributes, the decision making matrices $R_k = (r_{ij}^{(k)})_{5\times 3}(k = 1,2,3)$ are as follows:

$$R_1 = \begin{pmatrix} s_{-1} & s_0 & s_2 \\ s_{-2} & s_1 & s_2 \\ s_{-1} & s_{-2} & s_2 \\ s_2 & s_1 & s_{-1} \\ s_1 & s_1 & s_0 \end{pmatrix}, \quad R_2 = \begin{pmatrix} s_0 & s_{-1} & s_1 \\ s_0 & s_{-1} & s_2 \\ s_0 & s_1 & s_0 \\ s_2 & s_0 & s_0 \\ s_0 & s_2 & s_1 \end{pmatrix}, \quad R_3 = \begin{pmatrix} s_{-1} & s_{-1} & s_2 \\ s_{-1} & s_0 & s_1 \\ s_{-2} & s_0 & s_2 \\ s_1 & s_0 & s_1 \\ s_0 & s_2 & s_{-1} \end{pmatrix}.$$

Step 1. Utilize the LWAA operator to aggregate the decision matrices $R_k(k = 1,2,3)$ respectively to derive the individual overall aggregated values $z_i^{(k)}(i = 1,2,3,4,5)$ of the alternatives $x_i(i = 1,2,3,4,5)$:

$$z_1^{(1)} = s_{1.06}, \quad z_2^{(1)} = s_{1.18}, \quad z_3^{(1)} = s_{0.54}, \quad z_4^{(1)} = s_{-0.06}, \quad z_5^{(1)} = s_{0.40},$$

$$z_1^{(2)} = s_{0.34}, \quad z_2^{(2)} = s_{0.94}, \quad z_3^{(2)} = s_{0.26}, \quad z_4^{(2)} = s_{0.28}, \quad z_5^{(2)} = s_{1.12},$$

$$z_1^{(3)} = s_{0.54}, \quad z_2^{(3)} = s_{0.46}, \quad z_3^{(3)} = s_{0.92}, \quad z_4^{(3)} = s_{0.74}, \quad z_5^{(3)} = s_{-0.08}.$$

Step 2. Utilize the GLWOWA operator to derive the overall aggregated values of the alternatives $x_i(i = 1,2,3,4,5)$. In order to compare the GLWOWA operator with the LHAA operator, we use the same weighting vector $w' = (0.2429, 0.5142, 0.2429)^T$ as that was used in [6]. With $w' = (0.2429, 0.5142, 0.2429)^T$, we obtain the function

$$W^*(x) = \begin{cases} 0.7287x, & 0 \le x \le \frac{1}{3}; \\ 1.5426x - 0.2713\,, & \frac{1}{3} < x < \frac{2}{3}; \\ 0.7287x + 0.2713\,, & \frac{2}{3} \le x \le 1. \end{cases}$$

With $\lambda = (0.2, 0.5, 0.3)^T$, we get the associated weighting vector $v^{(i)}(i = 1,2,3,4,5)$ of the GLWOWA operator according to the alternatives $x_i(i = 1,2,3,4,5)$:

$$v^{(1)}{=}(0.146, 0.354, 0.500)^T, v^{(2)}{=}(0.146, 0.635, 0.219)^T, v^{(3)}{=}(0.219, 0.281, 0.500)^T,$$

$$v^{(4)} = (0.219, 0.635, 0.146)^T, v^{(5)} = (0.500, 0.281, 0.219)^T.$$

Thus, the overall aggregated values $z_i(i = 1,2,3,4,5)$ of the alternatives $x_i(i = 1,2,3,4,5)$ are as follows:

$$z_1 = GLWOWA_{\lambda,w'}(z_1^{(1)}, z_1^{(2)}, z_1^{(3)}) = s_{0.516},$$

$$z_2 = GLWOWA_{\lambda,w'}(z_2^{(1)}, z_2^{(2)}, z_2^{(3)}) = s_{0.870},$$

$$z_3 = GLWOWA_{\lambda,w'}(z_3^{(1)}, z_3^{(2)}, z_3^{(3)}) = s_{0.483},$$

$$z_4 = GLWOWA_{\lambda,w'}(z_4^{(1)}, z_4^{(2)}, z_4^{(3)}) = s_{0.331},$$

$$z_5 = GLWOWA_{\lambda,w'}(z_5^{(1)}, z_5^{(2)}, z_5^{(3)}) = s_{0.655}.$$

Step 3. Using the overall aggregated values $z_i (i = 1, 2, 3, 4, 5)$, we obtain the ranking of the alternatives $x_i (i = 1, 2, 3, 4, 5)$:

$$x_2 \succ x_5 \succ x_1 \succ x_3 \succ x_4.$$

Xu [6] utilized the LHAA operator to aggregate the linguistic information of these five alternatives and obtain the ranking of alternatives:

$$x_2 \succ x_1 \succ x_5 \succ x_3 \succ x_4.$$

In these two aggregation methods, we obtained x_2 is the best alternative.

6 Concluding

In this paper, we have defined a GLWOWA operator, which overcomes the drawback of the LWOWA operator. Then we studied the properties of the GLWOWA operator and compared it with the LHAA operator. We obtained the result that GLWOWA operator is an averaging operator while the LHAA operator is only a scoring operator. Finally, we have utilized the GLWOWA operator to solve multi-attribute group decision making problem with linguistic information and provided a practical example to illustrate the developed approach.

References

1. Bordogna, G., Fedrizzi, M., Passi, G.: A linguistic modeling of consensus in group decision making based on OWA operator. IEEE Transaction on Systems, Man, and Cybernetics 27, 126–132 (1997)
2. Herrera, F., Herrera-Viedma, E., Verdegay, J.L.: A model of consensus in group decision making under linguistic assessments. Fuzzy Sets and Systems 78, 73–87 (1996)
3. Herrera, F., Nartinee, L.: A 2-tuple fuzzy Linguistic representation model for computing with words. IEEE Transaction on Fuzzy Systems 8(6), 746–752 (2000)
4. Herrera, F., Martinez, L.: A model based on linguistic 2-tuples for dealing with multi-granularity hierarchical linguistic contexts in multi-expert decision making. IEEE Transactions on Systems, Man and Cybernetics-Part B 31(2), 227–233 (2001)
5. Xu, Z.S.: EOWA and EOWG Operators for Aggregating Linguistic Labels Based on Linguistic Preference Relations. International Journal of Uncertainty, Fuzziness and Knowledge-Based Systems 12, 791–810 (2004)
6. Xu, Z.S.: A Note on Linguistic Hybrid Arithmetic Averaging Operator in Multiple Attribute Group Decision Making with Linguistic Information. Group Decision and Negotiation 15, 581–591 (2006)
7. Wei, C.P., Feng, X.Q., Zhang, Y.Z.: Method for measuring the satisfactory consistency of a linguistic judement matrix. Systems Engineering Theory and Practice 29(1), 104–110 (2009)

8. Xu, Z.S.: Linguistic aggregation operators: an overview. In: Bustince, H., Herrera, F., Montero, J. (eds.) Fuzzy Sets and Their Extensions: Representation, Aggregation and Models, pp. 163–181. Springer, Berlin (2007)
9. Torra, V.: The Weighted OWA Operator. International Journal of Intelligent Systems 12, 153–156 (1997)
10. Delgado, M., Verdegay, J.L., Vila, M.A.: On aggregation operations of linguistic labels. International Journal of Intellifent Systems 8, 351–370 (1993)
11. Yager, R.R.: Priotized aggregation operators. International Journal of Approximate Reasoning 48, 263–274 (2008)
12. Bryson, N., Mobolurin, A.: An action learning evaluation procedure for multiple criteria decision making problems. European Journal of Operational Research 96, 379–386 (1995)

Group Polarization and Non-positive Social Influence: A Revised Voter Model Study

Zhenpeng Li and Xijin Tang

Institute of Systems Science, Academy of Mathematics and Systems Science,
Chinese Academy of Sciences, Beijing 100190, P.R. China
{lizhenpeng,xjtang}@amss.ac.cn

Abstract. In this paper, we analyze how the non-positive social influence affects group polarization by adding influence factor into the classic voter model. Through model simulation, we observe that a group would self-organize into two-polarization pattern, under no imposing intervention, which is entirely different from the result of drift to an extreme polarization dominant state in the classic voter model.

Keywords: group polarization, non-positive social influence, social identity, voter model, opinions dynamics.

1 Introduction

Research on collective emergence patterns has a long history [1,2]. It is widely studied in management science [3], social psychology [4, 5, 6], economics [7], socio-physics [8], system science [9] and computer science [10] etc. Recently, with the booming of Internet and information technology, especially when it entered into the Web 2.0 era, more and more collective behaviors are observed via Web 2.0 tools, which also provides great opportunities and challenges for this research. With this background, now the topic is maturing into the spotlight for social psychology, social risk emergency management, computer science, marketing and nearly all aspects of Web-based application or online emerging collective behaviors.

In this paper, we focus on one of the important aspects of human collective behaviors—opinions dynamics. We study what's the role that the three kinds of social influence would play for the group polarization, and the intrinsic relationship between three kinds of social influence factors and the group polarization. The rest of the paper is organized as follows: in section II, according to social identity, we discuss three kinds of social influence implication. In section III, we add three types of social influence into the classic voter model. By simulation computing we find an interesting conclusion that a group opinions with binary states could evolve into two-polarization steady pattern. Section IV is our conclusion remark.

B. Hu et al. (Eds.): BI 2011, LNAI 6889, pp. 295–303, 2011.

2 Three Types of Social Influence

Social influence refers to the way people are affected by the thoughts, feelings, and behaviors of others. Like the study of attitudes, it is a traditional, core topic in social psychology. It studies the change in behavior that one person causes in another, intentionally or unintentionally, as a result of the way the changed person perceives themselves in relationship to the influencer, other people and society in general [11]. Social influence occurs when an individual's thoughts, feelings or actions are affected by other people. Social influence takes many forms and can be seen in conformity, socialization, peer pressure, obedience, leadership, persuasion, sales, and marketing. In 1958, Harvard psychologist, Herbert Kelman identified three broad varieties of social influence [12]. Latter development contributors mainly include French (1956) [4], Latané,B.(1981) [5], and Friedkin, N.(1998) [6].

Social influence theory is one important theoretical basis in social science study. Most social simulation literatures consider the principle of homogeneous influence (attraction and social influence, the principle is similarity leads to interaction, and interaction leads to still more similarity). The basic premise is that the more similar an actor is to a neighbor, the more likely that the actor will adopt one of the neighbor's opinion. The homogeneous influence could be considered as "herd behavior" [19] or "information cascade" [20], which means individuals don't consider their own subgroup identity ("do as most people do"). For example, based on the single interaction principle of homogeneous influence, Axelord[13] observed a local convergence and global multiple polarization pattern, the voter model show one polarization opinions dominant result with any initial binary opinions percentage [14,15,16].

However, in respect of mutual influences, heterogeneity repulsion and unsocial attitude can not be ignored in a social system. In other words, individuals' opinions not only depend on homogeneous similarity, but also are influenced by heterogeneous repulsion and unsocial attitudes. We may refer to these three types of influence as "social identity" [17], which assumes that individuals have their own social identity that may belong to different specified social community or tagged social subgroup. Individuals within the same subgroup, share the same tagged consensus, such as beliefs, interests, education or other similar social attributes[18]. Since they share the common social tag (identity), when they face group decision making, homogenous positive influence will play vital role for achieving the group consensus. In this paper, in order to classify different influence factors, this kind of within group homogenous impact is called homogeneous influence.

Individuals within different subgroups find it difficult to gain the agreement when they face group decision making even under the pre-condition that they share the same initial opinions, since they have different social subgroup unified interests, emotions, actions and value orientation. This impact for individuals opinions selection can be named heterogeneous repulsion. The third one, unsocial phenomena is a type of special individuals attitude, in which the individuals do not belong to any tagged subgroup. Members in this group have no common social identity, no firm position about some social opinions and in a state of neither fish nor fowl.

3 Description of The Model

3.1 Classic Voter Model

The voter model [14,15,16] is a simple mathematical model of opinion formation in which voters are located at the nodes of a network, each voter (individual) has an opinion (in the simplest case, -1 or +1), for a randomly chosen voter, its opinion have the chance of being affected by the opinions of its neighbors. It is often used to see how ordered states can appear in systems originally in a state of non-equilibrium. This has several applications in a variety of disciplines including chemistry (reactions between different chemicals), physics (interactions between particles) and social systems (interactions between agents). The model formula is shown as Equ (1)

$$\varpi(-\sigma_i|\sigma_i) = \frac{\beta}{2}(1 - \frac{1}{k}\sum_{j\in n(i)} \sigma_i\sigma_j). \tag{1}$$

Where β is a constant adjustable parameter, $\sigma_i = +1, -1 (i = 1, ..., N)$, N is the group size, voter i opinion "+1" means "for", "-1 " means "against", $n(i)$ denotes for voter $i's$ neighbors, k is the neighbors size. The left term of Equ (1) is the probability that individual i might change it's opinion from ± 1 to ∓ 1 . There is a large number of literatures on the relationship between voter model and different topologies, such as scale-free, small world, lattices [16,21,22]. Especially in lattices, the voter model presents simple non-equilibrium dynamics with nontrivial behavior, hence this model has been extensively studied, most notably by the mathematicians and condensed matter physicists, from various aspects.

3.2 Voter Model with Three Types of Social Influence

In order to further understand the relationship between non-positive social influence and group opinions polarization quantitatively, we adopt three kinds of social influence mechanism on the classic voter model (see Equ (2)) in the topology of lattices. Individuals (voters) are impacted by others and also influence others, as conditioned by valence of the social identity tie:

(A) "+" implies attraction (homophily, similarity) and imitation,

(B) "-" stands for xenophobia (hetereophily instead of homophily) and differentiation (instead of imitation),

(C) "0" denotes for unsocial attitudes.

$$\varpi(-\sigma_i|\sigma_i) = \frac{\beta}{2}(1 - \frac{1}{k}\sum_{j\in n(i)} I_{ij}\sigma_i\sigma_j), \tag{2}$$

where $I_{ij} \in \{-, 0, +\}$. To illustrate how the revised voter model works, an example is given: voter i has the opinion $+1$ while its eight neighbors are all of opinion -1. By setting these values into the equation, considering different social influence cases, when all $I_{ij} = -$, means agent i and its neighbors have no common social identity, the probability that it will change its initial opinion state is 0. When all $I_{ij} = +$, means agent i and its neighbors share the common social identity, the probability that it will change its initial opinion state is 1. when $I_{ij} = +, -$ half half or all equal to 0 , means agent i and its neighbors share half of the common social identity or no firm position, the probability that it will change its initial opinion state is $1/2$. If we don't consider the social identity, we can see that the probability of voter i switching to the opposite state is always equal to 1, this particular case means $I_{ij} = +$, and corresponding to the single homogeneous influence scenarios, the classic voter model. Next, through simulation, we would like to find out what result come out if we consider the three types of social influences on the classic voter model in a closed lattice community.

3.3 Simulation Implementation

The revised voter model simulation is implemented as the followings pseudo-code: Fix β, T (final step of simulation)and group size N.

```
Step I: initial each voter i's opinion state, and social influences matrix I
for i = 1 : N
            initialize σ_i = ±1;
     for j = 1 : N
            initialize I_ij = +1, 0, −1;
      end
end
Step II: compute Equ (2), obtain voter i's opinion possible commutable
      probability Pr_value;
Step III: update voter i opinion state at each time step t
for t = 1 : T
      given threshold τ_I = rand();
            if Pr_value > τ_I and σ_i = ∓1
                        σ_i = ±1;
            else if Pr_value > τ_I and σ_i = ±1
                        σ_i = ∓1;
            end
            if Pr_value <= τ_I and σ_i = ∓1
                        σ_i = ∓1;
            else if Pr_value <= τ_I and σ_i = ±1
                        σ_i = ±1;
            end
end
```

3.4 Simulation and Discussion

In our simualtion we set $\beta = 1$, the neighbor size $k = 8$, the topology is 100×100 periodic boundaries lattices, $T = 10^4$. Fig. 1 show that the classic voter model final "+1" percentage fluctuation against time step t, in the end, it is

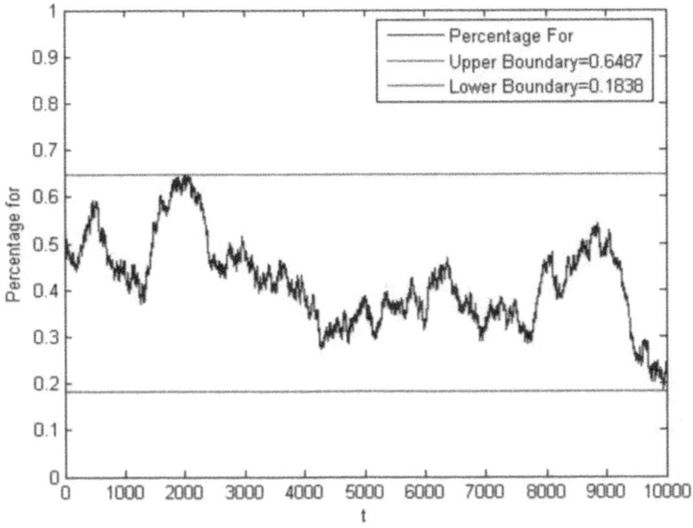

Fig. 1. Classic voter model one polarization dominant state with time evolution (50% for or "+1" initialization)

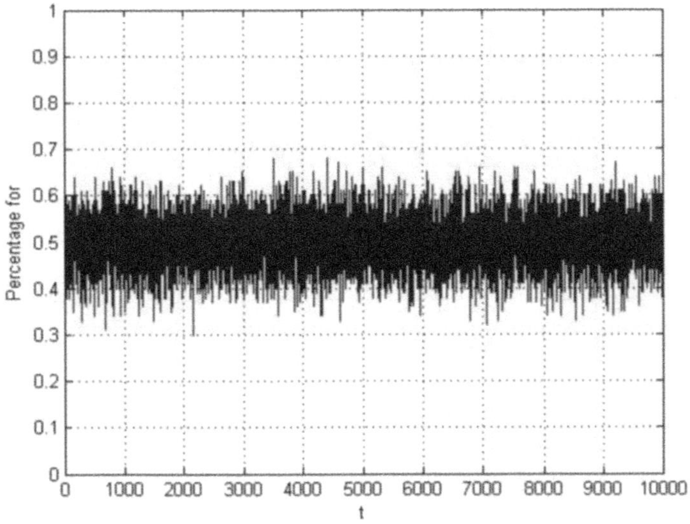

Fig. 2. Revised voter model two polarization steady state against time t (10% for or "+1" initialization)

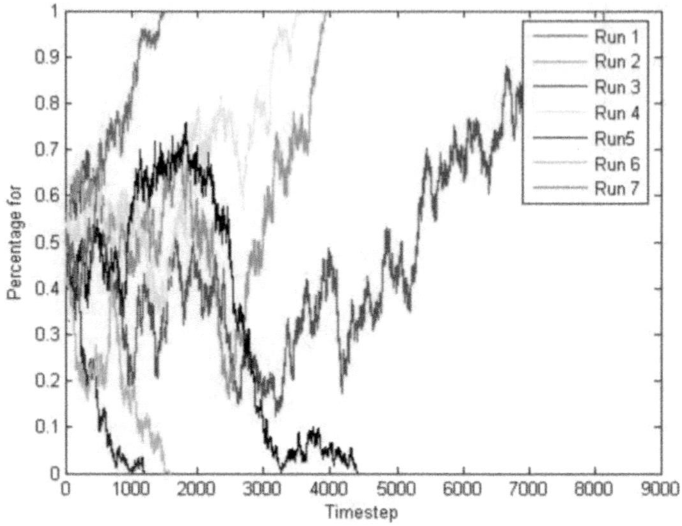

Fig. 3. Classic voter model one polarization dominant trend. Percentage for "for" variation in 7 times runs. Each of the runs was initialized under the same conditions (50% for initialization).

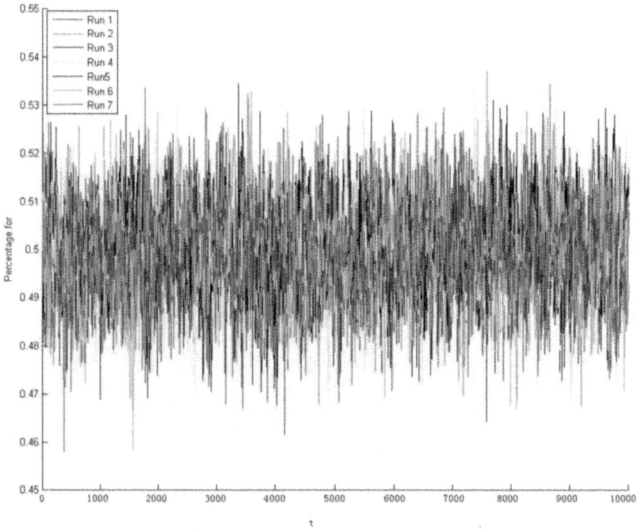

Fig. 4. Revised voter model opinions dynamics two polarization steady states. Percentage for "+1" variation in 7 times runs. Each of the runs was initiated under the same conditions (50% for initialization).

prone to reach one polarization steady state even with 50% "+1" initialization. Fig. 2 show the revised voter model with 3 kinds of social influence final "+1" percentage tend to 50%, although in the case with initial 10% "+1 ".

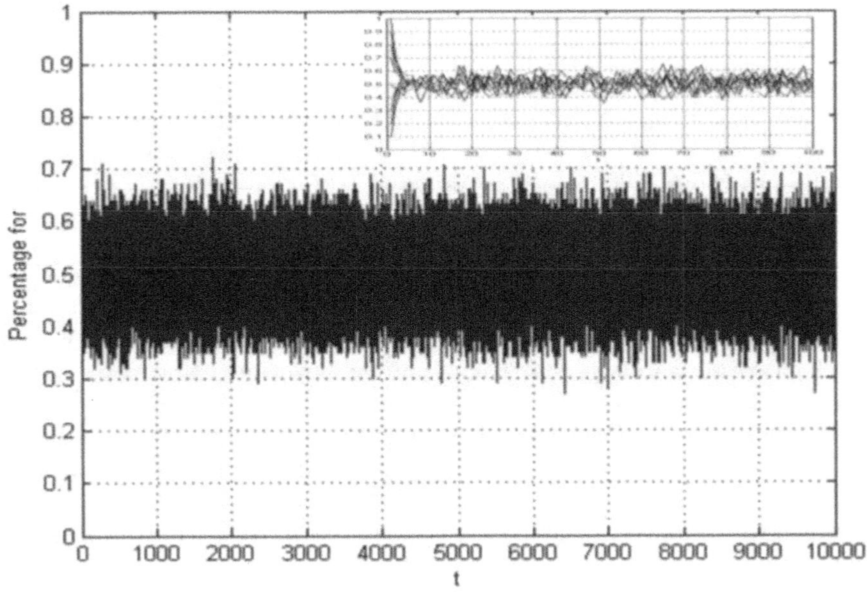

Fig. 5. Population for over time for 10 different initial for percentage

Further model analysis as shown in Fig.3, even with the initial percentage for "+1" is 50%, multiple runs still saw the classic voter model reach an "absorbing" or one polarization dominant state. On the contrary, we observe the two polarization opinions well-matched steady equilibrium in Fig. 4, that interesting result we can not obtain in the original voter model.

In addition, Fig. 5 shows percentage "for" (state=+1) variation in 10 times runs. Each of the runs was initialized under the conditions of "for" from 10% to 100%. The inset plot show that two antagonistic well matched cliques appear easily and convergent to stable soon. This result illustrate that even at a very low/high 'for" percentage the revised voter model still reverse direction and move back to a steady state of two-polarization equilibrium. moreover the convergent rate of reaching two polarization steady equilibrium is very soon, nearly within 10 time steps. That important simulation result tell us the social homogeneity is highly brittle.

With heterogeneous exclusion ("-") and unsocial ("0") factors into the classic voter model, we clearly see that a group opinions homogeneous consensus could not be realized, except the non-positive repulsion impact is eliminated.

4 Conclusions

In this paper, we consider three kinds of social influences implication based on social identity theory. Especially, after we add the three types of social influences into the classic voter model, simulation observes one fascinating result: a state of two-polarization equilibrium will appear soon even at a very low/high percentage "for", which is completely different from the result of drift to a single "+1/-1" extreme one polarization dominant state in the classic voter model. It is also shown that the consensus could not occur with considering the non-positive social influence as does on regular two-dimensional lattices, instead the system settles in a stationary state with coexisting opinions two-polarization. This result also well agrees with the conclusion drawn by Castellano et al[16], and is consistent with the earlier work on structural balance [23].

The original voter model emphasized the global stability of social homogeneity, where convergence to one leading polarization is almost irresistible in closely interacting populations. However, the voter model with some "influence ties" to be negative or zero suggests that social homogeneous stable state is highly brittle.

This study also demonstrates that in-group/out-group differentiation and rejection antagonism are the emergent properties of social network self-organization, and are labelled in the voters' cognitive architectures as assumed by social identity theory, our argument is different with the conclusion that agents' cognitive are not inscribed in Macy's work[4] .

We contribute to this literature by looking into "facet" of self-identity of group members. Our findings indicate that the voting behavior of heterogeneous group is, in fact, different from that of homogeneous. The prism of social identity theory, which holds that people maintain an "us" versus "them" portrait during the processes of the collective behaviors is the explanation of heterogeneous group voting result.

Acknowledgments. This work is supported by the National Basic Research Program of China (973 Program) under Grant No. 2010CB731405 and was supported in part by the Project of Knowledge Innovation Program (PKIP) of Chinese Academy of Sciences, Grant No. KJCX2.YW.W10.

References

1. MacKay, C.: Extraordinary popular delusions and the madness of crowds. Harmony Books, New York (1980) (1841, reprint 1980)
2. Le Bon, G.: The crowd: A study of popular mind, Larlin, Marietta, GA (1896)
3. Simon, H.A.: Bandwagon and underdog effects and the possibility of election predictions. Public Opinion Quarterly 18, 245–253 (1954)
4. Latané, B.: The psychology of social impact. American Psychologist 36, 343–365 (1981)
5. Friedkin, N.: A structural theory of social influence. Cambridge University Press, Cambridge (1998)
6. Blume, L., Durlauf, S.: The economy as an evolving complex system III. Oxford University Press, Oxford (2004)
7. Stauffer, D.: Sociophysics simulations II: opinion dynarnics. In: AIP Conference Proceedings, Granada, Spain, vol. 779, pp. 56–68 (2005)

8. Hummel, R., Member Manevitz, L.A.: Statistical approach to the representation of uncertainty in beliefs using spread of opinions. IEEE Tranactions on System, Man, Cybernetics-Part A: System and Human 26(3), 378–384 (1996)
9. Segaran, T.: Programming Collective Intelligence: Building Smart Web 2.0 Applications. O'Reilly Media, Sebastopol (2007)
10. Asch, S.E.: Effects of group pressure upon the modification and distortion of judgement. In: Guetzkow, H. (ed.) Groups, Leadership and Men. Carnegie Press, Pittsburgh (1951)
11. Kelman, H.: Compliance, identification, and internalization: Three processes of attitude change. Journal of Conflict Resolution 1, 51–60 (1958)
12. Axelrod, R.: The dissemination of culture: A model with local convergence and global polarization. Journal of Conflict Resolution 41(2), 203–226 (1997)
13. Clifford, P., Sudbury, A.: A model for spatial conflict. Biometrika 60(3), 581–588 (1973)
14. Holley, R., Liggett, T.: Ergodic theorems for weakly interacting infinite systems and the voter model. The Annals of Probability 3(4), 643–663 (1975)
15. Castellano, C., Vilone, D., Vespignani, A.: Incomplete Ordering of the voter model on Small-World Networks. Euro. Physics Letters 63(1), 153–158 (2003)
16. Tajfel, H.: Social identity and intergroup relations. Cambridge University Press, Cambridge (1982)
17. Prentice-Dunn, S., Rogers, R.W.: Deindividuation in aggression. In: Green, R.G., Donnerstein, E. (eds.) Aggression: Theoretical and Empirical Reviews, vol. 2(issues in Research), pp. 155–177. Academic Press, New York (1983)
18. Raafat, R.M., Chater, N., Frith, C.: Herding in humans. Trends in Cognitive Sciences (2009)
19. Bikhchandani, S., David, H., Welch, I.: A Theory of Fads, Fashion, Custom, and Cultural Change as Informational Cascades. Journal of Political Economy 100(5), 992–1026 (1992)
20. Suchecki, K., Eguiluz, V., Miguel, M.: Voter model dynamics in complex networks: role of dimensionality, disorder, and degree distribution. Physical Review E 72, 036132 (2005b)
21. Barabsi, A.L., Albert, R.: Emergence of scaling in random networks. Science, 286–509 (1999)
22. Cartwright, D., Harary, F.: Structural balance: A generalization of Heider's theory. Psy. Rev. 62, 277–293 (1966)
23. Macy, M.W., Kitts, J., Flache, A., Benard, S.: Polarization in Dynamic Networks: A Hopfield Model of Emergent Structure. In: Dynamic Social Network Modeling and Analysis. National Academy Press, Washington, DC (2003)
24. French Jr., J.R.P.: A Formal Theory of Social Power. The Psychological Review 63, 181–194 (1956)

On-Demand Dynamic Recommendation Mechanism in Support of Enhancing Idea Creativity for Group Argumentation*

Xi Xia and Xiaoji Zhou

China Aerospace Engineering Consultation Center
No.16 Fuchen Road, Haidian District, Beijing, China
xiaxi@amss.ac.cn, zh_xj@sina.com

Abstract. Versatile computerized aids for group argumentation for idea generation during problem solving process is becoming highlight research. In this paper, we propose a novel recommendation mechanism in the context of group argumentation, called On-demand Dynamic Recommendation Mechanism, which extracts user preferences from implicit and explicit feedbacks and provides personalized recommendation based on users' utterances and demands. The valuable reference provided by the mechanism could be accumulated to form a knowledge immersion environment to satisfy ever changing demand of users in support of facilitating idea creativity during the process of group discussion.

Keywords: Meta-synthesis, Group argumentation, On-demand recommendation, Dynamic recommendation, Knowledge creation.

1 Introduction

In early 1990s, Chinese system scientist X. S. Qian proposed the concept of Hall of Workshop for Meta-synthetic Engineering(HWMSE), which is utilized to solve unstructured problem by integrating qualitative and quantitative knowledge and by means of human-machine collaboration [7]. HWMSE, expected to enable knowledge creation and wisdom emergence, emphasizes the active roles of human beings during human-machine collaboration. Moreover, HWMSE could be treated as a more advanced form than group decision support system for group argumentation [11].

Group argumentation, especially held in most expert meeting, academic seminars, etc, is regarded as a convenient and efficient way to acquire ideas or knowledge from participants for new option or solutions towards complex problems. In this context, it often demands for collaboration with experts from various fields to carry out communication and innovative thinking. Versatile computerized aids for group argumentation for idea generation during problem solving process are developed in many researches[12], ranging from visualization of participant

* Sponsored by China Postdoctoral Science Foundation.

B. Hu et al. (Eds.): BI 2011, LNAI 6889, pp. 304–315, 2011.

opinions structure to text-mining of external information, from clustering of contributed opinions to evaluation of subjective participation.

Nevertheless, less quantitative analysis on the effect of those aids on knowledge creating process. Besides, in the course of discussion, a participant needs a lot of pertinent knowledge for reference. The valuable reference could be accumulated to form a knowledge immersion environment, thus facilitate idea creation for participants. Then, it is becoming an interesting and important problem — how to play a value-added feature for HWMSE such as knowledge creation to improve the efficiency of complex problem solving; specifically, how to better understand participants needs and integrate the knowledge for customization service to recommend information matching participants' inner demands during the problem solving process.

There are several intuitive strategies to attack this problem. One approach is to apply models from other recommendation systems[5,9] straightforward. However, this is intractable, since there is no previous rating for recommendation at the beginnings of discussion and recommendation should be dynamic because participant requirements may change along with progress of the discussion. In addition, the most preferred reference may not be the most needed. For example, as the authority of a field, an expert may be much more familiar with the reference of the field than others, and what he or she talks about are mainly within the field, then neither interest-based recommendation nor recommendation based on similarity between topic and expert's opinion can be an effective choice. Particularly, when he or she, as an expert, but not an expert in the field of discussion topic questioned the topic, information in the field related to the topic is more needed to answer his or her question and thus more conducive to the progress of discussion than that most relevance to his or her research field.

In this paper, we propose an on-demand dynamic recommendation mechanism for enhancing idea creation during the process of group argumentation as an effective aid for HWMSE. This mechanism allows us to recommend documents iteratively to satisfy participants' changing needs during the whole discussion process, which is supposed as a course of knowledge creating.

The rest of the paper is organized as follows. In the next section, we propose the recommendation mechanism. In section 3, we create profiles for both users and documents. In section 4, preference and demand is extracted through user-document similarity, user-document rating and demand analysis. In section 5, we generate a hybrid recommendation that considers utterance, response and demand of users. In section 6, a recommendation metric and updating are presented. Finally, we conclude the paper and give some future works.

2 Proposed Recommendation Mechanism

In this study we develop a recommendation mechanism in the context of group argumentation, called on-demand dynamic recommendation mechanism(ODRM), which extracts user preferences from implicit and explicit feedbacks and provides personalized recommendation dynamically based on users' utterances and ever changing demands.

2.1 The Motivation of ODRM

Our motivation of proposing on-demand dynamic recommendation mechanism in group argumentation environment is to produce valuable, dynamic and measurable recommendations, and consequently to form a knowledge immersion environment in support of knowledge sharing and facilitating idea creation.

To produce customized recommendations, we propose to analyze the demands of user by considering both internal and external factors, and to treat feedbacks of interest preference of users after recommendation, to construct the next recommendation list based on users' preferred information and inner demands, so it allows for better understanding of users needs, increasing users satisfaction and as a result, the progress of discussion is improved.

To make the recommendations dynamic, we consider to generate user profile by user current utterance and recommend though utilizing the attributes of documents to match user profiles. As utterances express participants' current standpoints and ideas which may change during group argumentation process, the more similar between utterance and document, the more common interests they share. This ensures recommendation recursive and iterative to satisfy ever changing demands of user.

To make the recommendations measurable, we estimate the impact of personalized recommendation every time. At the end of the meeting, measurement of the recommendation mechanism is the weighted average evaluation of recommendations for each user.

2.2 The Framework of ODRM

Fig. 1 graphically depicts the overall procedure of on-demand dynamic recommendation mechanism, which is divided into four phases: profile generation, preference and demand extraction, recommendation generation, and updating. The former three phases compose a recommendation process showed as the left part of Fig. 1, and the last phase ensures the recommendation dynamically updating to satisfy the changing demand of users, showed as the right part of Fig. 1.

In phase 1, user profile and document profile are created for two parts, respectively. In user profile, the one part is a vector of a user utterances, and the other is a rating vector of all keywords of documents. In document profile, the one part is vector of document attributes, the other is a binary vector that represents which keywords the document contains.

In phase 2, user preference is extracted from similarity between a user and a document, as well as response of user for recommendation. User demand is extracted by analyzing internal and external factors, such as topic of the discussion, user's attitude to the topic, etc.

In phase 3, two recommendation results are created from the two parts of profile through methods of Naive Bayes Classifier and Item-based Collaborative Filtering respectively. Demand-based recommendation result is generated by needs analysis in matrix form. The final recommendation list is offering in accordance with the weighted average value of ranking in the three results.

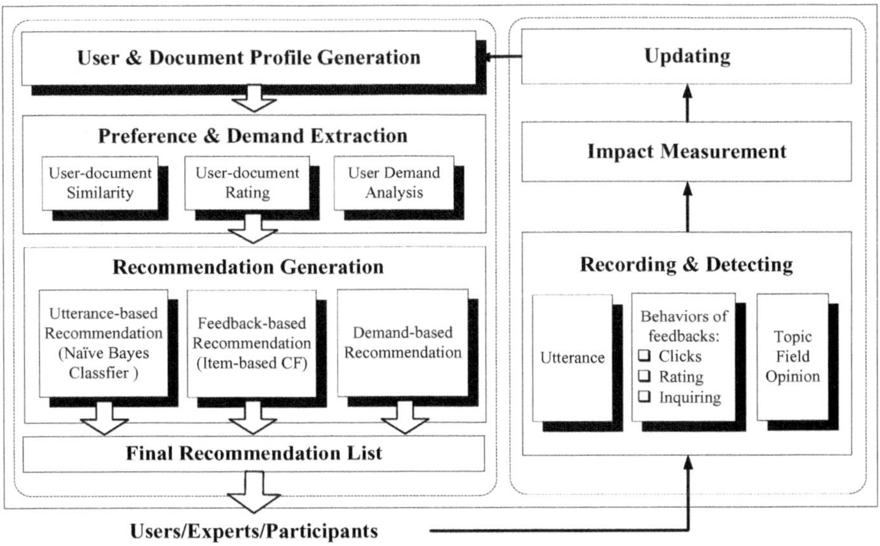

Fig. 1. Overall procedure of ODRM

In phase4, by recording and detecting the new topic, user standpoints and response for previous recommendation, we can measure the impact of personalized service, and updating information for the next recommendation process as long as the meeting or requirement for recommendation is not terminated.

3 Phase1: Profile Generation

In order to conduct a personalized recommendation process, it is necessary to understand users through profile building and deliver personalized recommendation offering based on the knowledge about the users and the documents[1], which signifies the importance of profile creation for both users and documents.

The utterance of participants express their standpoints and idea. User's profile can be established only when his or her view is presented. Additionally, user behaviors of feedbacks for recommendation reveal his or her interest preference, so the feedbacks can be an important component of user's profile.

We define (U, G) as a user's profile, which is consist of two parts: U that denotes utterances he or she has given, and G, rating feedbacks for recommendations.

A typical approach for representing the content of a document in information retrieval is to use a keyword vector or the abstract of the document if it has. If necessary, the full-text can also be used. Then, a document profile denoted as (A, B) involves two parts: A that denotes keywords, abstract, or words for full-text of the document, and B that denotes a binary vector representing which keywords the document contains.

3.1 The First Part of Profile Creation

Let $E = \{e_1, e_2, \ldots, e_n\}$ be the set of all participants and $D = \{d_1, d_2, \ldots, d_m\}$ be the set of all possible documents for reference. The first part of user profile is a union of the user's utterances he or she has given, which is denoted as $(U_i^1, U_i^1, \ldots, U_i^k)$, where U_i^k is the k-th utterance given by user e_i.

Keywords-Based. In this situation, we extract keywords from utterance to present its features. The profile of user e_i for the k-th utterance based on keywords is denoted as $U_i^k = \{u_{i,1}^k, u_{i,2}^k, \ldots, u_{i,m_1}^k\}$, where m_1 is the total number of keywords for U_i^k. The profile of document D_j based on keywords is denoted as: $A_j = \{a_{j,1}, a_{j,2}, \ldots, a_{j,l_1}\}$, where l_1 is the total number of keywords for D_j.

Full-Text-Based. The profile of user e_i for the k-th utterance based on full-text is denoted as $\hat{U}_i^k = \{\hat{u}_{i,1}^k, \hat{u}_{i,2}^k, \ldots, \hat{u}_{i,m_2}^k\}$, where m_2 is the total number of keywords in $\hat{U}_i^k$. The profile of document D_j based on text is denoted as: $\hat{A}_j = \{\hat{a}_{j,1}, \hat{a}_{j,2}, \ldots, \hat{a}_{j,l_2}\}$, where l_2 is the total number of words in D_j.

3.2 The Second Part of Profile Creation

We combine keywords from all over the documents for reference to construct a keywords set. The second part of a user profile is a vector of average preferred values for all keywords rated by the user. That is denoted as $(g_{i1}, g_{i2}, \ldots, g_{iS})$, where S is the total number of keywords set, g_{is} is the average value of the s-th keyword rated by user e_i. If a user e_i rated a recommended document d_j after reading it, then the keywords of the document share the same value of rating.

We define $(b_{j1}, b_{j2}, \ldots, b_{jS})$ as the second part of profile for document d_j, which is consist of a binary vector, depicted as equation(3.1):

$$b_{js} = \begin{cases} 1 & \text{if document } d_j \text{ has the } s\text{-th keyword} \\ 0 & \text{otherwise} \end{cases} \quad (3.1)$$

4 Phase2: Preference and Demand Extraction

We understand user preference by measuring similarity between a user and a document, and calculating the value of a document rated by a user. In order to identify and extract user requirements, we analyze internal and external factors that may leverage user needs, such as topic of discussion, view of use and his or her research background, etc.

4.1 User-Document Similarity

To construct the relationship between a user and a document, we need an approach to measure the affinity between them. We define the similarity measure between user's utterance and documents in two ways:(1) common words (2) a probabilistic way.

Common Words. The similarity between the view of user e_i and the concept of document d_j is measured by calculating the number of keywords that co-occur in them in the proportion of the number of their keywords union, $com_{e,d}$, which is given by

$$sim(U_i, A_j) = com_{e,d} = \frac{|U_i \bigcap A_j|}{|U_i \bigcup A_j|} \tag{4.1}$$

where U_i and A_j are row vectors of the first part of user profile and document profile respectively. Thus, $sim(U_i, A_j)$ is a number between 0 and 1.

A Probabilistic Way. In this way, we regard each user as a class, and the conditional probability of a text document d_j labeled in user class e_i as the similarity between them, which can be denoted as $sim(U_i, P_j) = P(e_i|d_j)$.

4.2 User-Document Rating

There exist three popular methods for extracting user preferences: direct, semi-direct, and indirect extraction[8], which are based on explicit, semi-implicit, and implicit feedbacks respectively.

Explicit Feedbacks. The direct approach asks the user to tell the system explicitly what he or she prefers, and user preference is extracted directly from what his or her query or searching during the process of discussion.

Semi-implicit Feedbacks. The semi-direct approach asks the user to rate all documents he or she has read, and user preference is extracted from the relevance feedback provided by ratings.

Implicit Feedbacks. The indirect approach captures user preference from browsing behavior recorded by the computer, such as recommendation clicks or time spent on reading a document[4].

The feedbacks mentioned above can be integrated to measure the rating of a document with a user.

4.3 User Demand Analysis

To better grasp demand of user, relevance factors need to be analyzed. Documents that is most relevance to topic of discussion is valuable, which can help for further understanding the issue. Additionally, standpoint of user is necessary to extract user demand. The research background of a user also reveals information in which areas needs least or most to be concerned about.

We propose a sort of demand analysis method for user in group argumentation environment, called $ANSO$ to analyze the current state for both external and internal, including current topic of the discussion, user current viewpoint to the topic—support, dispute or objection, the relationship between the field of topic and user research area, etc. $ANSO$ presents *Advantage*, *No advantage*,

Support and *Objection* respectively. Advantage means that a user who is the expert within the field of topic, has authority and advantage for discussion. No advantage means that the user who is expert outside the field of topic, has no advantage for argumentation. Support means that the user support for the topic. Objection means the user oppose to the issue.

The method enables us to extract four kinds of demand for internal and external matching, that is, AS-demand, AO-demand, NS-demand, and NO-demand.

***AS*-demand.** When a user who is professional in the field of topic holds supportive attitude, he or she knows well about the knowledge in the field thus needs information in different opinions to broaden thinking.

***AO*-demand.** When a user who is expert in the area of topic holds opposing or questioned views, what he or she demand most is not materials to support his view, but reference from other perspectives to enhance critical thinking.

***NS*-demand.** When a user support to a topic, to the field of which he or she has no advantages, the user firstly needs more information most pertinent to the topic to learn more knowledge about the area for reference. Moreover, to better understand the knowledge in the area and to facilitate divergent thinking for creation, the user need the reference closely related to his or her familiar or proficient area.

***NO*-demand.** When a user oppose to a topic, but he or she is not the expert of the field, the most popular documents may satisfy his or her demand during the process of group argumentation.

5 Phase3: Recommendation Generation

Our recommendation principle is that a document the closer related to user utterance, the more should be recommended; the higher rated, the more should be recommended; the more needed, the more should be recommended, since the similarity reveals common interest, high rating demonstrates interest preference, and demand reflects the value of information. Those documents that have been recommended and rated previously should be excluded from the reference for the user.

We make utterance-based recommendation by the first part of profiles, and feedback-based recommendation by the second part, respectively. Besides, demand-based recommendation is developed according to discussion process and user proposition. The choice from or the combination of the three recommendation is the final recommendation.

5.1 Utterance-Based Recommendation

Utterance-based recommendation uses attributes of the document to match user utterance profiles. If the user-document similarity is defined in common words way, as calculated by equation(4.1), then the recommendation of the top-N most similar documents is produced. If it is defined in a probabilistic way, the multinomial model of Naive Bayes Classifier can be employed for utterance-based recommendation[6].

In this approach, we regard each user as a class. A document is an ordered sequence of word events, drawn from the same vocabulary V. We assume that the lengths of documents are independent of class[3]. We again make a similar naive Bayes assumption: that the probability of each word event in a document is independent of the word's context and position in the document. We use the first part of document d_j profile which is assumed as $A_j = (a_1, a_2, \ldots, a_{l_2})$, where a_t is a word on the t-th position of document d_j. Then, the posterior probability of a document d_j labeled in class e_i is given as equation(5.1):

$$P(e_i|d_j) = \frac{P(d_j|e_i)P(e_i)}{P(d_j)} \tag{5.1}$$

where class prior parameters are calculated as equation(5.2):

$$P(e_i) = \frac{|e_i|}{\sum_{s=1}^{n} |e_s|} \tag{5.2}$$

With the naive Bayes assumption mentioned before, we have equation(5.3) as follows :

$$P(d_j|e_i) = P(a_1, \ldots, a_{l_2}|e_i) = \prod_t P(a_t|e_i) \tag{5.3}$$

Define N_{it} to be the count of the number of times word w_t of document d_j occurs in utterances labeled in class e_i, N_i to be the sum of the word positions in class e_i, $|V|$ to be the sum of the number of different words. Then, the estimate of the probability of the word a_t in class e_i is:

$$P(a_t|e_i) = \frac{N_{it} + 1}{N_i + |V|} \tag{5.4}$$

For each class e_i, we regard the union of other classes as $\overline{e_i}$. Then, according to the Total Probability Formula, we have:

$$P(d_j) = P(e_i, d_j) + P(\overline{e_i}, d_j) = P(e_i)P(d_j|e_i) + P(\overline{e_i})P(d_j|\overline{e_i}) \tag{5.5}$$

where, $P(\overline{e_i})$ and $P(d_j|\overline{e_i})$ denote the probability of other classes except for class e_i, and the conditional probability $P(a_1, a_2, \ldots, a_{l_2}|\overline{e_i})$, respectively.

Hence, the similarity between U_i and A_j is given by equation(5.6):

$$sim(U_i, A_j) = P(e_i|d_j) = \frac{P(d_j|e_i)P(e_i)}{P(e_i)P(d_j|e_i) + P(\overline{e_i})P(d_j|\overline{e_i})} \tag{5.6}$$

We recommend the top-N most similar documents to a user by means of title and keywords, which helps the participants to find common interest, stimulate further thinking. We define the recommendation list 1 as $RL_1 = (rl_{11}, rl_{12}, \ldots, rl_{1N})$.

5.2 Feedback-Based Recommendation

For the feedbacks, item-based collaborative filtering approach[10] is employed to make a recommendation list by the second part of profiles.

The rating of documents that has not be given can be predicted by the rating values of other documents, which can be calculated by following formula:

$$H_{i,j} = \sum_{s=1}^{S} b_{js} \times g_{is} \tag{5.7}$$

Then the rating of documents d_j by user e_i is:

$$R_{ij} = \begin{cases} H_{ij} & \text{if } r_{ij} = 0 \\ r_{ij} & \text{otherwise} \end{cases} \tag{5.8}$$

Hence we recommend the Top-N maximum rating documents to user e_i as the k-th recommendation. We define the recommendation list 2 as $RL_2 = (rl_{21}, rl_{22}, \ldots, rl_{2N})$.

5.3 Demand-Based Recommendation

We construct demand-based recommendation in accordance with the four kinds of demands extracted by $ANSO$ analysis. Different recommendation modes are matched for distinct demands.

As long as the user is the expert within the filed of topic, we conduct reverse recommendation. That is, materials support to the topic are recommended to users with counterview to the topic, and vice versa. For the AS-demand, recommendation should be associated with the theme of discussion but support for an opposite point of view to the topic. For the AO-demand, recommendation should be both topic related and supported. For the NS-demand, recommendation should be the most popular in the topic area and most relevance to the user research area. For the NO-demand, recommendation that is the most popular or with the highest rating score in topic area would be valuable reference for the user.

The recommendation mentioned above can be integrated into a matrix form illustrated as Fig. 2.

5.4 Final Recommendation

For the two parts of user's profile, we construct two recommendation lists respectively by steps mentioned above. Additionally, a recommendation based on user demand is built. Final recommendation result can be a choice of recommendations based on utterance, feedback or demand, as well as a hybrid one of the three.

Each document to be recommended has a weight in accordance with the ranking placed in recommendation list, so the final value of the document that should be recommended is the weighted average of its rankings. Then the hybrid final recommendation list is produced.

External / Internal	Advantage	No advantage
Support	**AS-demand recommendation:** • Topic related • Opposite to topic	**NS-demand recommendation:** • Most popular or with the highest rating score in the topic field • Most relevance to user research area
Objection	**AO-demand recommendation:** • Topic related • Support to topic	**NO-demand recommendation:** • Most popular or with the highest rating score in the topic field

Fig. 2. Recommendation matrix

6 Phase4: Updating

In this phase, user behaviors of reaction on recommendation are detected and recorded by the system, impact of personalized recommendation is measured, user profiles are updating, and analysis on user demands is renewing.

6.1 Impact Measure

Measurement of personalized recommendation impact is conducted to quantitatively analyze extent of attentions paid by participants for information recommended. To evaluate the quality of the recommendation list, F-measure have been widely used in recommender systems research[2]. F-measure that gives equal weight to both recall and precision is employed to estimate our performances of recommendation. The formula of F-measure is depicted as follows:

$$F_{ki} = \frac{2 \times Precision_{ki} \times Precision_{ki}}{Recall_{ki} + Precision_{ki}} \tag{6.1}$$

$$Precision_{ki} = \frac{m_{ki}}{N} \tag{6.2}$$

$$Recall_{ki} = \frac{m_{ki}}{M_k} \tag{6.3}$$

where, F_{ki} is the impact measurement of the k-th recommendation for user e_i, $Precision_{ki}$ is the precision metric, and $Recall_{ki}$ is the recall metric. m_{ki} is the number of documents that user e_i interests for the k-th recommendation, N is the number of documents in recommendation list, M_k is the total number of documents that are about to be recommended for the k-th time.

Hence, the measurement of the total performance for personalized recommendation is the average value of the measurement or all recommendations. The formula is given as equation(6.4):

$$F = \frac{\sum_{k=1}^{K} \sum_{i=1}^{n} F_{ki}}{K \times n} \tag{6.4}$$

6.2 Recommendation Updating

Along with the process of group argumentation, user profile is updating or changing by his or her latest statement, interest preference of the recommended documents, and the behavior of the relevance information inquiry. We use the updating profile and renewed demand analysis to assess the potential interest and requirement of the user in various documents, thus to make a new on-demand recommendation for the user during discussion.

7 Concluding Remarks

In this paper, we presented a recommendation mechanism in the context of group argumentation, which can extracts user preferences though his or her implicit and explicit feedbacks and provides personalized recommendation service based on user's utterance and demand to satisfy ever changing need of users. The valuable reference provided by our recommendation mechanism could be accumulated to form a knowledge immersion environment, thus facilitate idea creation for participants.

Our current work is still at very initial stage from both research and practice. We will keep trying to improve the system to facilitate knowledge sharing and idea creation. Lots of further work are under exploration, such as better human-machine interaction, optimization of recommendation efficiency, and evolving process of group preference and demand changing to detect the path way of knowledge creation, etc. More experiments will also be undertaken for verification and validation of recommendation mechanism in practice.

References

1. Adomavicius, G., Tuzhilin, A.: Personalization techiniques: a process-oriented perspective. Communication of the ACM 48, 83–90 (2005)
2. Cho, Y.H., Kim, J.K., Kim, S.H.: A personalized reommmender system based on Web usage mining and decision tree induction. Expert Systems with Applications 23(3), 329–342 (2002)
3. Domingos, P., Pazzani, M.: On the optimality of the simple Bayesian classifier under zero-one loss. Machine Learning 29, 103–130 (1997)
4. Liang, T.P., Lai, H.J.: Discovering user interests from web browsing behavior: an application to Internet news services. In: Proceedings of the 35th Annual Hawaii International Conference on System Sciences, Big Island, Hawaii, USA, pp. 203–212 (2002)
5. Liang, T.P., Yang, Y.F., Chen, D.N., Ku, Y.C.: A semantic-expansion Approach to Personalized Knowlege Recommendation. Decision Support Systems 45(3), 401–412 (2008)
6. McCallum, A., Nigam, K.: A comparison of event models for naive Bayes text classification. In: AAAI-1998 Workshop on Learning for Text Categorization. Tech. Rep. WS-98-05. AAAI Press, Menlo Park (1998)

7. Qian, X.S., Yu, J.Y., Dai, R.W.: A new Discipline of Science - the Study of Open Complex Giant System and its Methodology. Chinese Journal of Systems Engineering & Electronics 4(2), 2–12 (1993)
8. Sakagami, H., Kamba, T.: Learning personal preferences on online newspaper articles from user behaviors. Computer Networks and ISDN Systems 29, 1447–1455 (1997)
9. Sarwar, B., Karypis, G., Konstan, J.A., Riedl, J.: Analysis of recommendation algorithms for e-commerce. In: Proceedings of the ACM E-Commerce, pp. 158–167 (2000)
10. Sarwar, B., Karypis, G.: Item-based Collaborative Filtering Recommendation Algorithm. In: Proceedings of the 10th International World Wide Web Conference, Hong Kong, China (2001)
11. Tang, X.J.: Towards Meta-Synthetic Support to Unstructured Problem Solving. In: Chen, G.Y., et al. (eds.) Proceedings of the Fourth International Conference on Systems Science and Systems Engineering, pp. 203–209. Global-Link Publisher (2003)
12. Tang, X.J., Liu, Y.J., Zhang, W.: Computerized Support for Idea Generation During Knowledge Creating Process. In: Khosla, R., Howlett, R.J., Jain, L.C. (eds.) KES 2005. LNCS (LNAI), vol. 3684, pp. 437–443. Springer, Heidelberg (2005)

Utilizing Knowledge Based Mechanisms in Automated Feature Recognition Processes

Hao Lan Zhang[1] and Christian Van der Velden[2]

[1] NIT, Zhejiang University
haolan.zhang@nit.zju.edu.cn
[2] BAE Systems Australia
christian.vandervelden@baesystems.com

Abstract. Modern engineering design, analysis and manufacturing activities rely heavily on software to handle increasing volumes of data and model complexity. Automated Feature Recognition (AFR) technologies are highly demanded by manufacturing sectors since AFR can efficiently improve the performance of Computer-Aided Design (CAD) processes and reduce costs. Nevertheless, most existing FR applications are confronting various problems of processing CAD models in the manufacturing industry, such as aerospace and automobile industries. The missing link between CAD models and knowledge-based tools is one of the major obstacles. This research project investigates the feasibility and benefits of bridging the gap between knowledge based mechanisms and CAD models, and suggests a knowledge-based AFR approach for tackling AFR problems occurring in the computer-aid manufacturing design process. The AFR system significantly reduces time and costs of analysing CAD models for downstream design processes.

Keywords: Knowledge-based Systems, Feature Recognition, Enterprise Information System, CAD.

1 Introduction

The demands for reducing time consumption and improving the efficiency for analysing CAD models design have been rising in the past two decades. Nonetheless, current development in the CAD area cannot fulfil the requirements from the industry sector due to the missing link between CAD model design and knowledge based tools [1]. The application of AFR mechanisms to the CAD model design process has been embraced by researchers and system developers. The AFR systems have the potential to reduce the development costs through facilitating the automated construction of analysis and manufacturing models, and reducing workloads [2].

This paper describes a knowledge-based AFR system, which is based on a set of classified CAD entities and their topological and geometrical details. The AFR system incorporates the knowledge-based mechanisms into the feature recognition process, which efficiently bridges the gap between CAD models and knowledge based tools. The knowledge-based AFR system mainly focuses on feature recognition and extraction of common aerospace structural components, in particular stiffened panels.

B. Hu et al. (Eds.): BI 2011, LNAI 6889, pp. 316–326, 2011.

The AFR knowledge base developed consists of three major layers, i.e. the knowledge editor layer, knowledge representation layer, and knowledge inference layer. These three layers refer to the three levels of knowledge including domain, task, and process knowledge, respectively.

The knowledge editor layer (domain level) enables system users to define and modify rules, constraints, and domain knowledge, which can be used in the other two layers. The knowledge representation layer (task level) focuses on acquiring specific topological and geometrical knowledge from CAD models based on domain knowledge, and generating structured knowledge representation. The knowledge inference layer (process level) focuses on processing and generating the AFR results based on existing inference techniques and the information from the other two layers. The remainder of the paper is organized as follows. The next section reviews existing FR methods. Section 3 introduces the AFR design framework. Section 4 illustrates the knowledge-base design of the AFR system. The last section concludes the research methods and reveals the experimental results.

2 Related Work

Various FR methods have been developed in the last two decades. Five FR methods have been adopted widely in various FR applications, which include rule-based FR, hint-based FR, graph-based FR, volumetric decomposition FR, and neural network-based FR. These FR methods are briefly described as follows.

The rule-based FR method is the most common and efficient solution for various FR systems [3, 4]. It has proven to be a robust method, which can handle more recognition objects than other syntactic methods [5].

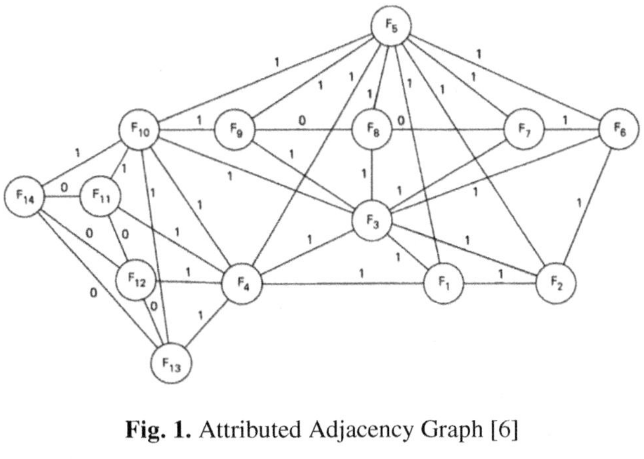

Fig. 1. Attributed Adjacency Graph [6]

The graph-based FR often refers to Attributed Adjacency Graph (AAG) method, which is one of the most common FR methods as shown in Fig 1. The AAG approach is a data-driven procedure and avoids the exhaustive search [6], hence resulting in drastic reduction in execution times for recognizing the features.

The general structure of rule-based systems separates rules and facts, which enhances the system flexibility and rationality. The hint-based FR can deal with complex feature intersections. It is generally integrated with other FR methods, such as the rule-based and volumetric FR methods, to improve the accuracy and efficiency of FR processes [7, 8]. Other FR methods such as graph-based FR, volumetric decomposition FR and ANN methods have also been applied extensively to a variety of applications [6, 9, 10, 11]. The developed AFR system skeleton applies the rule-based FR method as the main FR method; and it will investigate the feasibility and benefits to incorporate the graph-based and hint-based FR methods as the supplementary solutions to improve the system accuracy and efficiency. The significance of the AFR system can be summarized as below:

(1) Knowledge-based AFR systems utilise knowledge-based tools to solve the problems in the recognition processes based on existing FR methods. Numerous FR applications have been developed through incorporating existing feature recognition methods into knowledge-based systems [4, 5, 12, 13].

(2) The AFR system advances rule-based FR through separating STEP files from the actual recognition processes. This increases the flexibility of recognizing various CAD models based on a certain number of rules. In other words, the AFR rules can be reused in recognizing different CAD models. The rule-based mechanism is the primary approach for the AFR inference process that can maximise the system flexibility and extensibility.

3 Design AFR System Framework

3.1 Structuring AFR System Framework

The AFR system is developed based on the working process of an enterprise analysis tool, i.e. SPAT (Stiffener Panel Analysis Tool). A work process flowchart has been developed as a guideline for the AFR system. The AFR work process flowchart consists of five phases including the knowledge interpretation phase, AFR initialisation phase, AFR extraction phase, AFR recognition phase, and finalisation phase.

The knowledge interpretation phase involves in managing AFR rules, domain knowledge, and constraints. In this phase, domain experts can define, modify, and update AFR rules that can be further used by the feature extraction and recognition phases. The AFR initialisation phase is focused on setting the initial parameters for the AFR rule-based system. This phase also allows system users to import CAD models to the AFR system.

Several knowledge based methods have been incorporated into the AFR extraction and recognition phase to replace the human-based recognition process. In this phase, the domain expert knowledge is converted to AFR rules, fact bases, and other knowledge-based forms. The inference process will search and match the classified CAD entities against AFR rules and constraints to identify the domain specific components. The finalisation phase generates user-friendly outputs, which will provide detailed topological and geometrical information to system users.

Another essential method employed for analyzing and constructing the AFR system framework is AFR Data Flow Diagram (DFD). Based on the AFR work process flowchart, the DFD of the AFR system can be generated for clarifying the system structure and design processes. The DFD entities in the AFR system mainly consist of domain experts and system users. The illustrations of these two types of DFD entities help AFR system developers to understand the desired inputs and outputs. Thus, the AFR system can be designed more efficiently to accommodate the needs of these two types of external entities.

3.2 Typical Cases Description

Several domain-specific cases have been tested in the AFR system, in particular the CAD models for stiffened panels. The AFR system can separate stiffeners and panels from common aerospace structural components in particular, stiffened panels. A stiffened panel mainly consists of panels, stiffeners, fillets, holes, cut-outs, pad-ups, and pockets. Panels and stiffeners are the major objectives for the AFR system.

The other components are briefly described as follows. Fillets are radius of curvature connecting features, e.g. panels to stiffeners, panels to pad-ups, stiffeners to stiffeners, etc. Fig 2 illustrates a stiffened panel surrounded by curved fillets.

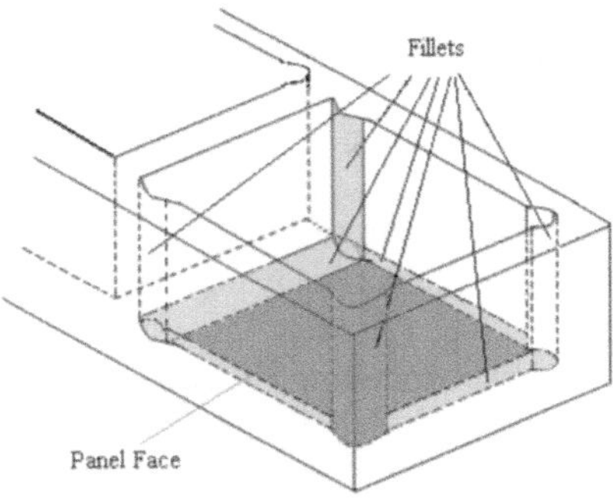

Fig. 2. Stiffened Panels Surrounded by Curved Fillets

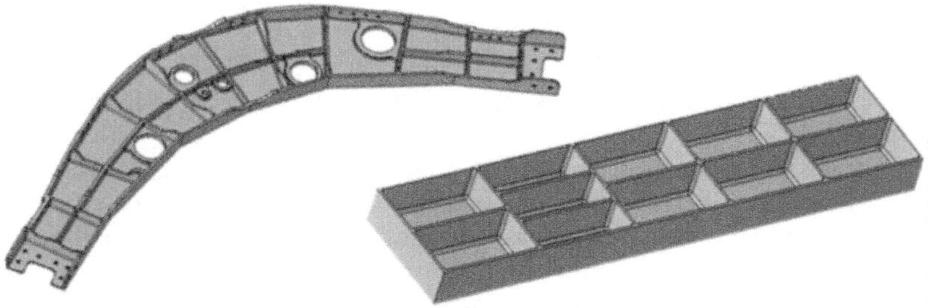

Fig. 3. Two Typical Test Cases for the AFR System

Fig 3 illustrates two typical test cases for the AFR system. These test cases are generated based on certain guidelines; and these guidelines can be incorporated into rules and used by the AFR rule-based system.

4 AFR Knowledge Base Design

The knowledge base design is the core part in the AFR system. The AFR-based knowledge is derived from CAD models and domain experts' knowledge through utilising several Knowledge Acquisition (KA) techniques. The acquired knowledge will be represented in three levels of knowledge include domain, task, and process levels knowledge. Once the three knowledge levels are represented, the external inputs (generally user inputs) can be delivered to the AFR inference for generating FR results.

4.1 AFR Knowledge Acquisition and Representation

Several KA techniques have been applied to the AFR knowledge base design process [14].

- Questionnaires and interviews: the questionnaires and interviews technique is the fundamental KA technique used in this project, which is primarily based on regular meetings and discussions with *GKN* domain experts. The constant discussions between project team members have been conducted as informal interviews and questionnaires.
- Data flow technique: the DFD method is a major KA technique adopted in the AFR knowledge base design process. It helps to identify the flow of data process and the major functionalities of the AFR system. DFDs can efficiently illustrate the process of identifying key components of a CAD model; and indicating the data store procedures.
- The ER (Entity Relationship) Modelling Process: ER diagrams have been used as one of the major KR techniques in the AFR process. It is also a main KA technique to acquire topological details from CAD models. Based on the discussions and informal interviews with the domain expert, the ER diagram of the AFR system has been generated. ER diagrams are the essential method to generate a systematic view of the AFR database, which stores the information on extracted CAD models.

Three major KA techniques have been used in the AFR system analysis and knowledge base construction process that help the system designers to understand the design processes.

ER diagrams are the major Knowledge Representation (KR) methodology for the AFR knowledge base design. ER diagrams have been adopted in both KA and KR processes in the AFR knowledge base design. The AFR ER diagram effectively describes the domain entities and their relationships. CAD models can be classified into a set of general entities, which can be referred to data tables in the AFR knowledge base. The relationships between entities place certain constraints on the knowledge base operation. The attributes of entities represent the detailed information of each entity, such as entity ID, surface type, edge number, etc.

The AFR ER diagrams as the major KR method avails to improve the organisation and operation of the CAD model data in the AFR knowledge base; more specifically in the AFR database that stores facts for the inference process.

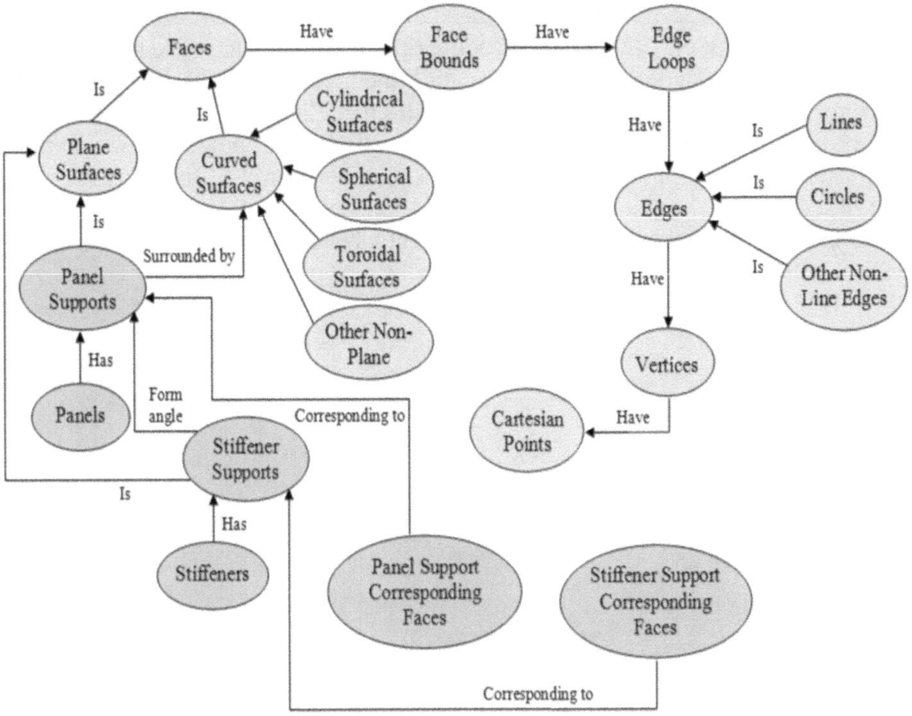

Fig. 4. AFR Semantic Network Based on STEP

Semantic Network Diagram method is one of the most comprehensive and efficient KR techniques. Individual concepts in a semantic network are linked by named associations that exist between pairs of concepts. The links can represent causal or functional, spatial, and class membership relationships, and so on. In many cases, this characteristic makes semantic networks more useful, flexible, and efficient than other KR methods. Based on the ER diagram, the AFR semantic network for can be generated as shown in Fig 4, which is based on the CAD models of stiffened panels. This semantic network consists of two types of entities include CAD-based entities and domain specific entities. The entities shown in orange colour in Fig 4 represent the domain specific entities, such as panels and stiffeners; and the entities shown in blue colour are the CAD-based entities. Semantic networks loosely provide more information than ER diagrams in terms of describing the variety of knowledge and flexibility.

4.2 Three Level of AFR Knowledge Base

Based on the AFR ER diagrams and semantic networks, the AFR knowledge base can be categorised into three levels of knowledge, i.e. domain level, task level, and process level. The domain level knowledge defines domain specific components, such as stiffeners, panels, etc., and domain specific rules and constraints. The task knowledge specifies what facts and associated information should be generated, which include the structures of neutral CAD format files, STEP files in particular, and the modelling rules. The process knowledge specifies detailed functions and processes for obtaining information specified in task knowledge level. The three level of the AFR knowledge base design is based on several test-case CAD models. Fig 5 illustrates the example inputs of the AFR knowledgebase and the outputs are identified in the unification process, which is shown as Panel_Face_List in the next page.

Domain Knowledge (feature definition, rules, etc.)

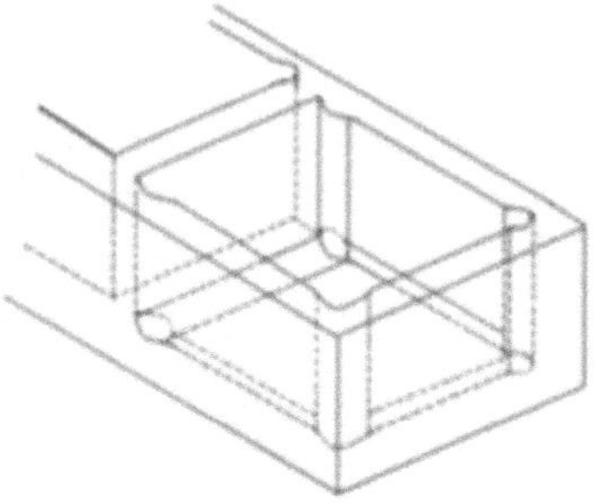

Feature Definitions

Feature Name	Property	Data Type
Panel	Edge Count	Long Integer
Panel	Thickness	Double
Panel	Adjacent Fillets	Integer
Panel	... ...	... ...
Panel Support	Face ID	Integer
Stiffener	Edge Count	Double
Stiffener	... ...	... ...
Stiffener Support	Face ID	Integer

Domain Specific Components Rules

Plain Language Description	Formatted Description (based on STEP file)
(1) Adjacent to fillets	(1) [Entity type]: {Fillet-Adjacency} [Attribute]: {Adjacency-Status} [Operator]: {=} [Value]: {True}
(2) Tangent to fillets	(2) [Entity type]: {Fillet-Tangency} [Attribute]: {Tangency-Status} [Operator]: {=} [Value]: {True}

Fig. 5. An Example of AFR Domain Knowledge

The AFR knowledge base system adopts the unification processes, which are essential for rule-based systems, which mainly deal with pair-wise matching procedures. The unification process of the AFR rule engine is based on classified STEP entities as indicated in the previous section. The substitutions of the AFR unification process are from the AFR fact base.

A logic resolution process applies inference rules to logical formulas in clause forms, and generates inference results. The resolution process of the AFR rule engine illustrated as the follows:

$$(cad\_F_1\ (F_1S_1, F_1S_2, F_1S_3, F_1S_4, F_1S_5, F_1S_6)\times\theta_1,\ List_{f1}).$$

$$PanelFace\ :-$$

$$(Member(List_{f1})\ \ ->$$

$$(cad\_F_2(F_2S_1, F_2S_2, F_2S_3, F_2S_4, F_2S_5, F_2I_1, F_2I_2, F_2S_6, F_2R_1, F_2S_7, F_2S_8, F_2S_9, F_2S_{10}, F_2R_2)\times\theta_{2-1},\ List_{adj1})$$

,

$$(cad\_F_2(F_2S_1, F_2S_2, F_2S_3, F_2S_4, F_2S_5, F_2I_1, F_2I_2, F_2S_6, F_2R_1, F_2S_7, F_2S_8, F_2S_9, F_2S_{10}, F_2R_2)\times\theta_{2-2},\ List_{adj2})$$

$$(cad\_F_2(F_2S_1, F_2S_2, F_2S_3, F_2S_4, F_2S_5, F_2I_1, F_2I_2, F_2S_6, F_2R_1, F_2S_7, F_2S_8, F_2S_9, F_2S_{10}, F_2R_2)\times\theta_{2-3},\ List_{all1})$$

,

$$(cad\_F_2(F_2S_1, F_2S_2, F_2S_3, F_2S_4, F_2S_5, F_2I_1, F_2I_2, F_2S_6, F_2R_1, F_2S_7, F_2S_8, F_2S_9, F_2S_{10}, F_2R_2)\times\theta_{2-4},\ List_{all2})$$

$$(\ \ (List_{adj1} = List_{all1}),$$

$$(List_{adj2} = List_{all2})\ \ ->$$

$$assert(Panel\_Face\_List(List_{f1})$$

)

).

cad_F₁: $(F_1S_1, F_1S_2, F_1S_3, F_1S_4, F_1S_5, F_1S_6)$ represents the STEP entity -- cad_face: (string ID, string STEPID, string BoundRef, string SurfaceRef, string SurfaceType, string Orientation), same as ***cad_F₂***. θ denotes unifiers for substitution.

The AFR rule engine acquires different θ from the fact base. For the above example, the resolution results are:

$$List_{f1} = \{\ 605,\ 610,\ 613,\ 614,\ \ldots\ ,\ 1305\ \};$$

$$Panel\_Face\_List =$$

$$\begin{Bmatrix} 605,\ 610,\ 613,\ 614,\ 618,\ 620,\ 624, \\ 626,\ 629,\ 658,\ 815,\ 818,\ 819,\ 997 \end{Bmatrix}.$$

The above unification process can be interpreted as descriptive rules as follows:

IF (FaceX's *Surface_Type* = "Plane") **AND**

(All Faces Adjacent to FaceX satisfy:

Surface_Type = "Plane" &

Adjacency_Number = 1 &

Loop_Number = 0 & *Formed_Angle* = 90 &

Concave_Status = "True" &

Fillet_Connection = "False" &

Connected_By_Fillet = "False")

THEN FaceX $\subset$ Panel Faces.

The AFR rules can be formulated based on the structure of AFR rules and the basic rule elements. The following example illustrates the formulations of AFR rules as shown in Table 1.

Plain Language Description	Formatted Description (based on STEP file)
Primary definitions:	*Primary definitions:*
(1) A face is plane.	(1) [Entity type]: {Advanced Face} [Attribute]: {Surface Type} [Operator]: {=} [Value]: {Plane}
(2) Faces bounded by curved faces.	(2) [Entity type]: {Curved Face Surrounding} [Attribute]: {Surrounding Status} [Operator]: {=} [Value]: {True}
(3) Area size is greater than 100	(3) [Entity type]: {Advanced Face}[Attribute]: {Area} [Operator]: {=>} [Value]: {100}

Table 1. Rule Formulation for Panel Face

The formulation for panels is according to the common design guideline based on typical cases. The rules describing a particular CAD model can be reused in other similar types CAD models, for instance stiffener-panel structure CAD models. Therefore, time consumption for generating rules can be minimized in the process of recognizing numerous similar types of CAD models.

5 Conclusion

This research addresses the specific problem occurring in the aircraft design analysis process, which mainly relies on the human-based FR process. A knowledge-based system approach has been adopted in order to tackle various problems in the recognition processes. The three-level AFR knowledge base provides an efficient solution to integrate the FR process with a CAD database that contains geometry and topological details.

Several test-case CAD models have been analysed and examined by the AFR prototype system. The results show that the prototype system can successfully identified simple CAD models (as shown in Fig 6) based on the three-level AFR knowledge base; and demonstrate the system can successfully identify the domain specific features, i.e. panel and stiffener analysis features. The following figures show geometry of a detailed test case, and results for panel features (Fig 7 below) and stiffener features (Fig 7 above).

The AFR system solves the problems occurring in existing CAD design processes, which mainly rely on manual data manipulation. The AFR approach bridges the gap between automated feature recognition procedures and downstream processes of CAD based design. It significantly improves integration efficiency; and reduces time and costs of analysing CAD models for downstream design processes.

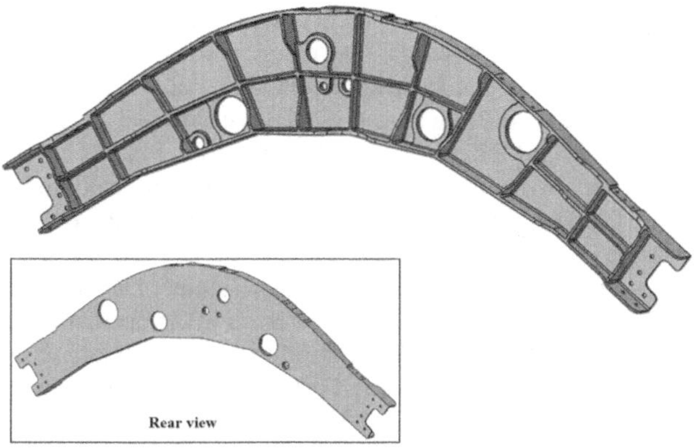

Fig. 6. Example Curved Frame CAD Model

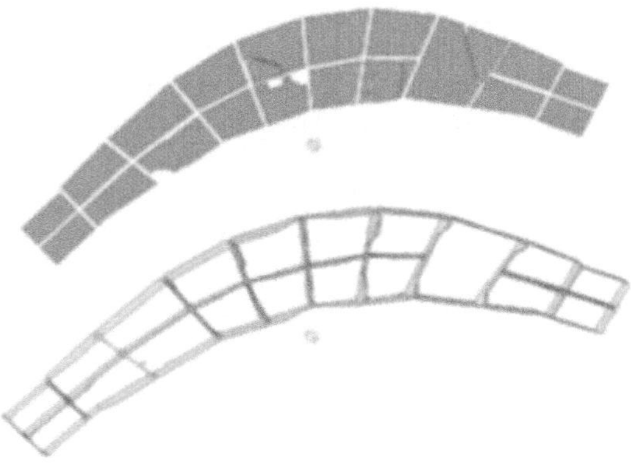

Fig. 7. Recognized Results based on Example

Acknowledgments. This research was supported by AutoCRC, GKN and RMIT University.

References

[1] Lockett, H.L.: A Knowledge Based Manufacturing Advisor for CAD. PhD thesis, pp. 23 –40. Cranfield University (2005)

[2] Zhang, H.L., Van der Velden, C., Yu, X., Jones, T., Fieldhouse, I., Bil, C.: Developing A Rule Engine for Automated Feature Recognition from CAD Models. In: Proc. of IEEE IECON, Porto, Portugal, pp. 3925–3930. IEEE Press, Los Alamitos (2009)

[3] Sadaiah, M., Yadav, D.R., Mohanram, P.V., Radhakrishnan, P.: A generative CAPP system for prismatic components. Int. J. of Ad. Manu. Tech. 20, 709–719 (2002)

[4] Bouzakis, H.K.-D., Andreadis, G.: A Feature-based Algorithm for Computer Aided Process Planning for Prismatic Parts. International Journal of Production Engineering and Computers 3(3), 17–22 (2000)

[5] Babic, B., Nesic, N., Miljkovic, Z.: A Review of Automated Feature Recognition With Rule-based Pattern Recognition. Computers in Industry 59, 321–337 (2008)

[6] Joshi, S., Chang, T.C.: Graph-based Heuristics for Recognition of Machined Features from a 3D Solid Model. In: Computer-Aided Design, vol. 20(2), pp. 58–66 (1988)

[7] Dimov, S.S., Brousseau, E.B., Setchi, R.: A Hybrid Method for Feature Recognition in Computer-Aided Design Models. Journal of Engineering Manufacture 221, 79–96 (2007)

[8] Subrahmanyam, S., Wozny, M.: An Overview of Automatic Feature Recognition Techniques for Computer-Aided Process Planning. In: Computers in Industry, vol. 26, pp. 1–21. Elsevier, Amsterdam (1995)

[9] Kailash, S.B., Zhang, Y.F., Fuh, J.Y.H.: A Volume Decomposition Approach to Machining Feature Extraction of Casting and Forging Components. In: Computer-Aided Design, vol. 33(8), pp. 605–617. Elsevier Publication, Amsterdam (2001)

[10] Ding, L., Yue, Y.: Novel ANN-based Feature Recognition Incorporating Design by Features. In: Computers In Industry, 55, 197–222. (2004)

[11] Marquez, M., Gill, R., White, A.: Application of Neural Networks in Feature Recognition of Mould Reinforced Plastic Parts. In: Concurrent Engineering: Research and Applications, vol. 7(2), pp. 115–122. SAGE Publication, Newbury Park (1999)

[12] Chen, Y.-M., Wen, C.-C., Ho, C.T.: Extraction of geometric characteristics for manufacturability assessment. In: Robotics and Computer-Integrated Manufacturing, vol. 19(4), pp. 371–385. Elsevier Publication, Amsterdam (2003)

[13] Yuen, C.F., Wong, S.Y., Venuvinod, P.K.: Development of a Generic Computer-Aided Process Planning Support System. Journal of Materials Processing Technology 139, 394–401 (2003)

[14] Liebowitz, J.: Knowledge Management and its Link to Artificial Intelligence. In: Expert Systems with Applications, vol. 20, pp. 1–6. Elsevier Publication, Amsterdam (2001)

The Order Measure Model of Knowledge Structure*

Qiu Jiangnan, Wang Chunling, and Qin Xuan

Dalian University of Technology, Dalian, 116024

Abstract. The recent researches on Knowledge Structure mainly focused on the connotative, components and evolution process of it, but little is known about its order. For the sake of knowing the process of growth and the degree of order of Knowledge Structure, this paper has introduced the Structure entropy to calculate the degrees of extension and richness of it which are used to build the order measure model in the view of the order. As the basis of studying the process of growth, the order measure model enables the evolution rules and influencing factors of Knowledge Structure.

Keywords: Knowledge Structure, Order, Entropy, Order Measure Model.

1 Introduction

Knowledge Structure that coming from Pedagogy field at the earliest mainly refers to the structure of individual's or subject's knowledge, then extends to group, enterprise and even organization. At present, researches on Knowledge Structure have focused on the connotative, components (individual[1], enterprise[2] and organization[3]), construction[4] and visualization[5] and so on. While the evolution of Knowledge Structure pays attention to components[6] and developing processes[7] which are relative to academic system[8] . According to SECI proposed by Nonaka, the evolution of Knowledge Structure has risen in a spiral with the knowledge promotion in both quality and quantity. The essential of knowledge promotion is the process of state changing from out of order to order or one order to another order of Knowledge Structure. While the present studies is lack of considering the aspect of order, research methods (such as citation analysis[9], altogether word analysis, cluster analysis[10] are not suited for the study Order in spite of being used for constructing academic system and Knowledge Structure. Therefore, this paper studies the Knowledge Structure in the view of order and analyzes deeply the relatively stable states of Knowledge Structure. The development of Knowledge Structure formed either by individual's development or by collaborative groups is essentially the process

* Supported by "The Fundamental Research Funds for the Central Universities"(DU-T11RW306).

B. Hu et al. (Eds.): BI 2011, LNAI 6889, pp. 327–332, 2011.

of changing the state of knowledge structure. This paper focuses on the order degree of knowledge structure in collaborative groups in order to study the stability of knowledge structure with coordination. Entropy considered as a dual concept of the degree of order is usually used as the core scale for measuring systems evolution. This paper proposes the Order Measure Model of knowledge structure by calculating the degrees of extension and richness of it based on the method of structure entropy from the perspective of order. This model helps us to deeply understand the self-organization mechanism of knowledge structure evolution and provides a measurement basis model for further research.

2 Concept and Evolution of Knowledge Structure

2.1 What's Knowledge Structure

Knowledge Structure is the hierarchical knowledge system of knowledge elements and the relationships among them. Meta-knowledge is unit possessing a complete knowledge representation. Knowledge Structure is tree structure with a unique root node and other nodes belonged to subtrees. Every node has a parent node except root node and every node has one or more child nodes except leaf nodes. Knowledge Structure can be formalized as $KS = (K, E)$. $K = (k_1, k_2, \ldots, k_n)$ is set of knowledge elements, and k_i is one of it; $E = \{(k_i, k_j) \mid \theta(k_i, k_j) = 1\}$ is set of the relationships of knowledge elements, and $\theta(k_i, k_j) = 1$ means that there is parent-child or superior-subordinate relationship between k_i and k_j with k_i being k_j parent.

2.2 Evolution of Knowledge Structure

In the processes of growth of Knowledge Structure, there is not only generating new knowledge (such as adding new nodes or relationships), but also changing former structure (such as deleting nodes or changing relationships) and even improving nodes' quality (such as changing information contained in the nodes). From the growth way of Knowledge Structure, it is related to the path length between two nodes and the centrality of a node. For example, generating new node would effectively extend the its depth and deleting node would shorten; while improving node's quality or changing node's weight would affect the centrality of adjacent node in varying degree. Hence, this paper considers the path length between two nodes and the centrality of a node as main factors impacting the developing of Knowledge Structure, namely the degree of extension and the degree of richness respectively.

3 The Order Measure Model

Path length between Knowledge nodes and node's centrality degree are the key indicators of measuring knowledge structure. The degree of extension and the degree of richness are defined to reflect the order degree R of knowledge structure.

There is a need to define path weight and knowledge node weight to calculate the degree of extension and the degree of richness. As antithesis concept of the degree of order and taken as core scale of system evolution, entropy is introduced to be the main basis for measuring the degree of order. The existing methods of structure measurement contain network structure entropy model[11,12,13], negative entropy evaluation model[14,15] and the time effect-quality model[16,17,18]. Network structure entropy model focuses on node's centrality degree without considering the path length between nodes; negative entropy evaluation model is fit for fewer nodes without considering node's centrality degree. The time effect-quality model pays attention to both the path length between two nodes and centrality of a node. On account of the comparison, this paper chooses time effect-quality model to be foundation of measuring knowledge structure. The degree of order is formalized as follows after gaining the degree of extension and the degree of richness.

$$R = \alpha R_y + \beta R_f \tag{1}$$

Where R_y is the degree of extension, R_f is the degree of richness,α and β are the weights coefficients of R_y and R_f respectively, here $\alpha + \beta = 1$.

3.1 The Degree of Extension

The degree of extension reflects the impact of path length between knowledge nodes on the overall knowledge structure. The entropy value reflects the uncertainty of the growth of knowledge along different paths. The formula is as follows:

(1) Path length L_{ij}. Path length between two knowledge nodes is defined as the shortest path between nodes of knowledge structure. Path length directly connected is given to 1, and plus 1 for every transit time. Based on the specific formation of knowledge structure, count micro states of each node, that is, the shortest length between the nodes of the upper and lower levels in knowledge structure L_{ij}, where i and j are the number of nodes.

(2) The total number of micro-states that the degree of extension of knowledge structure A_y.

$$A_y = \sum_{i=1}^{n}\sum_{j=1}^{n} L_{ij} \tag{2}$$

(3) The largest entropy of the degree of extension of knowledge structure.

$$H_{ym} = \log_2 A_y \tag{3}$$

(4) Set the path weight w_y, and calculate the probability of micro-states of the degree of extension P_yij. The node at the deeper level of knowledge structure will affect the efficiency of searching knowledge and also be detrimental to the overall growth of knowledge structure. So the longer the search path is, the smaller the weight of path is set where the degree of extension is higher.

$$\frac{w_y(k)}{w_y(k-1)} = \frac{k-1}{k-2} \tag{4}$$

Where k_i is the maximum length of the search path.

$$\sum_{k-1}^{n} w_y(k) = 1 \tag{5}$$

$$P_y(ij) = L_{ij}\frac{w_y(k)}{A_y} \tag{6}$$

(5) the entropy of the degree of extension between two knowledge nodes in vertical and horizontal levels of knowledge structure H_yij.

$$H_yij = -P_y(ij)\log_2 P_y(ij) \tag{7}$$

(6) The total entropy of the degree of extension of knowledge structure H_y.

$$H_y = \sum_{i=1}^{n}\sum_{j=1}^{n} H_y(ij) = -\sum_{i=1}^{n}\sum_{j=1}^{n} P_y(ij)\log_2 P_y(ij) \tag{8}$$

(7) The degree of extension of knowledge structure R_y.

$$R_y = 1 - \frac{H_y}{H_{ym}} \tag{9}$$

3.2 The Degree of Richness

The degree of richness of knowledge structure reflects the impact of node's centrality degree on the overall knowledge structure, and the value of its entropy reflects the uncertainty of the knowledge gathering. For the overall knowledge structure, the higher node's centrality degree is, the more important the node is, the more knowledge users can connect through the node. The formula of the degree of richness is as follows.

(1)Node's centrality degree K_i . Node's centrality degree is defined as the number of nodes directly linked to the node in knowledge structure. Based on the specific formation of knowledge structure, K_i of every node are gotten to determine micro states of the degree of richness (where i is the number of nodes.).

(2) Total number of micro-states that the degree of richness A_f.

$$A_f = \sum_{i=1}^{n} K_i \tag{10}$$

(3) The largest entropy of the degree of richness of knowledge structure H_{fm}.

$$H_{fm} = \log_2 A_f \tag{11}$$

(4) The weight of knowledge node $w_f(i)$ and the probability of micro-states of the degree of richness $P_f(i)$. The weight of knowledge nodes is influenced by the quality of the knowledge nodes itself. The more pages a knowledge node contains, the more information the page has, the higher information quality is, and the greater the impact on other knowledge nodes is. The formula of the weight of knowledge node is as follows.

$$w_f(i) = \frac{Q_{ki}}{\sum_{i=1}^{n} Q_{ki}} \tag{12}$$

Where Q_{ki} is the information quality of a knowledge node. Different carrier of knowledge has a different method to measure quality. In practice, the value of quality can be directly substituted in Q_{ki}.

$$\sum_{i=1}^{n} w_f(i) = 1 \tag{13}$$

$$P_f(i) = \frac{K_i w_f(i)}{A_f} \tag{14}$$

14 (5) The entropy of the degree of richness of every knowledge node in knowledge structure $H_f(i)$.

$$H_f(i) = -P_f(i) \log_2 P_f(i) \tag{15}$$

(6) The total entropy of the degree of richness of knowledge structure H_f.

$$H_f = \sum_{i=1}^{n} H_f(i) = -\sum_{i=1}^{n} P_f(i) \log_2 P_f(i) \tag{16}$$

(7) The degree of richness of collaborative knowledge structure R_f.

$$R_f = 1 - \frac{H_f}{H_{fm}} \tag{17}$$

4 Conclusion

The degree of order could be gotten by calculating the degree of extension and the degree of richness respectively. After analyzing the values of R, the growth of knowledge structure can be known. Values of R continuing arising indicates the growth of knowledge structure. The higher value of R, the degree of order is better. Declining in the value indicates that knowledge structure is in a relative unstable condition at some point, but it could recover in a short time with the value going up. If the change of value is getting smaller and smaller, it indicates that the knowledge structure is growing slowly and slowly. This paper has proposed the Order Measure Model of Knowledge Structure in theory. The next step will take experiments of simulation and practice to test and modify the model. In the experiments, analyzing the influencing factors of the stability of the growth processes of knowledge structure and concluding the evolution rules of knowledge structure would be done.

References

1. Dorsey, D.W., Campbell, G.E., Foster, L.L., et al.: Assessing Knowledge Structures: Relations with Experience and Posttraining Performance. Human Performance 1, 31–57 (1999)
2. Zhang, X., Wang, W., Chen, S.: Research on the Constitution and Devolvement of the Knowledge Structure System of Enterprise and Organization Learning. Journal of Dalian University of Technology (Social Sciences) 27(4), 23–28 (2006)
3. Anand, V., Clark, M.A.: Team Knowledge Structure: Matching Task to Information Environment. Journal of Managerial Issues 1, 15–31 (2003)
4. Song, G., Wang, X., Feng, R.: The Rise of MOT and Establishment of Its Subject System. Science of Science and Management of S. and T. 4, 116–120 (2008)
5. Sun, J., Zhang, P.: Visualization of Researcher Knowledge Structure Based on Knowledge Network. Information Science 28(3), 395–399, 480 (2010)
6. Chen, L., Liu, Z., Liang, L.: Study on the Structure of Mechanics Based on the Titles of Mechanics Papers. Journal of the China Society for Scientific and Technical Information 29(2), 305–313 (2010)
7. Leydesdorf, L.: The delineation of nanoscience and nanotechnology in terms of journals and patents a most recent update. Intellectual and Laboratory Dynamics of Nanoscience and Nanotechnology, Paris (2007)
8. Liu, Z., Hu, Z., Wang, X.: Knowledge Mapping of The 30-year History of the Science of Science in China. For The 30th Anniversary. Science of Science and Management of S. and T. 5, 17–23 (2010)
9. Leydesdorf, L., Zhou, P.: Nanotechnology as a Field of Science:Its Delineation in Terms of Journals and Patents. Scientometrics 70(3), 693–713 (2007)
10. Liang, X.: Review of Mapping Knowledge Domains. Library Journal 28(6), 58–62 (2009)
11. Xu, F., Zhao, H., Ha, T., Zhang, Y.: Research on the Changing Principle of the Internet Standard Structure Entropy. Journal of Northe Astern University (Natural Science) 27(12), 1324–1326 (2006)
12. Zhang, W., Zhao, H., Sun, P., Xu, Y., Zhang, X.: Research on Internet Topology Evolution and the Fractal of Average Degree of Nodes. Acta Electronica Sinica 34(8), 1438–1445 (2006)
13. Xu, F., Zhao, H., Ha, T., Zhang, Y.: Research on the Robustness Based on the Internet Standard Entropy. Journal of Northeastern University (Natural Science) 27(11), 1208–1211 (2006)
14. Yang, B., Qiang, M.: Improvement of Evaluation Models of Order Degree of System Structure by Means of Negative Entropy. Systems Engineering 25(5), 20–24 (2007)
15. Li, W.: Order Degree of Complicated System Structure–Negentropy Algorithm. Systems Engineering Theory and Practice 8(4), 15–22 (1988)
16. Zhang, J., Li, J.: Range and Span of Management on Application Structure Entropy Analysis. Statistics and Decision 10, 164–166 (2007)
17. Yan, Y.: Evaluation Model of Order Degree of Asset Structure Based on Structure Entropy. Communication of Finance and Accounting (Financing) 6, 27–28 (2008)
18. Zhang, Z., Xiao, R.: Empirical Study on Orderliness Evaluation of Production System Based on Structure Entropy. Chinese Journal of Mechanical Engineering 43(6), 62–67 (2007)

Author Index

GPSR Compliance

The European Union's (EU) General Product Safety Regulation (GPSR) is a set of rules that requires consumer products to be safe and our obligations to ensure this.

If you have any concerns about our products, you can contact us on ProductSafety@springernature.com

In case Publisher is established outside the EU, the EU authorized representative is:

Springer Nature Customer Service Center GmbH
Europaplatz 3
69115 Heidelberg, Germany

Batch number: 10844619

Printed by Printforce, the Netherlands